THE
TROUBLE
WITH
LIONS

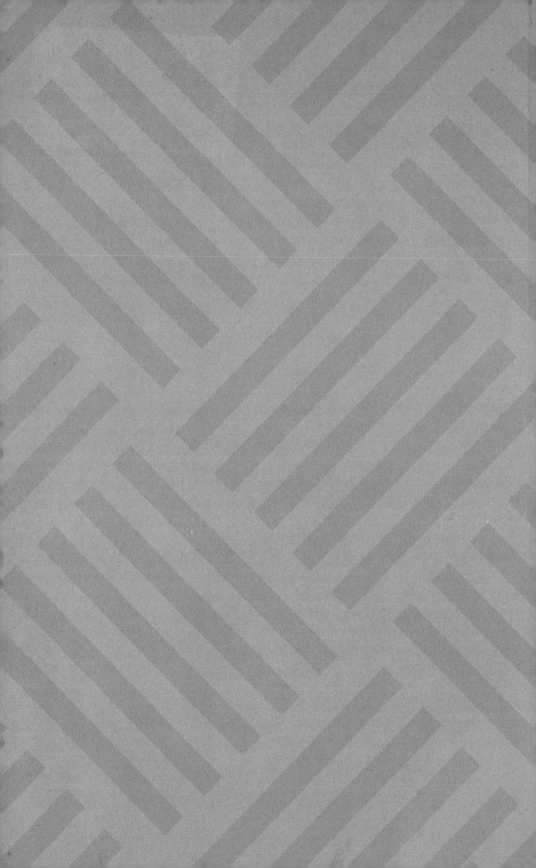

THE TROUBLE WITH LIONS

A Glasgow Vet in Africa

JERRY HAIGH

FOREWORD BY JANE GOODALL

 THE UNIVERSITY
of ALBERTA PRESS

Published by

The University of Alberta Press
Ring House 2
Edmonton, Alberta, Canada   T6G 2E1

Copyright © 2008

Library and Archives Canada Cataloguing in Publication

Haigh, J.C. (Jerry C.)
    The trouble with lions : a Glasgow vet in Africa / Jerry Haigh.

(Wayfarer)
Includes bibliographical references and index.
ISBN 978-0-88864-503-6

    1. Haigh, J. C. (Jerry C.). 2. Wildlife veterinarians—Africa—Biography.
I. Title. II. Series: Wayfarer (Edmonton, Alta.)

SF996.36.H34A3 2008   636.089092   C2007-907554-1

The University of Alberta Press is committed to protecting our natural environment.
As part of our efforts, this book is printed on Enviro Paper: it contains 100% post-consumer
recycled fibres and is acid- and chlorine-free.

The University of Alberta Press gratefully acknowledges the support received for its
publishing program from The Canada Council for the Arts. The University of Alberta Press
also gratefully acknowledges the financial support of the Government of Canada through the
Book Publishing Industry Development Program (BPIDP) and from the Alberta Foundation
for the Arts for its publishing activities.

Canada Council   Conseil des Arts
for the Arts   du Canada

Canadä

For my grandchildren, Sonia, Rachael,
Mathew and Gabriella, and their grandchildren's
grandchildren, and for the African children of
those generations, like Fifi in Uganda, who will
grow up in a very different world than the one
I have known. May they too thrill to the sight
of free-ranging lions, even if only in parks.

CONTENTS

FOREWORD
JANE GOODALL

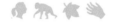

the Jane Goodall Institute

IN SEPTEMBER 2007 I travelled to Saskatoon, Saskatchewan, on the Canadian prairies, to meet with a group of Roots & Shoots youth—one of the hundreds of extraordinary and dedicated such groups around the world. Before my evening talk began, I met with Dr. Jerry Haigh of the University of Saskatchewan's Western College of Veterinary Medicine. Over tea at the Bessborough Hotel, we discussed our common conservation interests— chimps and Africa's bushmeat crisis in particular. Since then, Dr. Haigh has kept in touch with me, fascinating me with his stories about and interest in lion research in East Africa. One image is still vivid in my mind since it illustrates the conservation efforts the Maasai *morans* of Kenya.

The Trouble With Lions is about the complex relationships between people, livestock and wildlife. If you look on page 419 of this book you will see a photograph taken by researcher Leelah Hazzah, which even one year ago would not have been possible. This picture of a *moran* holding a radio transmitter, that allows him to track lions, illustrates the new direction of conservation efforts in East Africa. Dr. Haigh explains the reasons why the young Maasai warriors near Amboseli National Park have changed from being traditional ceremonial and revenge killers of lions to lion conservationists over a rather short period of time.

As Dr. Haigh has found from research done by Seamus MacLennan, between 2001 and the end of 2006 at least 116 lions were killed by people in Maasai lands, some within national park boundaries. Traditionally, a young warrior had to kill a lion to prove his manhood, but lions who killed or were suspected of killing cattle were also hunted. But then, in March 2007, a group of *moran* suddenly renounced the killing of lions, and instead vowed to be guardians of lions, conservationists, and community educators. How did this happen? Lion researcher Laurence Frank and his team made a powerful video explaining the issues. It was part of their outreach program, and its message reached the hearts of the Maasai community in the area. With these young men now working toward establishing and maintaining healthy lion populations in their traditional lands, the hope for a future that includes lions is burning brighter than it has in many years. The *morans'* commitment to conserve rather than kill the greatest of the predators, symbol of strength and courage, is extraordinary. It will demonstrate that protection requires as much or more courage than killing, these young men can legitimately feel proud. And they will have a job that will be respected. They will be a new kind of role model for the youth of their community, and it will effect others around the world.

The Trouble With Lions is not only about the plight of lions: Dr. Haigh regales us with stories about a variety of wild animals affected by humans and their livestock. He tells of the rhinos, threatened by encroaching human development, that he helped to translocate to parks or ranches in the 1970s. He describes the sanctuaries where dedicated African staff care for chimpanzees, orphaned mainly by the bushmeat trade, at Sweetwaters in Kenya and Ngamba Island in Uganda. Many of these youngsters have been so traumatized that they will be scarred for life. As Dr. Haigh points out, Africa is now a sea of human development and agriculture with mere islands set aside for wildlife—and even these fragmented remnants of wilderness are seldom completely safe because of the threat of illegal activities—poaching, plundering for firewood and so on—by surrounding people, often living in extreme poverty. And there is increasing danger from transmission of diseases from domestic animals. The human-livestock-wildlife balance in Africa is indeed a delicate one.

When I speak to Roots & Shoots youth around the globe, I always emphasize the power of the individual to make a difference in the world. Truly our planet is under siege, the problems and dangers can seem utterly overwhelming—but it is not too late to effect change. There is the amazing human brain, the resilience of nature, the indomitable human spirit. If only each one of us would learn more about the consequences of the choices we make each day—how they effect the environment and human and animal welfare—more and more people would start to make wiser and more compassionate decisions. Collectively this would lead to big changes.

We humans, unfortunately, are capable of inflicting great harm, either through ignorance or greed or apathy. But we are also capable of love, compassion and altruism. Young people who develop the right values, learn that this life is about more than just making money, and that by acting together, holding hands, we can make this a better world for all. Roots make a firm foundation, shoots seem small; together they can break apart the brick walls of environmental and social problems that confront us. Together we can and must find ways to live in greater harmony with each other and with the natural world.

Dr. Haigh has written a book that tells the interconnected stories of people, agriculture, and wildlife conservation, about species as diverse as rhinos, chimpanzees, domestic cattle, and Ugandan kob. In writing *The Trouble With Lions*, as in choosing a career as a veterinarian and teacher, Dr. Haigh made a decision to make a difference. His book will make you want to do the same. ✻

JANE GOODALL PH.D., DBE

Founder—the Jane Goodall Institute & UN Messenger of Peace
www.janegoodall.org
www.rootsandshoots.org

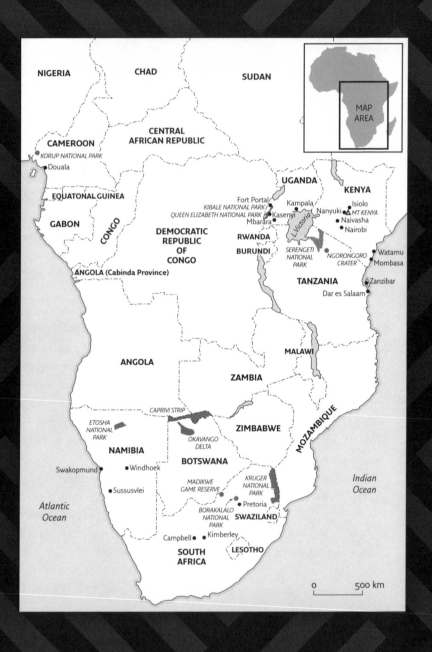

PREFACE

The lion is a beautiful animal, when seen at a distance.

—ZULU PROVERB

We carry within us the wonders we seek without us:
there is all Africa and her prodigies in us.

—SIR THOMAS BROWNE, *Religio Medici* (1643)

IN 2005 Canadian veterinary students travelling with me in Uganda were horrified to learn that villagers in Queen Elizabeth National Park had poisoned two lions. The lions had killed a cow, and there is nothing an African pastoralist values more highly than his cattle. What the students learned first-hand was that the killing was merely that latest skirmish in one of the longest running wars on the planet—the war between wild animals and humans. As one student put it, "That's not quite the same as the nature films we see on the TV at home."

There can hardly be a better example of the conflict between wildlife, on one hand, and livestock and humans, on the other, than the history of lion-human interactions. Jonathan Kingdon, whose magnificently illustrated, seven-volume *East African Mammals* is the pre-eminent text on many species, including lions, has described our relationship with lions as being governed by "the fact that for centuries lions have been predators of, competitors with and above all a source of symbolism for the human race." Each of these components of the relationship has created problems for the most charismatic of Africa's big cats. But, there are two other elements to our interactions with the so-called "King of Beasts" that are relevant to this particular story of the human–livestock–wildlife triangle. First, lion parts have long been used in witchcraft and for a variety of traditional medical practices. Second, within the last fifteen years a new element in the conflict has arisen as domestic animal diseases crossing into wildlife populations has become more prevalent.

Two hundred years ago lions ranged over most of Africa, the only exceptions to their large territory being a belt across the two great deserts, the Sahara and the Namib, and a swath of tropical rain forest stretching from the coastal regions of what is now the Ivory Coast across through to the Congo Basin. There were also lions in the southern part of the Arabian Peninsula, Persia, and across much of northwestern India, almost as far east as Delhi. As with most other wild species, today their range is much reduced and dwindling. The only wild population outside Africa lives in the Gir Forest of India's Gujarat state, where numbers are said to exceed three hundred, on a positive note up from the approximate twenty animals recorded a hundred years ago. More evidence of the former extent of lion presence, even beyond Africa and the Near East, was revealed when the Chauvet Cave in southeastern France was discovered in 1994. The cave is adorned with more stunning lion images than all other European art caves combined. It has been dated back about 35,000 years.

The symbolic significance of lions is pervasive. Indeed it is difficult to travel anywhere and not see the evidence of lions affecting the human imagination. The lion occurs everywhere in heraldry, notably for me perhaps as a Glasgow graduate, on Scotland's flag. Lions have been the subjects of countless works of art—paintings and statues, tapestries and so on—from those giants in Trafalgar square "guarding" Nelson to the New York Public Library Lions that sit at the library's entrance, from lions in Buddhist temples to those in ancient Egyptian works. Among

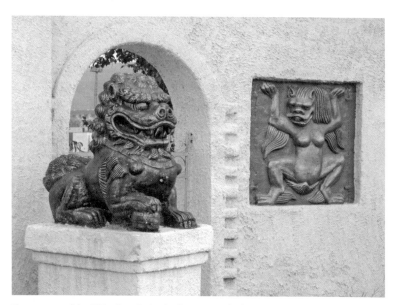

The gate posts of the children's garden in Ulaanbaatar, Mongolia, have this unusual piece of work in them.

the strangest images I have encountered involving lions is the chimera figure, a naked woman's body with lion's feet topped by a lion's head, which can be seen set into each of the gateposts of the children's garden in Mongolia's capital city, Ulaanbaatar. In Egyptian mythology there was also a lion-headed figure, the war goddess Sekhmet, who personified the fertilizing warmth of the sun and was later reduced in size to a cat. The ancient Babylonians also had a lion-headed deity, in this case an eagle named Imdugud. Still standing among the ruins of Babylon is a huge stone lion under whose feet lies the trampled figure of a man.

Kings, emperors and other leaders have been named for lions. Richard the Lion-Heart has been a hero for generations of schoolchildren in Britain and turns up at the end of the Hollywood version of the Robin Hood story. Who better to fill that cameo appearance than a bearded (maned?) Sean Connery? Emperor Hailie Selassie of Ethiopia was known as the Lion of Judah. Revered by some, the devil incarnate for others—Osama bin Laden's first name translates as "lion."

Lions have featured in most of the world's major religions. The Hindu god Vishnu appears in one of his avatars as a lion named Narasimha. The Old Testament prophet Daniel survived an ordeal in a lion's den.

The prophet Muhammad gave his first cousin and son-in-law Ali, the fourth Caliph of Islam, the title of Asadullah (Lion of God).

The first challenge for the Greek hero Heracles (Hercules to the Romans) was to slay the impossibly fierce and powerful Nemean lion, a competition immortalized (lionized?) by makers of ancient Greek vases and amphoras, Egyptian papyri, numerous mosaics, and by artists from the classical, Renaissance and Baroque eras, including works by Andrea Mantegna and Peter Paul Rubens. As Heracles won and wore the animal's hide as a cloak of immense power, it is small wonder then that so many of today's sports teams have the creature as a part of their name. They come particularly from most codes of football: rugby, the British Lions; soccer, the emblem of the English Premier League and the Indomitable Lions of Cameroon; Canadian football, the British Columbia Lions; and, in the American football code, the Detroit Lions and the Nittany Lions of Pennsylvania State University.

Then there is the most popular of British pub names: The Red Lion. It was James VI of Scotland (I of England) who, in 1603, when he assumed both crowns, ordered that the heraldic red lion of Scotland be displayed on all important buildings, including pubs. One of the more extraordinary manifestations of the royal lion obsession was recorded by John Hanning Speke, perhaps the first white man to see the source of the river Nile, who wrote somewhat scathingly about the gait of Mutesa, the Bugandan king, who walked on tip-toe in the belief that he was thus majestically representing the gait of the lion.

For ceremonial purposes several African tribes use lion headdresses or haloes imitating the mane. Tony Dyer records that in 1952, at the warrior's graduation ceremony of a Maasai clan in Kenya, twenty-two young men arrived, each wearing the mane of a male lion he had speared. It would be difficult to find a depiction of Maasai that lacked at least one image of warriors in a lion headdress, or *busby*, as author, artist and lion-lover Joy Adamson appropriately called them.

From a twenty-first century perspective, the use of lions in Roman circuses can hardly be believed. In many Roman circuses, at least one hundred lions were slaughtered per single event. The zenith (or nadir) of such slaughter was probably the massacre of six hundred lions in 55 BCE in the games organized by General Pompey. No wonder lions vanished from their former ranges in North Africa and on the northern shores of the Mediterranean. The reason for such slaughter could no doubt be attributed to both iconic and entertainment elements, as maned lions—the males—were much preferred in these shows. Perhaps the blood lust of the spectators and organizers of such events was a mere variation of that seen around the rings of the bull, dog and cock fighting shows that still occur today.

Now, with lion populations dwindling, in no small part because of humanity's love-hate relationship with them, lions are the key drawing cards in Africa's national parks. On one trip with friends to Kruger National Park in South Africa, we were struck by their obsessive counting of the creatures. By the end, our hosts had counted twenty-seven and considered the trip one of the best they had ever made, largely based upon this figure.

WHEN I WAS PLANNING THE STRUCTURE OF THIS BOOK, it seemed to me that the lion is symbolic of the entire gamut of wildlife species, not only in Africa, but worldwide. *The Trouble With Lions* might easily read *The Trouble With Rhinos*, or *Marmosets*, or possibly even the improbably named *Dromedary Jumping Slug* (threatened in Canada's British Columbia), not to mention the names of a host of other species. Of course a title such as *The Trouble with Jumping Slugs* or *Codfish* might not catch the potential reader's eye in quite the same way, and it would certainly not have excited a publisher. The type of trouble may differ between each of these species and humans, but it is undoubtedly there.

These days lions are principally considered trouble as livestock predators; but they are also *in* trouble, not only from humans defending their stock but also from massive declines in numbers of prey species and from newly emerged diseases. There are glimmers of hope that the trouble may not lead to the disappearance of the species in some areas, but overall numbers are way down and still declining.

The war humans are waging against lions shows no signs of stopping. As this book was being completed, a news item on the BBC website under the headline "Lion killer is killed by hyenas" related how Mr. Moses Lekalau, a Samburu herder in the Maralal area northeast of Nairobi, had been attacked by a lion and had somehow managed to fight it off, telling doctors "that it took him half an hour to spear and bludgeon the lion to death." Unfortunately he was subsequently attacked by a hyaena and died of blood loss, despite a seven-hour operation in Nairobi, where he had been airlifted.

I use the lion here as a symbol of the way that things have changed and are changing for wildlife in Africa, but this book is by no means limited to stories about these cats. As a wildlife vet, I have worked with numerous other species, and there are four chapters about my experiences with rhinos (perhaps appropriately enough, as one of my earliest medical cases required me to spend an hour evacuating a constipated rhino and then administering a four-gallon enema, with spectacular results). Other species whose stories I recount in the following pages include forest elephants, wild dogs, a variety of antelopes and other hoofed stock, several primates and a few species of bird. Most are in trouble because of humans, and some give people trouble in various ways that include attacks, crop damage and transmission of diseases, either to people or to their livestock.

A major theme of these accounts is the complicated relationship that exists between people, their livestock and the wildlife around them. In many ways this matrix defines the past, present and future of wildlife issues in Africa.

In this book I tell stories of working with wild animals and people over a forty-year span in Africa, from South Africa to Cameroon, and from early days in Kenya to recent activities in Uganda. All the stories are linked to my work as a wildlife vet and my fascination with the animal world. ✻

ACKNOWLEDGEMENTS

THERE ARE MANY OTHER PEOPLE TO THANK for their help and ideas over the time that this book was in its formative stages, and for allowing me to use their stories. Among them are old friends, farmers, and ranchers. Many of them were unfailingly generous with their hospitality and made us welcome in their homes on numerous occasions. They include Bea Anderson, Andrew Botta, Gordon Boy, Monty Brown, Liz Burroughs, Andrew Conroy, Linda Conroy, Miles Coverdale, Liz Coverdale, Batian Craig, Ian Craig, Rose Dyer, Tony Dyer, Don Hunt, Iris Hunt, Mark Jenkins, Muraya Kiai, Markie Kenyon, Susan Langford, Len Lemoine, Olwen Owles, George Murray, Irralie Murray, Anne Olivecrona, Court Parfet, Edward Parfet, Chris Parker, Ian Parker, Tony Parkinson, Annabelle Sayer, Nicola Sayer, Paul

Sayer, Simon Sayer, Christopher Sheehan, Wendell "Stevie" Stevens, Dorothy Tirima, Stanley Tirima, Nigel Trent, Muffet Trent, Jan van der Walt, Marie van der Walt, Gio van Eck, Hendrik van Eck and Hubert Wells.

Several biologists and veterinarians were kind enough to read sections or whole chapters and make useful suggestions, offer photographs and allow me to quote them. Some went even further and also gave us unstinting hospitality. In particular Ian Parker was a mine of information during numerous conversations and email exchanges. Laurence Frank, Seamus Mclennan and Leelah Hazzah shared a great deal of information about lion projects in Kenya. Others who contributed included Richard Burroughs, Colin Chapman, Sarah Cleaveland, Bob Cook, David Cumming, Markus Hofmeyr, Michele Hofmeyr, Peter Holt, Luke Hunter, Bill Karesh, John King, Richard Kock, Marie-Josée Limoges, David MacDonald, Becky Manning, Rowan Martin, Kay Mehren, Pete Morkel, Linda Munson, Steve Osofsky, Paul Sayer, Michael Somers, Tom Struhsaker and Rosie Woodroffe.

Jill Crawley-Low and her staff at the University of Saskatchewan's WCVM library were unfailingly patient in helping me find obscure reference material, and my sabbatical time from the university gave me enough space to get this project started.

There were also three unnamed readers who made many helpful suggestions and gave constructive criticism on early drafts. Thank you for that, whoever you are. I hope I have met your demands (or most of them).

In particular I wish to thank Peter Mehren who undertook to read through and early draft of the entire manuscript. For their faith in the work I thank the crew at the University of Alberta Press, headed by Linda Cameron and managing editor Peter Midgley. My editor Meaghan Craven made a huge difference to the text with her perceptive eye, inquisitive mind and dedication. Thanks also to Jane Goodall for writing the foreword with its hopeful message.

A special thanks to Karl Ammann, Patrick Garcia and Amy Howard, for the use of their disturbing pictures of the bush meat trade and dead lions. Others who helped by allowing the use of their photographs and with art references included Chris Bazeley, Jimmy Caldwell, my sister Brigid Cleaver, Marigold Cribb, Juliane Deubner, Trudy Janssens, Dick Neal, Cobus Raath, and Roger Windsor. I have mainly used my own photographs that accompany the last six chapters about work in Uganda, but hundreds of pictures were taken and shared by the 50 students who accompanied me over the years and the photographers were not always identified on the CDs that were circulated amongst us. Where I can I have acknowledged their work, but so many photos were taken, many of them indistinguishable from one another, that I may have missed some names.

My colleagues in Uganda have provided me with the most meaningful teaching and life experience of my career. Headed by the remarkable Christine Dranzoa they include Gil Basuta, Margaret Driciru, John David Kabasa, David Kahwa, Gladys Kalema-Zikusoka, Benon Kanyima, John Kasenene, Eli Katunguka, Denis Muhangi, Lawrence Mushiga, JB Nizeyi, Michael Ocaido, Innocent Rwego, Celsus Senthe, and Ludwig Siefert, and fifteen students who have joined us on our working safaris and made such a difference to the experience for the Canadian students.

A special thanks too to the many Canadian students who have joined Jo and me on those Uganda trips and have not only gained so much, but have given of themselves, not only to us, but to their Ugandan counterparts and especially to the children at Kasenyi and Equator Highway primary schools.

The members of my writers' group have been an enormous help in forcing me to clarify ideas and engage them in the narrative. They are Donna Bowman, Larry Gasper, Glen Kanigan-Fairen, Eve Kotyk, Murray Lindsay, Judy McCrosky, Joannie Savage, Br. Kurt Van Kuren, Jon Watts and Charlene Wirtz.

Ultimately, the perspectives, and any errors, are my own.

Of course none of this would have happened without Jo. ❀

1965–1975

KENYA THEN AND NOW

Soon we saw Mt. Kenya's serrated,
ice-draped peak clear and dark
against the northern sky.

—MARY JOBE AKELEY, in *Africa*

With regard to the decrease of
rhinoceros I cannot suggest any
remedy. It is undoubtedly an
impossible animal to preserve in a
settled district, and of course when
one wanders into or near such a
district he will be killed.

—RICHARD B. WOOSNAM,
Deputy Chief Game Warden, Kenya, 1910

1

MOVIE STAR RHINO

In the second half of my veterinary years in Kenya (1965–1975) I helped with a variety of rhino translocations. Here I recall a rhino capture recorded for posterity, a close call recorded for a Japanese audience, and the treatments of a sick rhino calf.

"I THINK SHE IS VERY SICK. She has not eaten for two days. Please come down as soon as you can."

The "she" was a half-grown Black rhinoceros calf that I had helped captured from a helicopter, using a dart and a mixture of very potent morphine-like drugs, ten days previously. She was waiting in her pen to be transferred to Meru National Park in about three weeks' time.

The call from Alexander Aaron, a Chagga from Moshi in Tanzania, was coming in from the frontier town of Isiolo over a crackling line that faded in and out. I knew right away that I would have to change the plans I had made to vaccinate three horses that afternoon. Alexander was a Grade A trapper with the Seago/Parkinson team of zoological collectors with whom I had been working for three years as they moved rhino out of areas where they were increasingly coming into contact with people.

It had not taken long for me and my assistant, a young Meru man named Mutua Mugambi, to organize my gear in the Peugeot 404 station wagon, registration number KPQ 144, and head out on the ninety-minute drive to the town of Isiolo, about 270 kilometres from Nairobi, north of Mount Kenya. Isiolo was more or less the "gateway" to the Northern Frontier District (known to one and all as the NFD). It was here where the rhino was being held in a *boma* (corral).

Mutua and I set out after lunch, first climbing from Nanyuki's 1,850-metre altitude, uphill most of the way past Timau, to Kisima at almost 2,400 metres, and then plunging down the steep incline that led to Isiolo some thirty kilometres beyond, but at an elevation of only just over 1,000 metres.

We passed many of the farms that made up my regular clientele and admired the fields of waving wheat on either side of the road. Grazing sheep and cattle also dotted the landscape, among them breeds such as Corriedale sheep at Embori, South Devon cattle at Ngushishi and Galloways at Embori and Kisima. As we dropped down, the landscape changed and the giant euphorbias became fever trees and small acacias scattered among the waving yellow grass. I stopped to admire the view as a group of reticulated giraffe obligingly posed in front of the mountain.

Alexander was almost certainly right. There was something wrong with the rhino. A newly caught rhino that does not move when someone enters its pen is certainly more than just a little off colour. The rhino was standing dejectedly, head down, ears uncharacteristically drooping as a steadily emptying plastic bag half-full of intravenous fluids drained into the vein in her ear.

Standing next to a half-grown sick rhinoceros in the middle of a high-walled wooden pen in Kenya was not exactly what I had envisioned myself doing when I entered veterinary school in Glasgow in 1959 and graduated six years later—after a slight hiccup and a year's delay when I accepted the invitation of the examiners to demonstrate better grades in pharmacology before proceeding. Had I not been

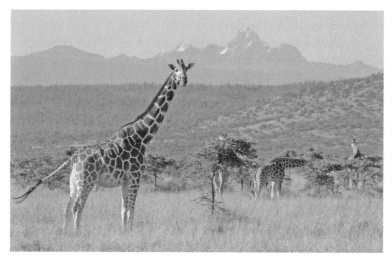
On the way to Isiolo, a view of Mount Kenya. A reticulated giraffe poses in the foreground.

given the opportunity to repeat my second year and delay my graduation, I would probably never have come back to my birth country or, much more important, met and fallen in love with Jo. It was a case of the Haigh family motto at work: *Tyde what may.* By the time I was approaching the sick rhino calf, Jo and I had been married for four years.

My father had been seconded to the King's African Rifles in 1939 and moved there from Fort William in the Scottish highlands, where he was stationed with his regiment, the Highland Light Infantry (City of Glasgow Regiment), and my mother joined him soon afterwards. I was born in Kenya in 1941. We left a couple of years after the war. After the typical itinerant life of a military brat—two years in one house, two years in another, and some time in Germany—I was admitted to the University of Glasgow's faculty of veterinary medicine in Scotland. At the end of that time I had a chance to return to Kenya as an intern at the new veterinary school, and I seized it.

My practice days in Kenya began in 1965 and consisted of a year's internship at the veterinary school at Kabete, near Nairobi. I then spent nearly five years as a government veterinary officer in the town of Meru, on Mount Kenya's northeastern slopes, before my five-year stint in private practice on the west side of the mountain at Nanyuki. While much of my work in Nanyuki involved cattle and horses, as well as a smattering of pets, I was increasingly involved with wildlife, particularly with rhino and their translocation. My early forays into rhino capture, allowing me to work with Markus Hofmeyr in South Africa much later in my career (see page 189), had come about because I was a keen tennis player (of course).

My very first day back in Kenya in 1965 ended with a game of tennis at the Vet Lab Sports Club courts where I met blond wavy-haired Tony Parkinson, one of several animal trappers and zoological collectors then working in the country. Within a few days I was at Tony's base compound in Lowe Kabete, about eight kilometres from the office, dealing with my first wild animal case as I had to climb up the side of the chute to inject the backside of the five-metre giraffe that had developed foot rot. Four years later, Tony and his partner, godfather and mentor, the skinny stooped John Seago, had asked me to join them as they switched from the old-fashioned method of catching rhino with a lariat to the more modern one in which drugs and darts were used.

Most of our work was carried out on the edge of the NFD, just north of Isiolo, where we captured the rhino and moved them out of the district in order to make room for a settlement scheme. Other than the basic biological imperatives of survival and propagation, nothing drives the lives of Kenyans more than ownership of a *plotti* (plot of land), so the settlement scheme was a high political priority for the local and very powerful minister, Jackson Angaine.

I went into the rhino work as a complete ignoramus, only knowing by hearsay that a few had been captured by the new method, but having no idea about the actual process. Tony and his team started each day by sending trackers out into the bush trying to find signs of the animals. At about mid-morning the trackers would return as the rest of us sat and hoped for good news. Then it was into the vehicles and off to the bush, often covering several kilometres across country. The cross-country driving was in itself hazardous, what with huge rocks hidden in the grass, truck-eating ant-bear holes, steep-sided *luggahs* (seasonally filled channels that carry water, sometimes raging torrents, during the rainy seasons) and thorns that could go right through tires often in groups. One puncture often meant several in the same inner tube.

I asked one of the trackers, named Meru, so nick-named as he was the only team member of that tribe, and with whom I could at least greet in my very rudimentary KiMeru (the Ki- indicates the tribal language, as in KiSwahili, the Ki- often being dropped), how he found the rhino. We chatted in Swahili.

"We search for the piles of manure where they have been to the *choo* and as those are always in the same place every day, we know the boundaries of their homes."

Later, I asked him to show me one such midden, and we stopped to look at one right beside a track.

"It looks as if he has kicked it around," I said.

"Yes," he replied with a grin. "Don't you know why?"

"No, tell me," I said, half expecting something weird, as I had already found out that he was a bit of a charming rogue, a *mkora* in fact. Meru at once launched into the following story:

> *The father of all rhino was once walking through the forest when he met an elephant and they had a fight. The rhino got the worst of it, and ran away with flaps of bleeding skin, all hanging down. After a while he met a porcupine and said to him: "Lend me one of your needles so that I can sew up my skin."*
>
> *"All right," answered the porcupine, "but you must be sure to give the needle back to me tomorrow."*
>
> *Rhino do not have thumbs,* [at this point Meru wiggled his right thumb about] *so his stitching job was not very neat and he had some places where there was too much skin, so he just put it together as best as he could, ending up with ridges. By the time he had finished he had forgotten all about returning the needle. Then one day he met the porcupine again.*
>
> *"Where's my needle?" asked the porcupine.*
>
> *The rhino couldn't remember, and thought he must have sewn it up inside himself. Ever since then he has been looking for it to return it to its owner and kicks his dung in case it has come out.* ❁

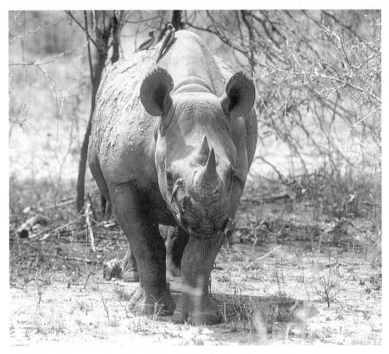

Red-billed oxpeckers not only seek out feed on the rhino, but they also act as his sentries.

After a few captures from the truck, with the inevitable damage to various parts of its body, not to mention the bashing about that I was getting standing in the back behind Tony as he drove, we had a confab, and decided that something better was needed, as we were taking too much time to achieve not much. A rhino every two or three days was not efficient. On my next trip to Isiolo I found a small red-and-white helicopter parked beside the camp. I soon met the pilot, solidly built Andy Neal, and we worked together on the project for the next four years.

After some more or less inevitable glitches, I established a very effective drug cocktail for rhino captures that was a great success. It was a mixture of two drugs: fentanyl, a potent morphine-like compound, and Azaperone, a very effective sedative, aptly named Stresnil because it did indeed reduce or eliminate stress in pigs, the species for which it had been first developed.

A darted rhino would begin to slow down and stagger about five minutes after the dart hit it in the rump. It would then begin to circle and soon fall over or come to halt against some trivial object, such as a tree. Only if the dart hit a rhino over bony areas, where drug absorption would be slow or even fail, did I have to consider administering top-up doses. These would ensure that the rhino did not stagger around for too long and exhaust itself.

While Andy and I waited for a darted rhino to slow down to a halt, we kept in touch with Tony over the two-way radio. Tony could usually keep quite close in his truck, often having the animal in sight as it blundered about. See the footage at www.jerryhaigh.com.

Once the rhino stopped, Tony and his team would park about thirty metres away from it, get out of the old Ford truck and gallop across the rough ground to it with hobbling ropes in hand. Once Tony had tied the rhino's legs together and the animal was on its side, it was an easy task to roll it onto a sled and winch the whole thing up onto a three-tonne lorry. From there it was usually no more than a couple of hours of rough cross-country driving back to camp.

My job, once the helicopter put me on the ground, was to keep a close eye on the animal's condition, making sure that it was breathing comfortably, that its pulse was steady and not too rapid and that its temperature did not escalate. In order to be able to give it the correct dose of antibiotics and other treatments that I felt it needed, I also had to calculate its weight from measurements of its length and girth.

The formula for calculating a rhino's weight in this manner had been developed by Cambridge veterinarian Dr. John King, who, when working with the Kenya Game Department had immobilized and weighed enough animals to be able to correlate measurements with actual weights with no more than a 5 per cent error margin. His formula, when one thinks about it, was elegantly simple and takes one back to high-school physics. A rhino is really no more than a cylinder with a few bits stuck on it. The volume of a cylinder is its length multiplied by the square of the radius of the circle. Using the girth as the circumference of the circle gives one the radius (using the knowledge of Pi, or Greek π, the roughly 3.141592653589793 multiple of the diameter). All John had had to do was add a constant to allow for legs and head, and—Presto!—he had a weight. The bigger challenge had probably been to devise a method of weighing a one-tonne rhino in the middle of nowhere with nothing

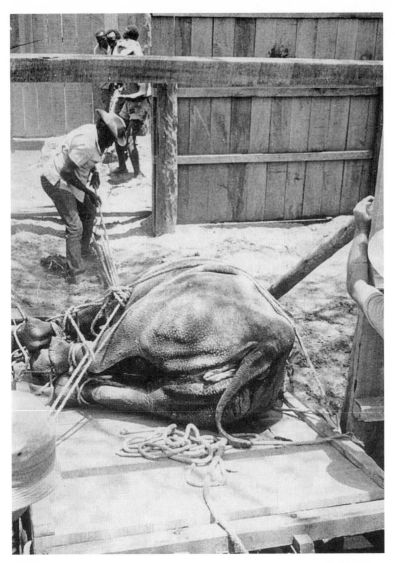

Unloading a rhino into the bomas at Isiolo.

more than a scale, a winch and some ropes, but this John had solved by rolling his charges onto a flat wooden palette and then hoisting the whole assemblage under a tripod.

Once back at camp, it was a simple matter of sliding the sled off the lorry into an empty and very robust pen, rolling the rhino off the sled and pulling his recent bed out of the pen before closing the heavy gate and administering the antidote to the fentanyl.

The animal would usually wake within a minute or two, no doubt surprised and certainly angry. Sometimes, especially if the air temperature was high and the animal remained on its side for too long after the antidote was given, we would pour twenty litres or so of water over it. The response was always immediate as the rhino leapt to its feet, which is quite a thing to witness when an animal has short legs and a big barrel of a body.

It usually took about four or five days to fill the eight pens that acted as the staging post before beginning the translocation to a park.

Tony and I had been working together for about two years, catching a new batch of rhino every four to six weeks, when a new twist to the program occurred. It was January 1972, and Tony had called, asking me if I was free to come down in ten days for a new capture session, adding that we would be working with a film crew.

As Mutua and I drove off the Isiolo-to-Marsabit road that day, and the fine white dust plume that had been blowing sideways behind us suddenly engulfed the car, we quickly closed the windows to avoid choking. We threaded our way between the acacias past the rhino bomas and up to the parking spot at the camp.

There were three vehicles that I didn't recognize—a fancy new Jeep and two Land Cruisers—parked alongside the company Land Rover and Tony's monster, a 1957 powder-blue, Bel Air Chevy, replete with fins and chrome fit for a space shuttle. There was also a small group of new tents erected away to the east and new faces round the dining table.

Tony introduced them, the names flying past in the usual blur, making them hard to remember. But one name did stick, both because it was the first name that flew at me and also because the man attached to the name had a distinct Hispanic look to him. He was somewhat overweight, although on his big frame it hardly showed. He was the first man I had ever met who carried Mexican blood in him. His name was Frank Zuniga, and I learned that he was directing a film that featured John, Tony and the crew, and that rhino capture and translocation were to be a part of the story. The film was being made for television and was to be called *The Biggest Bongo in the World*. (In the end, the TV movie was titled *The Track of the African Bongo* in two parts.) The bongo is a magnificent chocolate-coloured antelope, with large spiral horns and creamy vertical stripes on its body. Bongo live in the mountain forests of Kenya and farther west into the Congo and Cameroon. They are secretive and seldom seen in the wild.

The capture of some rhino was to be used as a way of introducing John and Tony to the story, which, I was told, involved a young boy's dream of seeing a huge bongo. It turned out that Frank worked for The Walt Disney Company, and he would be picking up the tab for all the rhino caught and also paying an extra daily fee to me while I was being filmed. It sounded alright to me!

"Jerry," said Tony, "Frank wants to film us catching a bunch of rhino, so I hope you've got several sets of the same clothes, so that they can develop continuity."

I thought for a moment. My shorts were all standard khaki, and I would be wearing the leather sandals called *chaplis*, so widely used in Kenya, so my shirts would be the only problem.

"I only have four shirts with me, and they are all of different colours," I responded. "I'll get pretty antisocial after a day or two, but I guess I can change just before we head out and then again when we get back to camp." Other than that, things went pretty much as usual, although there turned out to be some interesting differences to our usual capture routine.

While we continued to approach each animal using our now well-established team approach, Frank would now and again call for a pause and set up his cameras for a different angle. At first I was worried that this might create problems if there was some need for a specific treatment for the new captive; however, the film crew were very professional, and we simply got on with the job.

I had recently acquired my own movie camera, a Canon Super 8, which was of course dwarfed by the big professional equipment carried by the Disney crew, but it seemed to me to be a golden opportunity to enlist some help in improving my home movies. One thing I wanted to do was the get some film footage of the business of preparing and loading my darts. A young apprentice cameraman was quite willing to help, and so we set up the drug box on an upturned fuel drum and went through a couple of dummy runs of the procedure, during which I used water instead of my expensive, and dangerous, immobilizing drugs. Hoping to get some more footage later that day I was quite surprised and a little miffed to be told that the young man had been warned off helping me, and that he was not permitted to do any more shooting.

In his turn, Frank was not overly impressed with the intrusion of my very amateur camera efforts into his work, as witnessed on one occasion by his appearance in my lens using a well-known finger gesture of contempt as a tied-down rhino was winched on his sled up the ramp into the three-tonne truck.

The rhino immobilizations went smoothly, though, and after a few days we had the bomas filled up. The animals would be transferred, after the usual acclimatization period, either to Meru National Park or to the private game park at Solio that my client Mr. Court Parfet, the American chewing-gum millionaire, had established. However, the film was by no means finished with just this one series of captures, and so I found myself going to Isiolo on a regular basis for the next several months.

One afternoon, while everybody else was having a siesta, Tony and I sat chatting. "Frank made a film about wild horses," he said, "and one of his spectacular shots (in fact I believe that he made quite a name for himself with it), was taken when he put the camera in a trench and filmed the horses as they were let out of a corral and ran and jumped over the top of the film crew below them. He approached me about letting one of our rhino out to get the same shot, but I turned him down."

"Ye gods and little fishes, it would have been a disaster," I replied. "I doubt the beast would have seen the trench at all, and even if it had, rhino are hardly known for their cross-country jumping ability. Either way, there would have been a wreck. Dead cameramen and injured or dead rhino, as well." I heard no more about this idea, but I did get a brief speaking part. I have no idea if it made the final cut.

That culmination of my involvement in the film project happened when I was asked to act out a small part in the drama. The premise was that I was to "save" a rhino that had got into breathing trouble by injecting a small dose of antidote into its ear. Tony or John must have had the idea after seeing me use this technique to revive one of our early patients. My first "professional" acting slot involved running over a slight rise in the land and mouthing something to Tony about there being another rhino "just over there," and urging everyone to get a move on to catch it. Hardly a likely scenario in real life, but, as I was to learn, movies don't seem to take much account of reality, especially some of the so-called "wild animal" movies that I have seen over the years.

After being told not to worry about the other rhino, with an uncharacteristically scripted grumpy response from Tony, I had to get out my drug kit, pull up some emergency medication, and "treat" the rhino that Tony was monitoring. The fact that in real life it would actually have been me doing the monitoring, while Tony was fulfilling his part of the team effort (supervising the crew and ensuring that ropes were well tied), seemed to have slipped past the script writer.

We were in an open glade about seventy-five metres from camp. I did the running-from-over-the-hill thing half a dozen times, and then the syringe-filling thing about six more and, finally, the dramatic injection four times, with my face screwed up in concentration and my tongue half out between partially clenched teeth in a "characteristic" mannerism. All this for a needle insertion into a piece of three-centimetre rope. Of course, there was no rhino anywhere in sight.

I never did see the finished product. When I phoned the company to find out if I could have a short segment—no more than a couple or three minutes of the actual capture—to use as a teaching aid, I discovered that, at a dollar per foot of film, I was priced right out of the market. The film project did not run continuously because between each session of rhino captures there was usually a four- to six-week gap while the animals were acclimatized and moved to the their new destinations.

It was during this acclimatization period that careful monitoring of the newly captured animals took place under the supervision of Alexander and Mwaneki Kaundu, another Grade A trapper, a M'Kamba from Kitui district. Tony would check in regularly, but he had other duties and programs in various pars of the country, so he relied upon the two men to supervise everything at Isiolo.

There was no sign of Alexander in camp on that afternoon when I arrived to see the sick rhino calf, but Mwaneki was there, and he came out of his tent as we drove into camp in the station wagon.

"*Hujambo Daktari, habari yako? Hujambo Mutua,*" ("Good day doctor, what news? Good day Mutua,") he said. Although Mwaneki understood a great deal of English, he either preferred not to show it or was more comfortable in Swahili, so we continued in the latter as we moved over to one of the eight robust pens that had been constructed from camphor wood under the shade of a grove of flat-topped acacia trees. We climbed up the outside of the pen of the rhino in question and watched in silence as the rhino, not quite half grown, stood dejectedly in the middle of the pen, a pile of freshly cut acacia and other favourite food items only a metre or so away from her, but seemingly untouched.

"She has not eaten properly for five days," said Mwaneki. "I asked Alexander to call you two days ago, but he decided to wait."

"Where is he now?" I asked.

"He's in Isiolo," was the brief reply. I later found out from Tony that while this had been true, it may not have been the whole truth, as Alexander had a liking for beer.

It was obvious that I was going to have to get into the pen, but the key question was whether I would be able to do so without having to sedate, or maybe even immobilize, the animal. The first test to see if I would be in danger was easy. We put one of the five-metre-long bamboo poles that we carried in the ground vehicles into the pen. These poles had attached lassos, ready to snare and bring to a halt drugged rhino if they showed any inclination to get into dangerous terrain such as dry luggahs. Normally putting such an object in with a newly caught rhino would induce a quick and angry response. We saw nothing of the sort.

There was now only one thing for it. If I climbed in carefully, ready to exit with a record-breaking high jump if need be, I would get more information on the clinical status of the rhino.

As I gingerly descended the walls of the pen, there was no response from beneath, although I sensed a heightened tension from above as Mutua and Mwaneki watched over the wall. I stepped away from the security blanket of the rails on the inside of the vertical planks, which served as a ladder, and still there was no response. This told me that I could proceed, but more important, the lack of response told me a good deal about the condition of what was now very definitely my patient.

The first step was to take a blood smear from the tip of her ear, more important even than putting a thermometer where it would do its job, as so many animal diseases in East Africa are detected as blood-borne parasites. When I checked her temperature, it was a high 104° F (40° C). Next I completed a check of her eyes, in an attempt to see if she was anaemic. She at last showed signs of resentment, by moving her head away from me, but not enough to endanger me. I decided to let this ride, as it was a weak response, although I had already felt the effects of a rhino horn in my side after an accident filmed by a Japanese film crew the previous year.

I would love to have seen the Japanese footage, as the original included my somewhat abrupt somersault over the top of a rhino, propelled by its horn. I recollect very little of the details, except that I did manage a complete somersault as the horn speared me in the belly and flipped me about ten metres. I wonder what score for technical merit and artistic impression I would have been given by gymnastics judges. Not a ten, surely, unless one counts the unusual method of propulsion. Did the footage make it to the final cut? I've no idea.

Pushing thoughts of my previous horn encounter aside, I tried to listen to the sick rhino calf's breathing through my stethoscope, but as usual found this a frustrating exercise. If Meru's folk tale and Rudyard Kipling's *Just So* story "How the Rhinoceros Got His Skin" were a bit fanciful with their explanation of the irregular contours of a rhino's hide, and the Parsee's cake crumbs under the skin were not in fact the cause of the ridges, the thickness and roughness still made stethoscope work pretty futile.

Forewarned by Alexander's telephone call, I had packed some extra equipment in my car. My field microscope, basic equipment for counting the total number of cells in blood and some stain and glass vials for blood smears were on the rear seat, rather than in the luggage compartment, so we soon had a "laboratory" work table set up in the kitchen area. Tilting the mirror under the lenses so that the afternoon sun would reflect up through the stained slide was accomplished with the ease of long practice, and in no time it was plain that my instinct to bring the microscope and equipment had played an important role in diagnosing the animal's condition. The fiddly work of preparing and counting cells showed that the rhino had fewer of them than any I had previously examined, meaning that she was anaemic, although I had no published information of normal values on which to base this assumption. Many of the red blood cells contained the characteristic pear-shaped purple bodies diagnostic of the tick-borne fever known as Babesiosis.

Now to do something about it. The Babesiosis part was easy. Using my capture data from ten days previously, I checked on the weight estimation that I had made from the measurements of the rhino's length and girth.

Once I had a weight, I asked Mutua to mix up the correct amount of the German drug called Berenil that had proved so useful for the treatment of tick fevers, as well as sleeping sickness, in almost all the species with which I dealt. I had luckily heard of the disaster that had befallen a member of the Livestock Marketing Division who had, as an entirely sensible precaution, used the drug to treat a large mob of camels that he had had to move through country where sleeping sickness was known to occur. He had lost every single one of them to the "treatment." I had also had the luck to treat a single rhino with Berenil on a previous occasion and had not killed it. The two lessons have stood me in good stead to this day. If I have to treat animals of some species new to me using a drug that is not listed for that species, I will treat one beast only and then watch closely to see if the drug has any adverse effects.

After giving the rhino the Berenil, I treated her anaemia by giving an injection of iron solution and a multivitamin shot. It was also very important to try to give the animal something to boost its energy and give it a kick-start on the hoped-for road to recovery. I injected a healthy dose of energy-boosting corticosteroids and asked Mutua to bring several of sterile plastic bags from the car, each containing a litre of fluids that had both essential salts and a weak solution of dextrose in them, as well as the tubes needed to administer a drip and a forked stick about two metres long, on which to hang the bags.

As I stood there in the middle of the pen holding the stick, the drip solution running steadily, but not too rapidly, into a vein in the animal's ear, I heard Tony's voice and a moment later saw his hair sticking up over the top of the pen wall.

"Hi Jerry, what's going on?" he asked.

"She's got Babesiosis. Alexander phoned this morning and asked me to come down, and I've given her some Berenil. I think she needs a couple more bottles of fluids as well as the other stuff I've given her."

"Okay. I'll leave you to it, unless there's anything I can do. See you when you're finished."

A LITTLE WHILE LATER, I clambered out of the pen, the rhino's dejected attitude having changed very little, and went over to the mess tent where Tony had a welcome cup of tea on the go.

We talked of the rhino, and I told him of my guarded optimism for its future, being more concerned about its overall condition than the Babesiosis itself, now that the Berenil was on board.

"I knew that it was serious when I saw the drip," he said.

"I'll check her just now, but I think we'd better see how she is in the morning. So, I'll use my usual tent if that's okay." I had already warned Jo that I might not get back that night.

After chatting for an hour or so I went to check my patient by torchlight. She seemed much as I had left her. Then it was a hot shower under the stars and an early night to bed under the mosquito net in my tent. ❋

2

THE LAST OF THE ROANS

After checking on the rhino calf, I fall into conversation with Tony, who tells me about another translocation exercise in which he has been involved—this one being a long-term exercise (1968–1972) with roan antelope in the Ithanga Hills. It is not long before I find myself dealing with one of his former charges.

NEXT MORNING, as the dawn light started to make the stars vanish, a dove began its repetitive coo in the thorn trees near my tent, reminding me of the myth about the collared dove, whose descending rolling call is said to be the Greek word *dekaocto*, or eighteen. The story of this dove is part of the one of Jesus Christ carrying the cross to Calvary. When a Roman soldier took pity on him and tried to buy a cup of milk for him from a roadside vendor who told him it would cost eighteen coins. He only had seventeen and she would not budge even when he pleaded. When Christ was crucified, the unwilling vendor was turned into a dove and condemned to go about saying eighteen (*dekaocto*) for ever. If she ever says seventeen (*dekaepta*), she will be-come human, but if she ever says nineteen (*dekaennaea*) the world will come to an end.

My early-morning tea arrived dead on time at seven o'clock, and it was soon time to be up and about and check on my young rhino patient, who seemed to have perked up a bit. I hoped my observation wasn't just wishful thinking. She was certainly no worse and turned sharply as I began to come down the inside of the pen walls. It seemed best to stop before I reached the ground.

At breakfast, Tony and I chatted for a while.

"I've just come up from the Tana Ranch. We've been checking on another batch of roan," he said.

"How's that going?" I asked. "No more disasters?"

"No, everything has been going smoothly."

The whole roan translocation exercise had been well publicized and reported in several articles in *Africana*, the magazine arm of the East African Wild Life Society. The society had initially been consulted as settlement encroached on the ranch because there were known to be roan and several other wild species in the area. It was the society that had raised the funds, through public donation, for the exercise, and Tony had given me occasional personal reports over the three years up to 1972 as we sat and enjoyed the clear skies and night sounds of Africa.

Tana Ranch lay in the Ithanga Hills region south of the Tana River and the idea of translocating the roan had first been raised in 1968, when it was thought that only twenty-five of them remained on the land there. These were thought to be the last remaining herd of the species in Kenya, although herds in Tanzania and farther south were known to exist in fair numbers.

Miles Coverdale, a Thika coffee farmer and knowledgeable natural-ist, who was also an honorary game warden, had been the first to raise the alarm about the probable fate of the roan as a project was scheduled for African settlers to move into the area and develop smallholdings, which would inevitably destroy the habitat for wildlife. Tony, John and Mwaneki, with Miles as part of the team, had found out that there were more like eighty roan in the area, as well as other species such as eland and zebra, and all were under heavy poaching pressure.

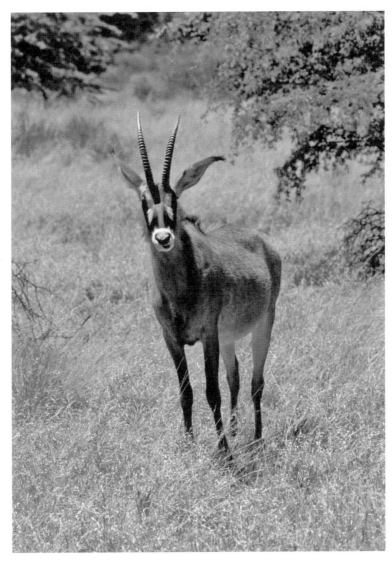

A healthy roan antelope checks us out.

Within eighteen months of the discovery of the large population of roan, the Seago/Parkinson crew had built a boma some three hundred metres in circumference that had a narrow entrance and wings stretching out in a long V down which the animals could be guided. The design was hardly revolutionary, as there is evidence of a similar construction in the Syrian desert that dates back to pre-Christian times, and similar capture structures that date back thousands of years were used in the bison cultures of North America. After a couple of near-miss attempts to herd the animals using Land Rovers and horses, the crew decided to bring in Andy Neal and his helicopter, which is where we had also gone with our rhino capture. The helicopter system improved the success rate at once.

The first roan capture success, of twelve animals, came in March 1970, but during the night poachers made a small opening in the walls and the inevitable happened. Tony had philosophically put this down to the fact that it was Friday the Thirteenth.

In May of that year Alexander had had a lucky escape. A roan breaking back against the chasers who had been hidden while the helicopter brought the roan into the wings of the trap, and who were trying to push them the last hundred metres or so into the boma, ran head-on into his horse. He flew clear, but both animals died instantly. The disaster was ameliorated by the fact that fourteen roan had been captured and seven more were driven into the trap that same day.

In September 1971 the ABC television network made a movie of the roan translocation process with Joe Kennedy, son of Robert Kennedy, as guest star, and during his Kenya trip he came to our house on Lunatic Lane with our friend Wilber James and then on to the Mount Kenya Rugby Club annual dinner. For the occasion I had to help him with his wardrobe, as the dress code called for a jacket and tie. Jacket he had, but his borrowed tie was that of the Glasgow University Union, to which I temporarily elevated him, albeit without any authority to do so.

It was during the after-dinner dance at this event that a senior member of the club showed her colours. An English schoolteacher who was of West Indian descent had come to Kenya with his pretty, very blonde, Caucasian wife, and had joined our team. He played and starred on the wing, having learned the game at Sheffield University. Not long married, the couple danced together (and I mean together), jiving, twisting and moving as a conjoined body, especially during the slow numbers when no daylight was visible between them. The senior, whose husband had been a keen rugby man between the two world wars, was outraged. When I saw her in the main street outside my office the next morning she said to me, "Did you see that nice white girl dancing with that black man? It was disgusting."

I replied that they were man and wife, and that he was, moreover, an Englishman. This seemed to stop her in her tracks. I was never sure if she was objecting to the racial mix or merely the very expressive dancing. Such an activity would raise no eyebrows today, but as Elvis Presley's hip gyrations had been banned on American TV in their time, perhaps the old settler was caught in some sort of time warp.

After our conversation I went back to the cottage for a mid-morning cup of coffee and found Wilber and Joe just struggling awake. As he retuned my tie, I asked Joe about the roan incident, but he seemed unphased by it after the passage of time, or maybe he had lost interest after the media circus.

Tony told me that over thirty roan had been taken to the Shimba Hills, south of Mombasa on the Kenya coast, and twelve had come to Solio, the private game ranch owned by Court Parfet, although no reason why these moves should have occurred has ever been offered. The habitats of both places are completely different than that of the Ithanga Hills.

I heard no more about the Solio roan and did not have contact with any of the translocated animals until several months after that conversation with Tony. In May 1972, Rodney Elliot, the gruff mustachioed ex-game warden, now the game ranch manager at the ranch, asked me to pay a visit and bring my immobilizing kit because he was concerned about a roan.

If you can imagine a row of hairy coat hangers on a rack, that is the nearest visual image that I can conjure up, short of an actual photograph, to convey the look of the ribs of the emaciated roan antelope that stood stock still in a daze. The animal was a gaunt outline against the backdrop of the Aberdare Mountains, standing about eight metres from the side of the Land Rover. We sat in the vehicle looking at the antelope and Rodney told me a bit more about the history of this, and the other eleven of its kind, that had arrived at Solio only a few months previously.

My challenge was to try to figure out how to deal with the animal, or even to find out what was wrong. Doing nothing was not an option.

"Look at his ribs and also at the bones of his pelvis and hips that are showing so clearly. He must have lost a huge amount of weight, and he seems to have very laboured breathing, as well," I said to Rodney as my assistant Mutua and M'Otoro Okuwam, Rodney's tough but ancient Turkana guard, looked on.

"Well, we can't leave him to die, and as far as I know none of the others are alive. There were three together ten days ago, but I haven't seen any trace of live ones, other than this one, since then. We did see a lion feeding on a carcass about a fortnight ago, but I couldn't tell what sort of condition it was in. What can you do?" Rodney asked.

"I don't like his chances much, but I suppose we shall have to immobilize him and carry out an examination."

Weight estimation, to use as a guide to correct dosage, was the first challenge, as the degree of emaciation made all my previous experience with other members of the antelope family almost irrelevant. I had never immobilized a roan antelope, but my fentanyl-based cocktail had worked safely, with no losses, on at numerous individuals of least fifteen other species, and I had become confident in its use. Some of those species had never been immobilized before, but at the quarantine station in Mombasa on the Kenya coast, I had injected fentanyl into several bongo and some Jentink's duiker, which are a rare, dark-grey, solid-bodied antelope about the size of a St. Bernard dog, weighing up to eighty kilograms. (My 1973 Christmas present copy of the *The Guinness Book of World Records* stated that the Jentink's was the rarest antelope known.) I settled on a dose that I thought the roan could survive and soon had a dart in the muscles of his hind leg (or what was left of them).

He moved only about thirty paces after the dart hit him, stood for a couple of minutes, and subsided gently against a nearby bush. Rodney and I were quickly out of the vehicle, followed promptly by Mutua.

Before I could even get a temperature reading, I knew that we had a problem. He was not going to survive. Within five minutes of going down he had stopped breathing, despite a dose of antidote directly into the vein and a general stimulant.

There was only one thing for it, and so I proceeded, with the others as very interested onlookers, to carry out a post-mortem examination.

In my field pathology notes, of which I have the carbon copies, I noted that the animal was covered in hundreds of ticks. The major finding inside the body cavity was in the lungs, which were dark red and hard, when they should have been pink and soft. There were between twenty-five and thirty dark cream-coloured masses throughout the lungs. They varied from about two centimetres in diameter to slightly larger than golf-ball size. Each mass consisted of numerous intertwined five- to eight-centimetre reddish-brown worms. The liver was also small and hardened. I sent samples of the lungs and other tissues to the diagnostic lab at the vet school at Kabete, as well as to the government labs.

Dr. Herbert Frank was one of the vet college pathologists and had lived in the flat next to mine when I had been an intern at the vet college in 1965. He kept a variety of venomous snakes in glass cages, which made potential visitors very nervous, especially when the odd one escaped, and thereby reduced his social life. Three weeks after receiving the roan samples, he reported to me that the entire lung tissue was inflamed and wrote that the worms were *Protostrongylus africanus*, the same worms that had been reported in roan in Tanzania's Serengeti. He therefore concluded that the animal had been infected when it left the Ithanga Hills.

In his report to the Director of Veterinary Services and to Mr. Parfet, Solio's owner, Rodney noted, even before the lab results were known: "I am satisfied cause of death was not the darting and animal would have definitely died anyway if no treatment tried."

Roan were not seen again on Solio, but they did survive for a while at the Shimba Hills, although it is not known for how long. There are none there now. Their disappearance could have been due to one or more of a number of factors. Rodney had seen lions feasting on a roan at Solio, so others might have gone the same way, especially if they were sick and therefore vulnerable. The moist conditions may not have been ideal and ticks may have played a role either as disease vectors or simply as bloodsuckers. In fact two roan were lost very early on in the Shimba Hills when huge numbers of ticks were found feasting on them in the release bomas.

Presumably the animals that were not translocated also died, but probably only one or two at a time as they became food for local people through the activities of "poachers" who may have been descendants of those who had hunted there for generations before the coming of settlers.

IN THE END, my rhino calf patient fared better than the translocated roan, at least at first. Within a few days she had recovered her appetite, no doubt somewhat helped by the euphorbia that Tony had arranged to be specially cut for her, knowing that it was as candy to a child. She was held for longer than usual at Isiolo, to allow her to fully recover her strength, and then loaded in her crate onto a lorry and taken to Meru National Park, a place to which many of our captured animals were shipped. If she survived the conflict that was sure to arise after being placed in another rhino's territory, she certainly did not survive the attentions of the poachers who cleaned out all the rhino at Meru National Park, both black and white species, within fifteen years.

The boma and wing-drive trapping techniques used by Tony and his team have been considerably refined in the thirty years since I worked with him and spoke with him about the roan captures. Many species are now captured using this basic system, and it has become the routine method for rounding up virtually all hoofed animals in Africa. In South Africa, many of the six thousand odd game ranchers capture and translocate surplus stock in this way, and they have had the benefit of the development of sophisticated drug cocktails to alleviate the stress on the animals. As a result, they achieve very high success rates with virtually no animal losses.

On the surface of it, translocation would appear to be a nice solution in all sorts of situations and later I will give examples of translocation as a conservation technique. The White rhino story that starts on page 189 is uplifting and shows clearly that translocation can be a huge success, especially when moving animals into areas where there is no competition. The wild dog story starting on page 207 is a little more complex, but for now it looks good. The roan antelope translocations from Tana Ranch, however, were a complete failure. For success to occur, one needs plenty of careful planning. The main things to think about include nutrition, competition, diseases, method of transfer and follow-up.

In the roan case many things went wrong. The coastal habitat and food supply at the Shimba Hills was very different than that of Ithanga, so this might have been a negative influence on the roan's survival. There was no competition from their own species at either destination, but the mass of ticks and the lung parasites' emergence as a major pathogen, no doubt increasing their effect when their hosts were under stress, was catastrophic.

The roan almost certainly took the lungworm with them, but there is also a risk for translocated animals to acquire a pathogen that they have never met before, upon arrival, which can be an even worse situation, as the animal will be naïve to the challenge of the new pathogen and will have no built-up resistance to it. For any translocation, anywhere, imported pathogens can be a particular problem if the pathogen the host brings in is unknown at the destination and proceeds to affect the native animals.

The best example of a disastrous translocation of animals that led to a disease outbreak occurred at the end of the nineteenth century when traders brought cattle infected with the deadly Rinderpest virus into Africa for the first time. Not for nothing is the disease it causes also known as cattle plague. Within a few years an epidemic had swept down the continent killing an estimated 90 per cent of all cloven-hooved animals, from cattle to buffalo, from tall giraffe to tiny dik-dik. Untold millions died.

The presence of competition among species at the destination site of a translocation once received scant attention from anyone, which is no longer the case. The competition is especially important if it includes members of the same species that have established home ranges that they defend. In such a case, battles are likely to ensue and battles mean losers, some of which are killed. In 2007 ecologist Laurence Frank put it to me succinctly about the species he has studied for over thirty years: "If you translocate lions, something bad will happen." He was echoing a report prepared for the then Kenya Game Department by long-time park warden Peter Jenkins, which urged that no lion translocation be conducted as it would be doomed to failure. The report has since been "lost," perhaps because it contains inconvenient truths.

Of course there is also the question of genetics relative to translocated animals. If the moved animals are of different genetic stock than closely related native ones at the destination, is it morally acceptable to bring them in? It becomes a question of degree and also one of per-ceived need. Are we creating hybrids, and if so, does it matter?

Only if due consideration is given to these and other factors can animal translocations be justified. ✳

3

ONE
SICK
LION

My first challenge dealing with a sick lion in April
1973. A British army major works with Jo on
cases of altitude sickness and then accompanies
me when I return to the lion.

ONE OF THE STRIKING DIFFERENCES between the clients during my
five years as a government veterinary officer in Meru and the subsequent 1970–1975 period of private practice in Nanyuki was the fact
that in the latter years I had two clients who ran private game parks.
Only one had lions in it, and only once was I called to deal with a sick
one. This was at Solio on the Laikipia Plains west and slightly south of
Nanyuki between Mount Kenya and the Aberdare Mountains, where
I had had to deal with the emaciated roan antelope. In 1968 the ranch
owner, Court Parfet, put a game-proof fence up around an area in
which it had proved impossible to keep cattle because of the swampy
ground and the heavy loads of disease-bearing ticks. Some species

like the beautiful reticulated giraffe with its dark chocolate and mustard patches, and the graceful impala, had simply not left the river valley and therefore became residents of Parfet's ranch by default. Mr. Parfet also started to stock the area with a variety of other animals, particularly rhino and some lions.

Rodney Elliott, the park's game warden, was a classic example of the ex-army type who might have been spoofed by Noel Coward in his excruciatingly funny, but bitingly satirical, song, "I Wonder what Happened to Him." Tall and straight-backed, Rodney's greying hair was swept back off his forehead and his upper-crust accent would have made him a natural for a movie part about the British Raj. He had been at Maralal in Kenya's Northern Frontier District for many years and upon retirement had been offered a job by Mr. Parfet. He called in at my office late one afternoon when I was relaxing and reading a fly-tying magazine.

"Good afternoon, Haigh," he said. "I wonder if you would be free to come and see one of Mr. Parfet's lions. He is a particular favourite, and one of my scouts found him this morning looking a bit groggy and not moving from under a thorn bush. I took some meat out this morning and the lion showed no interest in it, even when I dropped a largish lump right onto his foot. I tried to phone you at lunchtime, but the phones were out, so I thought I'd better drive in."

"Yes, I'm sure I can come tomorrow morning, first thing. It's probably a bit late today. I don't think we can get there before dark. How long has the lion been sick, do you think?" I asked.

"Well, he killed an impala four days ago and had driven a lioness off a kill the day before that."

"Nothing else?" I asked.

"He has been lame on and off for a few months."

The morning visit to the park had presented an interesting problem. If we were to get anywhere with the patient, I would have to make a more detailed examination. One choice would have been to get out of Rodney's Land Rover after testing the big cat with a prod, and just do it. This naturally was not my first choice. Despite the fact that he was not moving, I was not foolhardy enough to jump out of the vehicle to examine him straight away. He took no notice when

Rodney revved the engine, so we had moved and come in at a different angle. This time the lion lifted his head and had a brief look at us. That decided it.

"Rodney, if I'm going to get a closer look at him I shall have to immobilize him," I said. "He's obviously very ill, but I'm not brave or dumb enough to do it any other way. I've got my dart pistol here, and the drugs to go with it, but with an animal in that condition there's a real risk that he won't survive the anaesthetic."

"Of course," Rodney said. "Go ahead. We must see what's what."

More manoeuvring had allowed me to get a shot into the patient's right hip, at which he promptly sat up, but immediately flopped over again. After waiting ten minutes, I tested him by prodding his rear end with an umbrella that was handily available in the back of the vehicle. There was no response, so, cautiously, I climbed out of the Land Rover, and Rodney backed me up with his rifle.

It was at once apparent that the lion was quite out of it. Even a reluctant Mutua emerged from the back seat and was standing by.

We took blood samples, and while Mutua prepared the lion's ear for the smear, I began the clinical examination of my first lion patient. He was thin. Desperately thin. There was no fat on his body anywhere. His stomach was empty. One of his big canine teeth was broken off below the gum line, and grass and other debris were packed in the cavity. His right foreleg was swollen and hot almost all the way to the elbow. Closer examination of his foot revealed what was probably the source of his problem. His second claw was embedded deep into the pad, and an old broken nail was capped on top of the new one. When I tried to straighten it out, several gobs of creamy pus oozed from the hole, and my gloved finger, probing deep into the cavity, gave me the seriously grave message that the bones of the foot were involved.

I asked Rodney to write down some details as I called them out.

"Temp 104.5. Resp 5/min. Heart rate 60/min. Pulse full. Mms—that's mucous membranes—injected, a few small hemorrhages in the gums and conjunctiva."

I then stood up and turned toward the vehicle.

"Rodney, I'll take these samples back home and examine them. It may take a few days to get anything from the lab, but we can check the slide for tick fever, and I can get a rough idea about white cells from it, as well. However, with his history, and the overall picture, plus that nasty mess with his claw embedded like that, the swollen leg, and the infected bones, I think he may have a septicemia. His gums look pretty bad, and I don't like the blood spots there or in his eyes. He's got a fever, and I suspect that he has been sick for a few days at least. Then there's also the possibility of tetanus, either now, or in the near future, which would be very bad news. I'll start him on some antibiotics, give him an anti-tetanus shot, as well, and get some fluids into him."

Thinking that the drug I chose might need to get into his brain in case he had a form of meningitis, I selected chloramphenicol as the treatment of choice, and gave him a good dose, probably slightly overestimating his weight, which seemed safer than underestimating it. Mutua and I tag-teamed as we gave his infected foot a thorough clean-up with water and a dilute disinfectant, and I packed the hole with an antibiotic dressing.

I naturally discussed the case with Jo over a late supper after she had been called to see one of her patients at the Cottage Hospital. A medical doctor, she, as usual, offered helpful ideas as I tried to work out what to do next.

The lion's blood smear told me nothing other than that there was a severe bacterial infection, but our visit on the next day gave us a little encouragement. I did not have to use any immobilizing drugs, but we were able to get another good volume of fluids under his skin and more antibiotic into him. When I tried to give him an injection directly into his vein he objected with vigorous tail twitches and some leg movements. I needed no second warning and dove through the open door of the nearby Land Rover as the lion showed his displeasure by getting up and moving off about fifteen metres.

While I was with my patient that day, Jo had an interesting visitor to her clinic. He was Major Ken Hedges of the Royal Army Medical Corps, who had come out to Kenya with one of the many army units posted there for intensive training. The soldiers were always based at the Nanyuki Sports Club and had a semi-permanent camp set up at the Agricultural Show Grounds adjacent to the club.

The Nanyuki Sports Club was more than just a sports club. Founded just after the First World War, it was initially the centre of virtually all social activity for white people in the small market town. While membership fees, bar tabs—particularly the bar tabs of certain individuals—and meals were major sources of income that kept the club solvent and the staff paid, the adjacent showgrounds, property of the club, was also a vital part of the operation from its inception. For many years various regiments of the British Army had used the showgrounds as a base from which to launch training exercises. With the Mount Kenya forests less than fifteen kilometres away and the semi-arid deserts of the NFD only about forty-five kilometres in the other direction, Nanyuki provided an ideal mixed-training area. The fact that the club was also a great place for officers to mix with members, and that the town had restaurants and bars for the soldiers to visit, were added bonuses. The only time that the "officers only" rule for use of the club could be broken was on rugby nights, when we could—and did—recruit anyone willing to play for the always-a-man-short Mount Kenya team.

One of the training exercises for army units was a climb of Mount Kenya, which started from the forest edge high up the Naro Moru track. This had naturally been named for the river near which it ran, which was always well stocked with rainbow trout, no doubt descendants of those brought to the country by "Cape to Cairo" Ewart Grogan, the first European to traverse Africa from end to end. Technically, the climb of Mount Kenya was not really a climb but more of a walk. The third highest peak, named Lenana, which was the destination of most of the soldiers, rises to 4,979 metres and can be reached without any of the technical gear normally associated with mountain climbing. I have climbed it myself shod in Bata safari boots—the crepe-soled shoes worn so widely in Africa—wearing long wind-proof trousers over my shorts only for the last three hundred metres up the side of the Lewis Glacier from Top Hut. Only experienced or enthusiastic climbers attempt the higher peaks of Batian (5,199 metres) and Nelion (5,188 metres).

A problem experienced by many climbers and high-mountain walkers is altitude sickness. In its most benign form it consists of a fierce headache, while the more severe form can kill a person as the headache worsens, the breathing becomes laboured, the chest fills up with fluid and death quickly ensues.

Mountain Park Warden Phil Schneider had set up a medivac program, mainly to deal with this one condition, and his team had rescued numerous victims on stretchers, most of whom went to the Nyeri Consolata Hospital, but some of which came to Jo in Nanyuki. Part of the safety protocols for would-be climbers involved a clear order to get companions off the mountain as quickly as possible if they showed signs of altitude sickness and especially if they started to cough.

Almost all the army battalions had the odd soldier develop this condition. Many of these ended up as Jo's patients, as they would be closer to camp at the Cottage Hospital than if they went to Nyeri.

Altitude sickness and its implications for young soldiers was Major Hedges's main interest and his visit to Jo was, essentially, to talk about it.

"We seem to get it most commonly in these fit young chaps, nineteen- and twenty-year-olds, who practically run up the mountain. I wonder if you'd share your records with me, as I plan to write up a bit of a pamphlet for our people," Ken had asked.

Jo responded, "Of course. There is definitely something different about your soldiers. I wonder if it has anything to do with the fact that they have just arrived from sea level, or close to it, and before they've even had time to acclimatize to the six thousand feet [1,800 m] of Nanyuki they're off up the mountain. They're very fit, so they get to Teliki Hut at 13,000 feet [4,000 m] in one day and probably don't even rest or get more than a few hours of sleep before they go on up to 15,000 feet [4,600 m] to Top Hut. Perhaps the fittest do even more. I know that Phil Schneider's rangers can get to Top Hut in one day easily, but they're fully acclimatized and probably even fitter than the soldiers."

Jo and Ken sipped coffee as they conversed on the verandah of the hospital that jutted out toward the river. The verandah offered a view up to the mountain peaks through the podo trees along the riverbank. A thin trail of clouds hung to the north, seemingly attached to Batian by some sort of loose string. The conversation turned to other things, and Jo mentioned my unusual lion case. Ken immediately seized the chance to ask a professional, although cross-disciplined, favour.

"Do you think your husband would mind if I went along?" I think the chance to see a lion close-up, and to take some time off from his soldiering duties, was the driving force behind this request, although he may also have been interested in comparative medicine.

He was waiting for me at my office when I got there the next morning, and as we shook hands I was at once struck by his quiet manner and low-key approach.

"I'm interested in what you're doing with the altitude sickness," I told him as we drove out of town. "I can remember, only too vividly, the blinding headache that I had when I tried to climb Kilimanjaro. At about 17,000 feet [5,200 m] I was so affected that I hardly knew what I was doing. Luckily the fellows I was with sent me back down to Top Hut, where I lay in a daze waiting for them. The headache only improved after we dropped down toward our starting point. There's a similar condition in cattle, and I can clearly recall my first case. It was in a bull from up this way."

"That's interesting," he said. "Can you give me any material on it?"

"I'll have a look in my Jubb and Kennedy when we get back"

"Jubb and Kennedy?"

"Oh, sorry. It's THE veterinary pathology book. Two volumes. Glossy paper, expensive, but worth the money. I'm sure they'll have something on it."

As we drove out across the edge of the Laikipia Plains, toward Naro Moru, we could see the Aberdares range rising in the haze ahead and to our right.

"This seems to be a regular posting for you Brits," I said. "Where else have you been?"

"Oh, the usual spots. I did spend some time in the Arctic once, as well, which is a bit off the beaten track and quite a contrast to this place."

We turned at Naro Moru, crossed the tracks and took the left fork in the road. As we drove across the dusty plain, a few scattered small herds of kongoni and the odd Thomson's gazelle were grazing in the grass to our left.

"We are lucky it's not raining," I told Ken. "This road is mostly black cotton and quite impossible, and impassable, in the wet, especially in a station wagon like this, even a Peugeot 404. The ranch is fully fenced; those animals over there are free-ranging. We'll see the fenced area when we get to the ranch."

"What's the history of this place we're going to?"

"It's owned by an American millionaire, a Mr. Court Parfet. He's rumoured to have made his first million selling chewing gum to the GIS in France during the Second World War, but I don't know if that's true. Anyway, after buying Solio he found that he simply could not keep cattle alive in the tick-infested swampy areas in the middle of the place. He soon decided to fence in the swamp and some adjacent land and make a game park. The work started in 1968, and the fence was completed two years later. You'll see it in a moment. It's phenomenal. It's six feet high [1.82 m] page wire, topped with an overhang that makes it effectively seven feet [2.15 m]. He's already put in quite a number of rhino, and there are lots of giraffe, waterbuck, kongoni and other things in there. The bird life is interesting, as well. He also has this lion and at least one full pride that I know about. The manager is a retired game warden called Rodney Elliott, who was in the game department for years. Retired army man I think. A major like you."

"What about the lion?"

I gave him a synopsis of the case so far and continued, "It's ironic in a way because the lion was a cattle killer, and now he lives on a cattle ranch, albeit inside a fence, and Rodney shipped it from Maralal himself. Mrs. Parfet has given him a name. He's called Metternich, after an Austrian statesman who died in 1859. He was apparently responsible for negotiating the wedding of Marie Louise to Napoleon the First."

The open plains changed into bushier terrain dotted with the whistling thorn so often associated with black cotton soil. We turned right at a T junction where a ten-metre euphorbia reached up to the sky, and after dipping over a small stream lined with fever trees and tall gums, we turned right again into the ranch yards. I greeted Jimmy Caldwell, the manager of the cattle operation.

"Morning, Jimmy. We're going through to pick up Rodney and have a look at that lion again. How's that cow I saw last week? She didn't look very good"

"Morning, Jerry. She died, which was really no surprise. Please can you call in on the way back. There's a lame Charolais bull I'd like you to take a look at."

As I pulled up alongside the Kai Apple hedge, Rodney, his baggy shorts reaching almost to his knees, emerged from the verandah and greeted us in his deep and cultured voice.

"Good morning, Jerry. I'm afraid the lion is worse this morning. We went out at first light, and he doesn't seem to respond at all."

"Rodney, this is Ken Hedges. He's a medic with the British army in Nanyuki. Ken, this is Rodney Elliot. He runs the game park."

"Good morning, Rodney," said Ken. "I hope you don't mind me being here. Dr. Haigh said I could come along. He thought you wouldn't mind, and so I took the morning off."

"No. Quite delighted. Let's go in my Land Rover."

"*Hujambo Mzee*," I greeted the Turkana scout, M'Otoro, who had witnessed our efforts with the roan antelope and went everywhere with Rodney when he worked.

We went through the padlocked security gates of the game ranch, and Rodney drove us along the twisting path to where the golden-maned lion lay under a wait-a-bit thorn bush. He turned the vehicle so that I could look straight down on the animal, no more than two metres away, and cut the engine. The lion did not even move his head in response. He lay on his breast-bone with his head slightly to one side of his paws. A strand of tacky saliva was hanging from his mouth. His ribs stood out starkly and his hair lacked any of the sheen that one would normally associate with a healthy big cat. His rear end lay up against the trunk of the bush, well back and almost out of sight.

Ken stood back and used his camera from time to time as I carried out my examinations and took another set of blood samples, not needing any form of sedative or anaesthetic to examine the animal. He took one picture of me as I plunged my arm into the lion's mouth, all the way up past my elbow, while trying to check for any possible obstruction in the throat. After administering some more fluids we returned to Nanyuki, asking Rodney to continue his vigil with the patient.

A few hours later on that third day of the lion's treatment, at about 3:00 P.M., Rodney was able to persuade the cat to eat a little meat, and he drank some water. Rodney called me with the good news before he returned to his watch duty. As his meticulous notes showed,

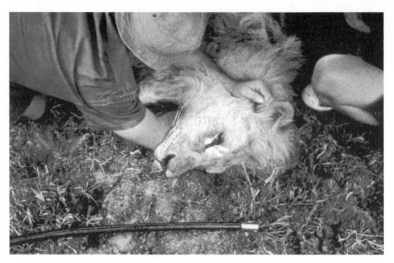

Hand in mouth. Checking an immobilized lion. (Photo by Ken Hedges, in possession of the author)

however, quite suddenly things took a turn for the worse. At 5:00 P.M. the patient went through a violent convulsion, and then a series more occurred every fifteen to thirty minutes for several hours as Rodney stayed awake watching his charge. I spent a brief while the next morning watching as the lion's fits increased in frequency. Each time they started with a slight shivering of the tongue. Next, his limbs started to shake, followed by his head. His neck arched back and then bent down between his forelegs. His pupils opened up wide throughout the sessions, and he took no breaths throughout.

Although I was now increasingly pessimistic about the outcome, I gave the lion a dose of the tranquilizer Valium, hoping at least to control the fits, which could not be doing him any good. I then gave him another set of intravenous fluids, so that at least we could keep his hydration in balance, if nothing else. At a quarter past five in the evening of the fourth day of treatment he was growling, and his tail was twitching, and the fits seemed to be under control. Rodney stayed on the job for a third consecutive night and told me the next morning that at 3:45 A.M. the lion sat up and focused his eyes on the Land Rover.

Despite the odd encouraging sign, the lion continued to go downhill. On the sixth day Rodney said, "Mr. Parfet, no doubt urged by his wife's concern, has requested a second opinion. Whom do you suggest?"

I responded, "I would think Dr. Paul Sayer, from the vet faculty would be best. He probably has more experience with lions than anybody else in Kenya."

Next day, a Saturday, Paul and I met at the ranch office. It was a pleasant surprise to see his wife, Elma, with him. Paul and I had shared a flat as interns, and although he may not remember it, I had encouraged him to marry Elma when it became apparent that he was spending much more time at her house than in our flat.

I had asked him to check at the lab in Kabete before he left, and he reported that there was still no news of the samples I had sent. Our own checks at my office in Nanyuki had given no further insights, so we still had no back-up to the clinical impressions I had formed on the first day.

"You have been invited to lunch at Mr. Parfet's house," Rodney told us as we finished examining the lion.

After we had seen the lion, which was unresponsive, we headed for the house. Paul discussed the case with Mr. Parfet and his elegant French wife, Claude. "Like Dr. Haigh, I don't think there's much hope of a recovery. I think that a septicemia may have been the major problem, tetanus is certainly a possibility, and it seems quite possible that he has meningitis. I would think that the pad injured by his claw may have been the place where it all started."

"Can you suggest any other treatments?" asked Mr. Parfet, as he sat at the head of the table in his neatly pressed safari outfit.

"Not really. If the chloramphenicol has not done the trick, I feel that not much else would be of use."

Eventually, when they realized that the prognosis was grave, the Parfets became gracious hosts and we stepped out from the drawing room onto the terraced lawn. The view was spectacular. Framed by two huge pepper trees, the mountain stood out majestically slightly to our right, wisps of cloud seeming to cling to its peaks. From this vantage point we could see all three of the highest of them, and the Lewis Glacier stood out against the black rock and the blue sky. On the left, a wild fig tree reached up, and the strange crowns of a cabbage tree intermingled with those of the right-hand pepper. Between the tiered and manicured lawns and the mountain slopes, a mixture of yellow-brown grass and green thorn bushes was dotted with Boran cattle.

"Mr. Parfet, did you build this yourself?" asked Elma.

"No. I came to Kenya in 1964 and bought the place from David Cole, Lord Enniskillin, in 1966. He sure had an eye for a location, didn't he?"

"It is beautiful," she responded.

We concentrated on the superb meal put before us. The Parfets had a French chef, and he did himself, and the reputation of his kind, proud.

"What about the Charolais? Presumably you brought those in," I asked during a lull between courses, mindful of Mrs. Parfet's nationality.

"We brought those in 67," said our host. "They were on the last boat through the Suez Canal before it was closed. I suppose that we were biased as they are from France, but we did some research and found that they were the fastest-growing breed anywhere at the time. As far as we could make out, no one had tried them before, with the exception of a few attempts at AI with imported semen. We've found that they make an excellent cross with the Borans. In a good year with plenty of grass, we can get the cross-bred steers to market in twenty-two to twenty-four months, which is at least a year sooner than the straight Boran." We all left after coffee and some more conversation, Paul and Elma heading back to Kabete as I headed out toward Nanyuki.

The lion died three days later, never having shown any signs of recovery. A Cambridge biologist studying waterbuck in the park, who had no experience with the requirements of such a task, carried out the post-mortem, and we never really got to the bottom of the riddle.

IN DUE COURSE Major Hedges wrote his report, "Acute Pulmonary Oedema at High Altitude," for the *Journal of the Royal Army Medical Corps*, duly acknowledging that the clinical cases were Jo's.

The following Christmas, when browsing through my new copy of the *Guinness Book of World Records*, I was astonished to find the terse report that a then thirty-four-year-old Major Ken Hedges RAMC had been a member of the four-man 1968 British Trans-Arctic Expedition that had spent an amazing 464 days crossing the sea-ice from Alaska to Spitsbergen. Appearances can be deceiving. The quiet-spoken soldier I had briefly known in Nanyuki hardly seemed to fit the mould of Arctic explorer, but here was the evidence. Ken's oblique reference to having "spent a bit of time in the Arctic" was something of a typically British understatement. ❋

4

A
MIXED
BAG

*I am called to help set a broken wing on a
beautiful bird in 1972. Then, Jo and I make a
trip to the Kenyan coast, especially "one of the
seven best beaches in the world," where I meet
local characters and recall an unusual treatment
I once received on that same stretch of coast for a
wound that involved a veterinary drug.*

MY USUAL MID-MORNING BREAK SPOT during those Nanyuki practice years was the Marina Café, almost opposite my office. As I sat
having a cup of tea and a samosa, my office clerk, Njeru Nyaga, whom
I had hired a year or so after taking Mutua on, appeared and told me
that there was a call for me from Mr. Burroughs, the manager of the
Safari Club. Abandoning the half-drunk cup and popping the rest of
the snack into my mouth, I headed across the road and picked up the
phone.

"Hello, Jerry Haigh here, what's the problem?"

"Jerry, glad I caught you. One of our cranes needs to be looked at.
His wing is drooping. It looks as if it's broken, and there have been a

couple of reports from concerned guests. Can you get here fairly soon? I've asked our man to catch the pair of them up in their night pen."

With the car already loaded with most of the basic gear, it took no time for Mutua to load up the more valuable bits and pieces that I usually kept locked away in the safe. Soon we were ready.

We headed on up the road, past the military barracks, and passed smoothly through the gate with its cattle grid base, into the grounds of the game ranch, through which one passed to get to the Safari Club.

My first case at the game ranch had been a wildebeest, but between the horses and birds at the club, and the varied wild species at the ranch, I had a regular patient list that ranged from Jonjon the chimpanzee through to rhino, lemurs, a leopard and a variety of antelopes such as impala.

The guard at the gate knew the car well by now, and the formalities of signing in were no longer considered essential. We drove slowly over the speed bumps, designed to slow traffic in the game ranch, and could not resist watching the antics of a rutting male impala as he tried his best to keep control of his harem, chasing females that wandered too far from the pack and thoroughly exhausting himself. As we pulled into the club's car park, with its spectacular view of the green lawns, the swimming pool and the forest beyond, I recognized Jo's white Ford Taurus station wagon, KMN 104. Before we could even start getting equipment out of the car, she came out of the main door of the club.

"Well, fancy seeing you here. Do you come here often?" I ventured.

"Oh, hi. I've got to run. What are you here for?"

I told her about the crane and, observing her smiling, asked what the grin was about.

"Can't tell you now. I'll tell you later. See you at tea time." Mutua and I moved off to the bird pens and found the keeper waiting for us.

After the club was built as a hotel in 1938, the original owners had set about obtaining a collection of birds that had assimilated into the mix of the native and exotic species that could be seen all over the grounds. All of the exotic ones had been pinioned, to prevent flight, but by the time I began to work with the collection in 1970, all of the native species, including both Sacred and Hadeda ibis, herons, marabou storks, Helmeted guineafowl, five species of duck and several pairs of Egyptian geese were able to fly. They didn't bother to go far, as there was almost nothing to harass them, and they were fed daily. Indeed, one of the main attractions for guests was the ritual afternoon feeding of this mixed bag, whose diets varied from the small fish that were thrown every afternoon into the gaping maw of the one remaining pelican, to the meat for the marabou storks and the mixture of fruit, table scraps and bread that went to feed the others. Not surprisingly, small native birds such as starlings and weavers had taken no time to join in the feasting and the lawn between the swimming pool and the big picture windows became a hive of activity every afternoon as the watching guests sipped their afternoon tea and nibbled on a variety of delicious cakes and the oh-so-British thin little crustless triangular cucumber sandwiches.

The most unlikely species of birds remaining from the original collection was a pair of Sarus cranes, whose native range includes the northern Indian subcontinent, southeast Asia and northeast Australia. Each area is said to have its own subspecies, but no one knew where the Safari Club pair had originally come from.

The beautiful blue-grey crane, the tallest of all its kind, almost as tall as my 1.82 metres (6 ft), with its red head and white neck, had somehow fractured its left upper wing bone, and the whole limb was drooping down as if paralyzed. The wing-tip feathers dragged on the ground, and the patient looked thoroughly unbalanced and out of sorts.

Linnaeus, the Swedish father of taxonomy, no doubt leaning on the classical education that would have been standard in his day, had given the Sarus crane the Latin name of *Antigone antigone* (later changed to *Grus antigone* to more neatly, but very prosaically, fit it into the crane family in general), which was testament to a heroine of Greek mythology: Antigone, Oedipus's daughter. She was unable to control her emotions on the death of her brother, Polynices, and in her struggle to secure funeral rites for him. Legend has it that pairs of Sarus cranes not only mate for life—a not uncommon phenomenon in the bird world—but that should one die, the other may haunt the scene, calling distractedly for weeks and may pine away in grief for its partner.

Telling the club manager what I planned to do, I took the bird down the hill back into town, Mutua holding it in his arms, neck tucked down, stopped off at the office for some anaesthetic and moved on to the Cottage Hospital, where the only x-ray machine in town, which I had repaired when we moved to Nanyuki, was located. Using my new short-term bird anaesthetic (which was called CT1341) that had worked so well for one or two pervious bird patients, including a pelican, I took a couple of x-rays of the damaged wing. These showed a long spiral fracture of the humerus, which meant that we had a reasonable chance of success with a pin.

I put on a figure-of-eight bandage, drove back up to the club and told the bird keeper to keep the patient inside until I could get back to it. Next, I contacted the manager again, and told him that we would either have to send the bird to Nairobi, as I needed professional help and was not equipped to do the job in my Nanyuki office, or better, I would try to ask a colleague from the vet college at Kabete to come and help. "I'll get back to you tomorrow. It's not an emergency, and the bandage will hold it for now," I told him.

Over supper that night Jo told me what had made her smile at the Safari Club. "Now I've seen it all," she said. "My patient, who had a mild strain, asked me if it was okay to dye her pubic hairs, as she had a new boyfriend and didn't want him to get any ideas that she was old."

"Hm, you live and learn," I commented with a smile.

After the meal I phoned Kabete, knowing that our long-time friend Paul Sayer was away on leave and hoping to contact the new surgeon at the faculty of veterinary science. His name was Peter Holt, and he, too, was a Glasgow graduate, albeit a few years later than me, whom I had met on the Kenya rugby field. A fair bit taller than me, he played in the second row. I explained the situation with the crane, and the problems of my inadequate clinic, and my inability to anaesthetize a bird for any prolonged procedure.

"Is there any chance you could get up here fairly soon?" I asked. "The bird needs attention, and I don't think I can transport him all the way to you."

"You've timed your call to perfection," he said. "We've just taken delivery of a new Australian portable halothane machine, and I can easily bring it up to Nanyuki. If you can manage it for Saturday, that would suit me well, as I have to work in the small animal clinic during the week."

"Saturday would be great," I replied. "Jo and I have plans to go to the coast next week. We're off to Watamu, so it would be just right."

By Saturday, everything was under control. At my request the manager had put the club sauna off limits and dedicated it to us for the day. Peter had brought up a collection of pins, all neatly sterilized in the autoclave, and I had prepared a package of sterile instruments.

Once again the CT1341 worked its magic. Before I had even finished injecting the clear fluid, the bird's head drooped and his entire body relaxed. We soon had the little gas machine fixed up, with a tube down the crane's windpipe and the portable tank supplying vital oxygen and the smidgen of halothane that kept the bird asleep. I doubled as nursing aid and anaesthetist as Pete carried out his pre-surgical scrub and then proceeded to make the incision, expose the broken ends of the bone and begin to insert the metal rod. It was all over in less than half an hour. For me, it was a joy to watch a good surgeon do his thing, which has many similarities to observing a fine woodworker. For both the surgeon and the craftsman, experience and an innate sense of touch are as important as a thorough knowledge of both the tools of the trade and the material with which one is working.

We took the bird back to the Cottage Hospital for a check x-ray and then returned him to the club where he would be most comfortable with his mate and would hopefully make a full recovery. The case had gone as smoothly as one could wish, the unusual surgical suite would make a nice story to tell over dinner and the bird would be fine for the few days that we would be relaxing at the coast.

The coastal trip had been planned some time previously, and we loaded the car with the usual paraphernalia, mostly stuff for Karen, our two-year-old, and headed off early in the morning, hoping to make the roughly eight-hundred-kilometre journey in one day. We stopped in at Hunter's Lodge, half-way to Mombasa, for a relaxed late brunch, after having travelled for almost six hours and needing to stretch our legs. It was John (J. A.) Hunter who had, by 1952, during his time in the game department, shot, by his own account, over

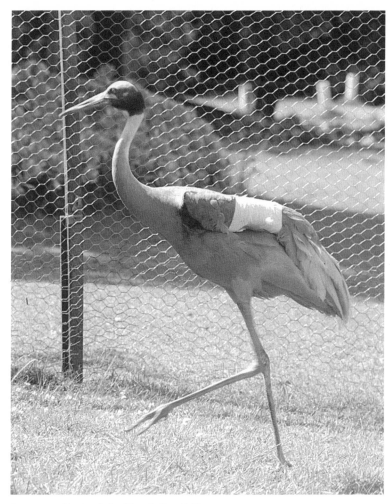

Sarus crane and bandaged wing. (Photo by Peter Holt)

one thousand rhino in order to clear the area around Makueni for a settlement scheme. His books give a fascinating insight into the history, especially the wildlife history, of his times. The lodge was set in a beautiful grove of fever trees and had a dammed-up stream beside which a seething mass of golden weavers were working nonstop on their nest construction, the males madly competing to see which one could gain mating privileges as the colony's females checked the actual construction.

Next stop was at the Mombasa Club for tea and then on to Watamu, where we had been offered the use of our friends', clients and some-time patients (Jo's not mine) George and Irralie Murray's, beach-front house. The house was about a kilometre along from the Ocean Sports Hotel, owned by our friends, Chris and Mary Nicholas.

I had first met the Nicholas family in my first year back in Kenya in 1965, when recuperating from an appendix operation, and they had allowed me to stay in their own home (the six bookable rooms at the hotel being full) for one night before I moved into the hotel proper. Chris, who features in Charles Chevenix Trench's *The Desert's Dusty Face*, a wonderfully entertaining account of life in Kenya's Northern Frontier District, had been a livestock officer before going into the hotel business. Chris was the nearest thing to a vet that could be found in the 250-kilometre stretch between Kilifi and Lamu and then on to the Somali border, and he had a small store of drugs on hand to treat the pet dogs in the area that seemed to get tick fever with great regularity. Mary had obtained her fine arts degree at Bristol University and had used her skills with the brush to decorate many parts of the hotel. The most striking example of her work was the wall that she painted with many species of fish that could be seen on the reef just off the beach.

The beach at Watamu has recently been rated as one of the top seven beaches in the world by a leading British Sunday newspaper, although I have no idea by what criteria, and seems to retain much of its charm, even forty years after my first visit. In 1965 one could be almost certain that one would see absolutely no one, unless one made the effort to do so, and to see more than two or three people along two-kilometre stretch of beach in front of the Murrays' plot and beyond would have been cause for comment. The sea was warm and shallow enough at low tide that even the most fearful swimmer could have fun, and the crabs shooting back into their holes, if one approached too closely, gave endless delight to small children. Fresh fish could be purchased daily from locals, as it took no time for them to figure out that someone was in residence. The highlight of a week at the coast would be the Sunday lunch buffet at the Ocean Sports, where a wonderful array of fresh seafood was always on offer. One could always head back to the hotel and book a glass-bottomed boat ride for some spectacular goggling or rent a small single-sailed boat for an exhilarating spin inside the reef.

One of the real treats of a coastal holiday was the availability of fresh fruit, especially fresh mangos. Some of the varieties of mangos available on the coast may well have come to Africa's coast from India, and we made sure that we got a plentiful supply from the vendors sitting under the shade of *makuti-* (coconut-leaf-) roofed stalls along the road. The usual method of eating a mango can tend to be a bit messy, especially if one cuts off the cheeks on either side first and then sets to on the large pip by holding it and biting and sucking off the delicious juicy flesh. It was time to introduce little Karen to this delicacy. For a delightful description of the proper hedonistic way to indulge in this prince of fruits there can surely be none better than that of Lowell Thomas who wrote: "You cannot eat a mango casually, just like that. You must take it to your bathroom, reverently disrobe, get into your bathtub, and then fall to. Only thus, in the twilight of an Indian ghuslakhana can you woo this mystic fruit as it should be wooed."

So following those instructions, which Jo had also had as a youngster in India, and Jo and Karen sat, stark naked, in the bath and enjoyed the feast.

That first trip I had made to the coast in 1965—before Jo, before Karen, before knowing about the proper way to eat a mango—when I was on sick leave to recuperate from surgery, had led to an interesting meeting with a real coast character. The sutures in my abdomen had not healed as well as I would have liked, and after a couple of extra days of attempted self-remedy Chris had suggested that I drive up the coast a few miles and visit Dr. Rossinger, whose office was in Malindi, just past the Blue Marlin hotel, on the left, as Mary told me.

As I had sat in the reception room, waiting my turn amidst a crowd of folks from every walk of Kenya's life, as well as some tourists who were speaking German, I reviewed what little I knew about Dr. Rossinger.

I knew that his name was Zultan, and he originally came from Hungary, with his wife, as a Jewish refugee before the Second World War. He had not been allowed to practice in the UK, although he had been given a British passport; he had also not been allowed to practice medicine in most of Kenya, but for some reason, possibly because there were precious few doctors on the coast, he had been allowed to put up his plate in Malindi. I also knew that he had a fearsome reputation for his attitude toward German tourists, who had a dubious reputation for their sexual behaviour. I had heard stories of them arriving on package tours, perhaps having won the trip in reward for extra industriousness. Upon arrival, the women promptly removed all the clothing above their waists. Being topless was not frowned upon at the time, as this was the common mode of dress among some coastal peoples, particularly the Giriama. The next step for the German tourists, however, was to find a courtesan who would provide the wished-for attentions for the duration of the brief holiday. Not surprisingly, as it has always been with human society under such circumstances, the tourists risked contracting social diseases that, before the advent of AIDS and herpes as major risks, could be treated with appropriate antibiotics. Those who fell victim to these complaints would often end up with Dr. Rossinger. The somewhat malicious rumour among Kenya residents had it that he would have not one whit of sympathy for them. He would, of course, treat them, but none too gently, using a large-bore veterinary needle.

Many years later in 1994, when talking to Dr. Stan Houston, an infectious disease specialist who had been working in Africa, I learned that the behaviour of those same randy European tourists along Kenya's coast had not changed much. However, the risks had vastly increased due to the arrival of HIV. When Dr. Houston had asked the tourists if they knew about AIDS, he received this startling reply, "Oh, we know about that, but we also know that it takes ten years for the symptoms to appear, and by the time that comes along there will be a vaccine and treatment." Talk about risky behaviour, and sadly, misinformation.

When my turn came that day in Rossinger's office, I was ushered into his consulting room only to find it empty. Within a couple of minutes I heard the "slap, slap" of leather ringing down the passage on tile, and he appeared, the noise explained by his enormous black formal shoes. Medium height and of dark complexion, he took a look at the seven-by-four-centimetre skin ulcer that was all that remained of my appendix scar and pulled down a large jar from the shelf behind me. It was full of pills of every imaginable shape and colour. He started to sort them out with his hand, paused a moment and shovelled them all back, higgledy-piggledy, into the jar. He then turned to another container and scooped out a white paste, which he deposited in a small wax-paper container and told me to apply it three or four times a day. The consultation was over in a couple of minutes.

When I returned to the Nicholases and recounted the unusual visit, Mary explained the pill jar by recounting that she had taken JJ, one of her children, to see Dr. Rossinger and had been somewhat astonished when he did exactly as I had described, pouring out a pile of the jar's contents and with his finger set aside six white tablets, and twelve red and yellow capsules, telling her to give the boy one tablet and two capsules daily.

My skin ulcer did not show any sign of healing over the next few days, and eventually Chris suggested a treatment that he had obviously used after reading the red lettering on the silver sachet of a veterinary drug called Berenil, which he kept for his canine tick-fever treatments. This is the same drug I use on other animals, such as the sick rhino I describe in the first chapter of this book.

"Try pouring some of the powder on the wound after a swim, or bathing, or at least twice a day. I've used it to good effect, but I don't know what's in it," he had said.

With a nothing ventured, nothing gained approach, I gave it a try. The powder stung for a moment or two after being applied, but within a couple of days the wound had begun to heal, and the messy-looking depression on my belly was completely covered in more-or-less normal-looking skin within a week. I have no idea why it worked so well, but have remembered it ever since and was able to recall the unorthodox treatment with Chris when we visited in 1972.

On our visit with Karen that year, Jo and I naturally relaxed and enjoyed the heat and cool evening breezes, as well as the early dawn light coming up over the reef. There was not another soul in sight when we went down to the beach and Karen got used to the gentle lapping waves. She soon got used to the idea of going for a dip as I walked out to midriff depth with her in my arms, and playing with bucket and spade in the sand was a huge delight.

On Sunday we went along to the Ocean Sports to greet Chris and Mary and enjoy the buffet lunch. I recalled my memory of my off-label

Berenil treatment as the four of us sat at the distinctive bar sipping a cold passion fruit juice or White Cap as Karen played in the sand under the watchful eye of her *ayah* (nanny). The bar was unusual because half of it was made from the front portion of a clinker-built boat, which jutted out into the main room.

To Chris I said, "You know, a couple of years ago Jo had a case of tropical ulcer that would not heal on a guy's leg in Meru. I told her about my success with your Berenil suggestion, and in desperation she tried it. It worked!"

After we laughed a bit, remembering my personal experimentation with the drug and my first encounter with Dr. Rossinger, Mary said, "Did you know that Dr. Rossinger is a world authority on stonefish poisoning? He has captured enough of these unpleasant characters to learn how to extract the poison and has developed an antidote. Because of this work he's been invited to present some his valuable information in Australia, where stonefish are also a danger."

These fish, as the name implies, lie well camouflaged on the reef, and woe betide anyone unfortunate enough to step on one and be injected by any of the spines. Death can easily follow, and excruciating pain peaking after sixty to ninety minutes and persisting for six to twelve hours is a certainty. It has been reported that the pain may be severe enough to cause delirium and may persist at high levels for several days. In a modern text on wilderness medicine, some thirty-four symptoms of stonefish envenomation are listed. Delirium, paralysis, seizures and heart failure are among the less attractive ones.

Mary also remarked, "You know, Dr. Rossinger goes up your way every year or so, and has a ten-day holiday with his wife at the Mount Kenya Safari Club. Have you seen him by any chance?"

We hadn't, or if we had, we had not recognized him.

There is no doubt a legion of stories about Dr. Rossinger. Another one that impacted friends of ours occurred when Judi Gamble, maker of our wedding cake and wife of my colleague, cricket and rugby teammate, Peter, had driven to Malindi from the Ocean Sports after being up all night with an excruciating earache that she put down to coral ear, an affliction all too well known to those who swim in tropical waters.

I added to the Rossinger lore and recounted Judi's experience as she had told it to us. "I was practically weeping with the pain, and had to wait for ages as he dealt with his waiting room. When he finally examined me it was very brief. He straightened up, put down his otoscope, and said 'Madam, there is nothing wrong with your ear.' I was absolutely furious and drove away in a rage. The weird thing was that by the time I got back to the hotel my ear was fine."

This account triggered a memory in Mary.

"There was a fellow from down the beach here—I wish I could remember his name—who had been unable to get hold of Rossinger and had gone instead to the chemist seeking something for coral ear. You're right, it can be nasty. The reply, from the slightly deaf old pharmacist, was 'Gonorrhea! You had better see your doctor about that.'"

AFTER A TEN-DAY BREAK, soaking up sun externally and whitecap or fresh fruit juice internally, we headed back to Nanyuki. Naturally, the first patient to see to was the crane, which was doing just fine. Two weeks later I anaesthetized the bird again and checked the wing under x-ray, and as the bone had healed I was able to remove the pin, a process made that much easier because the end of it was sticking out of the wing at the shoulder, so I could simply grasp it with a pair of pliers and gently pull it up and out. The wing held up and at least looked both comfortable for the bird and presentable for the guests, none of whom was ever likely to notice the very slight misalignment. Of course, as the cranes had been pinioned long before I saw them, he was never going to need a repair that would give him flight.

While I dealt with the satisfactory conclusion to the crane's injury, and the more mundane domestic animal cases, Jo had to get back to her duties at the hospital and we were soon back into the flow of our normal lives. ✳

5

THE
EYES
HAVE
IT

*The chimpanzee at the Mount Kenya Game
Ranch, Jonjon, damages an eye in an accident,
and I have to take it out. Things don't always
happen in threes. Another eye problem crops up,
this time a cancer in a beautiful palomino mare.*

"DR. HAIGH, THIS IS JOHN KARIUKI, AT THE ORPHANAGE. I'm calling about Jonjon, our chimpanzee. He has a sore eye, and I would like
you to examine him if you get a chance to come this way. When can
you come?"

The orphanage was an integral part of the Mount Kenya Game
Ranch, which had been founded in 1967 by film star William Holden,
safari guide and hunter Julian McKeand, and Don and Iris Hunt, who
lived on the ranch in a beautiful house located just a couple of hundred
metres below the Mount Kenya Safari Club. To get to the club one had
to drive through the ranch where a variety of hoofed stock, including giraffe, wildebeest, oryx, bushbuck, reedbuck, eland and impala, roamed

free. Appropriately there were strict rules about sticking to the roads. Don once related to us how Queen Beatrice of the Netherlands and her husband, Claus, who had honeymooned at the club, had been arrested by a zealous member of staff and locked in the gate house for breaking the rules when caught driving off-road in their VW Beetle.

Partners William Holden, Carl Hirschman, a Swiss banker, and Ray Ryan, a Texas oilman, owned the Safari Club itself. It has now gone through a few changes in the forty-odd years since its initial development, but at the time I worked there, it was a retreat for the rich and famous. Michael Caine, Barbra Streisand and David Niven were some of the film stars whom I saw in the bar or dining room. Niven had been in the same Scottish regiment as my father—the Highland Light Infantry—before the Second World War, but I don't know if they ever met. I did not bother the star, as he was probably there to get away from fans.

Set in beautiful grounds full of shrubs and flowers, with an immaculate bowling green, a nine-hole par-three golf course, numerous ponds stocked with fish and several discrete cabins, of which Holden occupied Number 12 when he was in residence and not filming in some exotic location, the club was the only place I knew where one could loll in the swimming pool and watch the moon or sun rise over the peaks of Mount Kenya. The golf course had its own special hazards in the form of the black kites that would occasionally swoop onto the third green and seize one's ball then disappear over the trees toward the mountain. None of the holes was particularly difficult, but a round that would finish in the gathering dusk had its special moments and Lee Tyler, a leading American golf travel writer, stated in the *Los Angeles Times*: "It's the most exotic 19th hole I know."

There was a thick hedge between the course and the animal orphanage, but guests at the club could go and see some of the animals, including Jonjon, by walking through a small gate set in it.

Within ten minutes I was on my way, as there were no appointments waiting, and this sounded more interesting and was certainly more urgent than office work and accounts. The chimp, which had been "donated" to Don and Iris when rescued from poachers as an infant, had grown steadily, and now, at eight years of age, was just becoming mature and therefore increasingly difficult to deal with. He had lately taken to picking up whatever he could lay his hands on and hurling it at visitors. Most unsavoury was his habit of collecting his freshly voided feces and using them as missiles. He had long since become unsafe to approach closely and demonstrated sexual excitement when Iris was around.

John, a tall slim handsome Kikuyu and James Mutuoto, slight and a good deal shorter, were waiting anxiously for me by the office, and at once we walked over to the railing that was supposed to keep the public out of Jonjon's range. John explained that a new member of staff had, that morning, been inside the rail to pick up a collection of small branches and debris that had blown down from the upper reaches of the tree that was Jonjon's home, as well as to give him his morning meal, when the chimp suddenly came for him on a dead run. An angry adult male chimp is an imposing sight, powerful of limb and very scary. In one of my old editions of *The Guinness Book of World Records* there is an account of an enraged chimp exerting a one-armed pull of over 350 kilograms!

Understandably, the staff member had quickly taken defensive action, moving backwards and at the same time throwing one of the sticks that he had picked up, more or less as a reflex response. By sheer bad luck he had hit the chimp in the eye.

John had thoughtfully brought a set of binoculars from the office, and I tried to take a look at the eye from long range. Jonjon was having none of it. He retired to his perch in the big acacia and turned his back on us. I had only had a brief look but was not able to make any kind of a diagnosis. Don and Iris were away in Nairobi, so John was nervous about letting me anaesthetize the animal. We compromised, and emphasizing that I needed to get closer to the chimp, I gave John a tube of antibiotic ointment in the hope that Jonjon's regular keeper could get it into his eye. We arranged that I would come back when Don had returned.

A few days later I was back, having taken out my darting gun, as well as some of the more dangerous drugs that I sometimes used for wild animals, out of the safe. Although I had never had to restrain a chimp before, I thought the best bet was a drug called Sernylan, also known on the streets of America as Angel Dust, which is a powerful psychedelic in people and would reliably immobilize a variety of animals. But how to get the anaesthetic into him? My options were to shoot him with the dart gun or possibly get him to take something in food or drink. While the gun would probably work, it was not a precision instrument, and accuracy could only really be guaranteed within eight or ten centimetres of the aiming point, which is absolutely fine for a rhino or an elephant, or even a wildebeest, but not adequate for an animal the size of a chimpanzee. There was also little likelihood of him obligingly bending over and offering his buttocks as a target. Even if he did, if the dart were to hit him over his kidneys instead of in his backside, it could do severe damage. All in all, I decided that darting was not an option as there were far more chances of causing severe damage than of getting a good hit.

It was this conundrum that later led me to work out how one might adapt some of the ancient techniques of the Aboriginal hunters of several societies and develop a blow-gun system that would get drugs into patients without risk of injuring them at all.

For now, though, I was left to my own devices. As John and I debated the options, it was James who came up with the solution that we eventually adopted and which worked like a charm.

"Doctor," he said, "can you give him something in an orange? He will take one of them very easily, and I can throw it to him. As he did not get his meal this morning he will be hungry."

I had never attempted such a technique before, but it seemed worth a try. I recalled a report of someone spraying Sernylan into a caged leopard's mouth as it snarled at him and having success.

Guessing the weight of the patient was my next adventure into the unknown. I could tell that he would be more than forty kilograms and less than eighty, but that left a huge gap for me to dive into, so I just guessed at sixty—half-way—and hoped.

The orange was soon turned into a Trojan horse, and James threw it in the general direction of the tree, where Jonjon sat in the lowest fork screaming defiance at the world as we approached again. He stopped voicing his displeasure as soon as he saw the fruit out of his good eye and, quick as a wink, he was down on the ground and digging his teeth into the tasty treat. I had not realized how long we would have to wait, but at last, after about an hour, when I was really beginning to worry, Jonjon began to show distinct signs of drowsiness, and a few minutes later he lay down, stretched out and appeared to be sunbathing like the most dedicated tourist.

We waited a few minutes longer, and finally I deemed it safe to approach, but not before I had commandeered a long bamboo pole to use as a testing rod. The examination made it immediately obvious that by the bad luck was even worse than anyone had imagined and that the end of the tumbling stick had gone deep into Jonjon's eye and destroyed it. This made the decision for action quite simple.

"John, I'm going to have to take what is left of this eye out and try to sew the lids together, or it will be very susceptible to infection and will almost certainly cause a lot of trouble. It looks as if he is anaesthetized deeply enough that we can go ahead right now and get it done, if that is okay with you. I've got my instruments along, and we can boil them in the orphanage kitchen."

I let him absorb that and, after a pause, continued, "Do you want to call Mr. Hunt about this, or shall we go ahead?"

While we waited for Don to come over from his house, Mutua got the instruments we would need boiling on the gas ring in the orphanage kitchen. Don recognized that there really wasn't any choice, and so we prepared the chimp, shaving an area around his eye, injecting a local anaesthetic behind the shattered remains of the ball itself. As there was already some sign of infection in the socket, I knew that this was not going to be a truly sterile surgery, so I drew up a syringe of antibiotic that I injected into Jonjon's hind end.

Half an hour of careful dissection later, the contents of the orbit, held by clamps, were lying in a handy kidney dish along with the edges of the of the lids, which I had also cut away in the normal fashion so that we could create a wound that would heal. Next came the more tricky part of stitching up the edges in such a way that Jonjon would not simply pull out the sutures and ruin our efforts to help him. There was only one thing for it, so I went through the fiddly business of inserting buried sutures, so that no loose ends were sticking out.

Jonjon's anaesthetized state had not changed at all. He was breathing deeply, but slowly, and there was no other movement of his body.

We sat and watched him for a while, and then, as there was still no change at all, I left Mutua in charge, instructing him to turn the chimp every half hour, and went back to the office for a while, returning in the afternoon to a still-sleeping patient.

It took him almost twelve hours to emerge from his coma, and he did so only gradually, his tongue being the first thing to show signs of movement; and then slowly and progressively he regained control of his limbs, arms first then legs. Even the following morning he was still somewhat dazed but otherwise fine and he had also left the stitches alone, which was a relief. I left some antibiotic tablets for John to grind up and add to the chimp's daily banana and we headed back to town.

Jo is convinced that things come in threes, and it was not long after Jonjon's surgery that she had to deal with a shard of metal that had found its way into the eye of one of her patients. He had been working with an electric grinding tool, trying to repair a broken tractor part, when a sliver shot up. He had been incredibly lucky in that it went into the corner, rather than the middle, of his eye. The pain must have been intense, but some anaesthetic drops had temporarily sorted that out. Luckily the metal piece, which was over a centimetre long, had come out easily and there had been no damage to the eyeball.

What at first seemed to be the third and final part of the equation happened when I examined a Hereford cow's weeping eye and saw that a small cancer had started in the third eyelid. This was easily dealt with, using a drop of the same brand of local anaesthetic as Jo had used, a short wait for it to take effect, a grasping of the tissue with a pair of forceps and a quick snip with scissors.

The coming-in-threes theory fell apart a day later, however, after I had finally seen that Jonjon was doing well. It was during one of my routine visits to Marania, which were mainly concerned with the herd health of the beef and dairy cows, that Irralie Murray asked me to look at Sahara, her beautiful palomino mare. Jonathan, the stocky *syce* (stable hand), brought her up to the front lawn of the house for me to examine. I had often admired the gorgeous creamy coat and pale mane and tail of this horse, but I had not been up close to her since I had tried to examine her hoof, about a year previously, and sliced the ball of my thumb wide open exactly a week before a tennis tournament. She lived in the small paddock just below the Murrays' house, and, as she had been retired from riding, she lived a pretty cushy and decorative life, coming over to Irralie whenever called, expecting to be offered some sort of treat: a carrot or a sugar lump, maybe.

Irralie was concerned about the horse's left eye, and it took no time to determine that she had a cancer, similar to but more severe than the one in the cow, which had spread deep into the tissues and was obviously causing discomfort. Again, there was really no choice on treatment. The eye would have to come out, and the sooner the better, under a general anaesthetic. However, I could not do it right away, as Sahara would have to be starved for twelve hours or more to reduce the risks associated with anaesthesia.

I promised to return early the following week when I would have a full morning free. Anaesthesia was again a challenge for this case. I had grown used to an injectable barbiturate for horse castrations, but this drug only provided about ten minutes before the patient would start to wake up, and I knew I would need more time than that. I had also tried my elephant-immobilizing drug, called Immobilon, on horses a few times. This cocktail was originally developed for horse work in England and was a useful product for short-term procedures, but I did not like it for any operation lasting longer than a few minutes. Horses injected with Immobilon tended to shiver uncontrollably during the whole procedure and their heart rates rose alarmingly. What I needed was a drug that would keep the horse quiet for as much as an hour, because I thought that the cancerous eye might be more difficult to extract than Jonjon's collapsed one.

Another important consideration in this case was where to carry out the procedure. I needed an open area, with a soft landing and plenty of room to control the situation. Fortunately the solution to this problem was not difficult to find, and we set up on the flat section of the lawn that doubled as a badminton court when needed.

With all the instruments safely prepared, and a collection of green drapes ready to place over the horse's face, I slowly injected the initial sedative into Sahara's jugular vein. I had chosen to use an old, but very reliable, drug called chloral hydrate. It would produce a very relaxed patient, and I knew that I could apply a local anaesthetic around the eye and so have both a sleepy patient and a comfortable one. I had placed ropes around her neck and legs, so as to be able to control her as she lost balance. I asked Irralie to hold her head, and I put Mutua and Jonathan on a leg rope each, as we waited to see what would happen. Sahara gently subsided on to the level grass as I removed the needle and helped Irralie to control her head to prevent her from banging it down and injuring herself. Soon after administering the local anaesthetic injections around the orbit, I was again concentrating on the basic anatomy of the eye and its associated muscles. The first task was to suture the two lids together, as they would be coming out with the eyeball and, hopefully, all of the cancerous tissue.

The basic anatomy of the eye of a chimp and a horse (and any other mammal) is the same. Even the size does not vary as much as one might expect from mammal to mammal, given the range of mammal sizes. The main difference that I had to deal with was Sahara's intact globe, which made for a little slower going than with the chimp, although when stitching up I did not have to place the buried sutures that had been called for last time. Nonetheless, about forty-five minutes later I was able to stand up, stretch my back, which was rebelling from its bent position, and, after getting Mutua to move all the equipment well out of the way, watch and wait for Sahara to wake up so we could help her to stand safely.

I took station at her head, where I could readily judge her responses. In fact, I sat on it for a while, as we had been taught at veterinary school that control of the horse's head is the key to most equine manipulations, and sitting on it would convince her she had nowhere to go. Once I felt that she was responding normally I stepped away and held on to her halter rope. She had obviously completely shaken off the effects of the chloral hydrate and rolled and stood almost in one movement.

After a few moments of discussion with Jonathan, and instructions on aftercare, we moved into the house where Kisuku, the Murrays' old African Grey parrot called his imitation of Irralie's voice from his cage near the front door. He was so good that he could call George, Irralie's husband, or either of the kitchen staff, Munene and Josiah, and quite frequently get them to respond. As we sat admiring the view down over the Northern Frontier District, George recounted a bizarre tale when I asked about their life on the farm, and the strange things that they must have seen.

"One of the oddest," he said, "was the time we had a dead bull at the foot of that round hill by what is now the airstrip. This was years ago now, and that area was a grazing paddock for some of the new Aberdeen Angus animals that we had started to breed. The tractor was being repaired, so we had not been able to move the bull, and one afternoon I looked out of this window and saw a line of what looked like ants climbing up from the carcass, which was the best part of a mile [1.5 km] away. When we went over we discovered that the ants were in fact vultures that were having trouble getting airborne. They seemed to have gorged themselves on the feast and were then climbing up the hill in a line, turning near the top, and running down, wings flapping. Most managed to get going, but the odd one would not make it, try to put on the brakes, and collapse in a tumbling heap at the bottom. I suppose that the warm air, in the early afternoon, did not give them enough lift, and their eyes had exceeded the capacity of their stomachs."

SAHARA RECOVERED COMPLETELY and went on to live her pampered life for several more years, as the cancer did not recur. She lived in the paddock just below the house, and her pale golden coat was an attractive sight against the dark green of the surrounding trees and hedges as one drove up to the farm.

Jonjon's end was not so happy. He became increasingly difficult, unhappy and disruptive, and one day Don asked me to put him to sleep. In order to soften the blow for John Kariuki, who had a established a bond with the ape, I told him some story about moving the chimp to a zoo in the States, and we once more decided to feed him a Sernylan-laced orange.

Even though he knew full well that he could not get near us, as we stood about five metres back from the rail, and his neck chain would stop him in his tracks, the chimp put on a full-scale charge. He seemed to associate me with bad things. He came at us with his mouth wide open, which exposed all his impressive teeth, and his hair was standing erect, which increased his profile considerably, all the while screaming loudly in an attempt to intimidate us. The hair on the back of my own neck stood up at this performance, even though I knew I was safe.

This time he was much more suspicious of the orange, and only ate about half of it, pulling a face as he bit into a section that must, I suppose, have had a bit more of the tart solution than he would tolerate. An hour after the first dose I injected some of the drug into a pawpaw (papaya), but he rejected this out of hand after only one sniff. About fifteen minutes later he began to get slightly drowsy, and I took the risk of giving him a dose with a syringe in his backside. He collapsed within a couple of minutes. We bundled him straight into the car, and I headed down to our house on Lunatic Lane.

The deed was soon done, as a lethal injection of powerful barbiturates entered his bloodstream. His body joined the other dead animals in the deep custom-dug pit at the edge of our garden. Sadly, Jonjon was testament to the inadvisability of raising pet wildlife, which, in so many cases, do not do well and come to a sorry end.

Other patients later joined him, or, more accurately, ex-patients, and I have often wondered what some future archaeologist will make of that pit, with its mixture of bones of chimp, baby elephant, a variety of birds and numerous household pets. ✳

6

CROP
RAIDERS

I see more of the problems of farming in a country where wild animals have free rein. Jo treats a man who has had a miraculous escape after being charged by a buffalo in 1973. Other examples of lucky escapes from buffalo wrath, including a particularly acrobatic one.

AS MUTUA EMERGED from the passenger door of the Peugeot station wagon, and I was opening my door, a battered old Toyota Land Cruiser pulled up behind us. A man I recognized as a dairy herd hand from Endarasha Farm, one of my major clients, got out of the vehicle and approached me with a sorry look on his face and a note in his hand.

"*Hujambo Daktari*," he said. "We have two dogs in the car. They were attacked by a big pig and have some sores on their sides." The note confirmed his statement, and clarified things a bit. It had been hastily scribbled on a lined pad, but the message was clear enough.

Jerry,

These two dogs got into a fight with a warthog this morning. Please can you fix? I'll be in later.

Buster

Buster Cook was the owner of Endarasha, a mixed farm halfway to Timau, and I made regular visits there to the dairy farm. It was Buster who had made up my rhino darts on his lathe.

The dogs were a mess. The driver's Swahili had not adequately described the situation. He had said sores, using the term *kidonda*. While this would also have been the only Swahili word I knew for what I was seeing, it was surely not the right one. They looked as if they had been attacked with razor-sharp knives.

Warthogs are a perfect nuisance for the grain farmer because they get into fields and eat some of the growing crop, but, much worse, they trample and root around, leaving a wide swath of destroyed ground behind them. Farmers thus wage war on them, and one of the only ways to hunt them is with courageous dogs, but a warthog's tusks are formidable weapons. These two patients were testament to just how dangerous the tusks could be. It was not uncommon for dogs to be killed by these cousins of the European wild boar, which also has a fearsome reputation. Almost ninety minutes after setting eyes on them, and with inventory depleted by several packets of suture material, a couple of bottles of penicillin and half a bottle of anaesthetic, I sent the dogs on their way.

But, this was not the only time I would deal with the aftermath of a warthog confrontation.

Next day, during our monthly routine visit to the dairy herd at Mureru Farm, where our friend Vagn Pedersen was the manager, we talked of problem animals and he passed on that Jean, his wife, had invited us for supper. A couple of afternoons later Vagn called, just as we were thinking of having tea and relaxing for an hour before getting changed to go out to the farm.

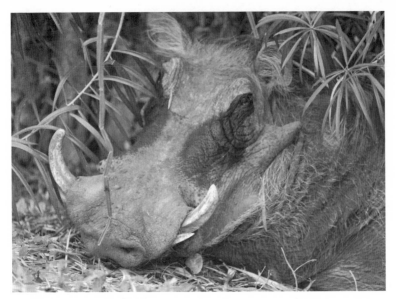

Beautiful in an ugly way. Warthog at rest.

"Jerry," he said in his distinctive Danish accent, "if you can get here a bit early we have a problem in the wheat. The warthogs have been in and are making a terrible mess. I want to go out and see if we can get one or two with the spotlight after dinner. We can eat early and then have time to go at about eight-thirty. They are usually here by then."

We did as bid, packing now three-year-old Karen into the car, as she would be able to play with Julie, Vagn and Jean's daughter, who was almost the same age. The two girls had stayed at one or other of our houses on several occasions and were firm friends.

A cup of tea had seemed to be a good idea as we sat on the verandah before our evening meal and watched the last of the sun's rays catch the top of the mountain and the few wisps of cloud that hung onto it.

As we sat there, Vagn and I revisited an unusual event that had occurred a few weeks previously but that stuck vividly in our minds. He had called me out to help with a cheetah that he had found in a snare. The animal was straining forward against the wire and at our approach began to struggle even more frantically. Despite the fact that I had had my immobilizing kit with me, something, a half-forgotten memory, stopped me from getting out the darts and other bits that would be needed if I resorted to a drugging solution.

"Have you got some wire cutters in the Land Rover?" I asked.

"Hang on a minute, I think so," he said as he turned back and lifted the cushion on the passenger seat. From the box beneath he produced pliers, rather than wire-cutters, but fortunately they were a stout pair. I looked at the cutting edge and decided to have a go, although they might not be ideal.

"Grab his tail and pull. When the pressure comes off, I'll give you a shout, and you let go," I said as the cheetah made no attempt to turn on us, but pulled away as hard as it could.

The very practical Vagn did not hesitate, and I was able to stand beside him, inch forward along the animal's body and reach farther forward to cut the wire. Everything happened in a blur, the wire parted, the straining cheetah pulled out of Vagn's grip and took off. We made no effort to measure and see if the kilometres per hour matched the claims about running cheetahs that every schoolchild knows, but the cheetah was moving at great speed.

Over a pre-dinner beer the conversation turned from the cheetah to our mutual love of fishing and on to the coming attempt at the warthogs. Then it was a feed of roast lamb with all the trimmings. Leaving Jo and Jean to chat over coffee, Vagn and I set out. We drove slowly, with all the lights off, around the field behind the house. After slipping along quietly beneath some of the tall eucalyptus that were so common all over the district, about eight hundred metres from the house, Vagn asked me to switch on the spotlight. There, rooting about on the edge of the wheat, were a small group of pigs, beautiful in their own ugly way, with the various bumps (warts) on their faces. Quickly, without speaking, Vagn was out of the truck and had nailed one before they took off.

In this case, with no dogs involved, the warthog confrontation led to a different and more delicious conclusion, as Vagn delivered a leg of pork to the house a few days later. We turned this over to our cook, Abuyeka, who dealt with it in his usual skilled fashion. This is the only time I have ever eaten warthog, but I'd be happy to try it again—it was excellent.

Another of the most serious pests on farms around the Mount Kenya area was also one of the most dangerous. While lions were often
shot as they preyed upon cattle, buffalo brought a parasitic disease
called "corridor disease" to cattle. The disease is caused by a blood-
borne organism known as *Theileria parva* that was named for one of
the great veterinary scientists of the late nineteenth and early twen-
tieth centuries, Sir Arnold Theiler. The buffalo carry it without ever
showing any clinical signs of it, and it is transmitted to cattle or other
cloven-hoofed animals indirectly through ticks, particularly the brown
ear-tick. If even one tick feeds on a buffalo, picks up the parasite and
then happens to fall off and move to cattle for another meal, the cow
(or cattle if there are more ticks) will surely die, having acquired the
Theileria from the buffalo via the tiny but deadly pests. There was, at
that time, no treatment or vaccine.

A herd of these very large ruminants can also create havoc in a
wheat field, especially one near maturity. As Tony Dyer, chairman of
the East African Professional Hunters Association, has succinctly written in *The Big Five*, "buffalo are the most persistent raiders of man's
crops. They use cunning, audacity and determination to get a bellyful of
stolen fodder." They will eat a good deal of the grain, but they will also
trample and ruin a great deal more, just like the warthog does. A large
herd will cause huge economic damage with a single night's visit. One
day in 1973 I had a chance to see and help deal with this menace when
our friend Frank Douglas, a powerfully built, mustachioed ex-South
African who had been the general manager at Marania for many years,
said to me, "If you are free this evening come up to my house about
eight o'clock and we will take you out on a buffalo control hunt."

After supper, leaving Jo and Karen at home, I went up to Marania
and met Frank and Eddie Fernandes, the crop manager from neighbouring Kisima farm.

Frank donned a leather helmet that made him look like a First World
War flying ace and climbed into the driver's seat of the old grey Land
Rover. Eddie and I stood up just behind the cab, each of us inside an
old tire, which had been bound onto the frame. The reason for the tire
was soon apparent as we bumped along on a rough track at the top
edge of the farm. Without the tires we would have been thrown all

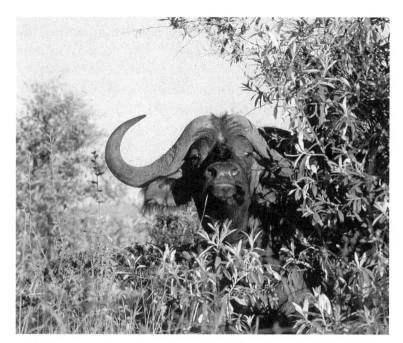

A buffalo bull checks us out.

over the place. Frank also had a powerful spotlight beside him, and Eddie and I had heavy rifles at hand. Mine was a beautiful double-barrelled .470 Rigby that belonged to George Murray, Marania's owner; Eddie's was a bolt action Winchester .375 magnum.

Frank's helmet was more than an eccentric expedition accessory. Attached on each side were tubes and earpieces that looked for all the world like a stethoscope. The tubes joined and a long extension tube ran up behind him through the sliding window to a mouthpiece, jigged from a small plastic funnel, the sort of thing one would normally see in a kitchen or vehicle workshop. The mouthpiece was tied to the side of the tire next to Eddie.

The reason for using the top track soon became obvious, as we had to get above the buffalo and intercept them if they broke back and headed for the forest from whence they had come. Eddie bent over and whispered into the funnel. I could only just hear him telling Frank to move forward slowly keeping the engine revs as low as possible. Inevitably the buffalo heard us and began to make a beeline for the break in the fence that they had created about fifty metres ahead of us when getting into the field. There was no longer any need for quiet or dark. The headlights came on; the Land Rover jerked forward and moved to intercept the panicked herd, which had been confronted with this situation before. We stopped when Eddie called to Frank, who quickly turned on the spotlight, and we were in the middle of a herd of over fifty buffalo intent on making their escape.

Before we had left the house, Eddie's instructions had been clear and simple, "When I tell you which animal to shoot at we will both fire at the same one. Go for the chest shot."

Not more than five metres in front of the vehicle a cow gave us a clear view, without any chance of hitting another by mistake, and possibly wounding it, which would have been a very serious problem, given the reputation of wounded buffalo. With one loud bang the two guns fired in the same split-second. The buffalo staggered for two strides and fell dead.

Acting upon experience and instinct the two farmers agreed to leave the body and we at once turned into the forest using the now generous the gap in the fence that the herd had created. I had no real idea what was happening, as we maintained our silence, but within twenty metres Frank, who was moving the spotlight slowly round, stopped with the beam pointing into the bushes. It took me a moment to see what had caught his attention. Eddie took no such time and raised his rifle.

"On three, put one straight up its Jacksie," he said.

I lifted my gun and saw the rear end of a big bull, more or less as a darker mass in the near black. "Ready?" asked Eddie. I nodded and he counted out the numbers.

At the report the animal ran off about ten metres, stood for a few seconds and collapsed.

In this manner the buffalo were deterred from ruining the crop until it was combined a couple of weeks later. We were not shooting for sport, just for crop protection.

When I next saw Eddie he told me that our bullets had done a good job. In the first animal, mine had driven through the ribs and destroyed the base of the heart, while his had been a few centimetres higher and had smashed the spine. The bullets in the bull had tracked all the way along from the back, destroying the aorta, tearing through the liver and heart and ending up, one on each side, buried in the muscles of the shoulder.

The mountain of meat had quickly ended up as a most welcome supplement to the Marania farm staff diets, all except the tongues, delicacies that went to Frank and Eddie.

At the time, deterrent parties were the most common means of controlling buffalo, and most of the time the humans ended up as only temporary winners. At Endarasha, Buster Cook's farm, for example, a deterrent party set out on foot in 1973, with dogs, after a buffalo herd that had been using the wooded Sirimon River valley as a base and coming up onto the grain fields at night. The valuable herd of Friesian cattle was at risk from diseases carried by the buffalo, never mind the damage to the grain.

All did not go according to plan. The Kikuyu under manager, Jackson Kamau, was part of the hunting party. He was at the back of the line when a wounded buffalo suddenly charged from a thicket that everyone had already passed, and he was too slow to dive into the underbrush as it came roaring up the track.

Kamau was smashed from the side as he turned to see what was coming. By sheer good luck the enraged and vengeful animal had continued up the path and was quickly dispatched by a single deadly shot before it could do any more damage.

The staff somehow managed to get Jackson out of the river valley as one man had run back for Buster and a vehicle. He arrived at the Cottage Hospital in the open back of the farm Land Rover just before lunch. Luckily Jo was in her office doing up her case sheets before heading off for home for lunch and her afternoon house calls.

The nurse knocked and entered all in one movement, Buster just behind her.

"Doctor, can you please come quickly. A man has been badly injured."

Outside by the ramp four men had each grabbed a corner of the sheet of plywood on which the patient was lying and had unceremoniously begun to haul him out. Each jerk of his improvised stretcher was followed by a deep-throated groan from the blanket-covered form.

"Steady, steady. Take it easy." said Jo firmly. "What happened?"

The men stopped and all started to talk at once in rapid, and to Jo, somewhat incomprehensible, Swahili. She turned to Buster, who explained the thing in measured tones.

"Wait a minute." She took the stethoscope from around her neck and moved over to the back of the vehicle. "Are you okay? Where does it hurt?" He was conscious and alert but in obvious pain.

"I can't move my leg. My side hurts."

Jo examined the leg, no longer covered by the blanket. The artery in his foot was pulsing strongly "Can you feel that?" she asked, pinching his toe. He nodded.

Turning to the nurse, she said, "Get me the blood pressure cuff, please."

Surprisingly the pressure was holding up.

"Let's get him onto a stretcher and take him gently into the x-ray room."

That done, the helpers went back to the vehicle, and Buster sat in the waiting area. He knew that he was now powerless to help.

The examination seemed to indicate that the man had been incredibly lucky. He was badly hurt, but there was no head or neck injury, no tenderness over the lower back and no sign of internal trauma. The only thing Jo could find was the broken left thigh bone. Just how severely broken would have to wait until the x-rays were developed.

Now came the next problem. Mr. Kamau was the largest Kikuyu man Jo had ever seen. Tall, probably almost two metres (6 ft. 4 in.)—but that was difficult to tell for sure with him lying down—and massive, weighing at least 135 kilograms (300 lb). Choosing a setting for the x-ray machine was going to be really tricky. The chart of settings based on our dog's weight, which I had taped to the wall, was useless. The textbook that a friend had loaned Jo did not cover anyone quite this large.

As Jo related the events to me at lunch, it seemed surreal. "I checked the book and our records. Then I took the longest exposure that we've ever used, and increased it by half. It just about did the trick. I've never seen anything like it. The whole middle of the femur and hip looks like bone meal," she said as she held up the films against the sitting room window for me to look at.

"What are you doing for treatment?"

"Oh," she said, "I called the Flying Doctor Service. I've got him in traction, but he's more than I can handle. We've got to get him to the airstrip at about four this afternoon and Buster's going to stay in town and help me get him out there. I can just about manage my house calls by then."

A year later, as Jo was about to leave the hospital at a run, her head down and covered by a file folder to protect it from the teeming rain, she almost ran into the bottom half of a figure entering just as hurriedly. Looking up, she stepped aside and was about to continue when the man said, "Good afternoon Doctor. Don't you recognize me?"

She looked and thought. The face was familiar, but no name came to mind. Before she could speak he saved her further embarrassment.

"You last saw me as you helped me onto the Flying Doctor plane to Nairobi twelve months ago. I'd been hit by a buffalo."

She could hardly believe her eyes. There was no trace of a limp. He was standing tall and firm.

"I'm delighted to see you. What happened after I saw you at Nairobi Hospital? It must have been about a month after the accident. They had you in traction."

"I was like that for four months, and then they started me on exercises, which were slow going. But everything has healed, and now I'm back at Endarasha."

Jo told me about this encounter over lunch and we marvelled at the man's luck and the power of good health in the healing process. I also thought that the fact that Jo had done exactly the right thing in the first place had been a vital element.

Mr. Kamau was not the only person to get away with being attacked by buffalo, of course. The nineteenth-century explorer Joseph Thomson, for whom the beautiful Thomson's gazelle, or "Tommie" is named, had a narrow scrape when he failed to take notice of the warnings issued by his guide, Brahim, after he had fired three shots into a buffalo and seen it collapse, as he thought, dead. As he approached in misplaced triumph the animal jumped up and tossed him in the air as he tried to run away. He was saved from a goring only by Brahim's presence of mind and quick thinking when he finished it off with yet another shot.

Another example of a close call with a buffalo, this time in my day and age, was related to me at the bar in the Nanyuki Sports Club by hunting guide Boet Danhauser. Danhauser told me how he had saved himself because he always carried a holstered pistol on his belt. He had been visiting Meru National Park on a busman's holiday, and when he got out of his Land Rover near a swamp, a buffalo knocked him down and started to trample him and gore him. As he lay under its belly he was able to extract the weapon and put it right against the animal's chest before pulling the trigger repeatedly and killing it.

Out friend Nigel Trent, whose dog Ranter I had treated for a dislocated hip, had an even more bizarre escape from buffalo, which must have looked like a Keystone Cops version of the bull leapers depicted in wall paintings from the ancient Minoan culture in Crete's capital, Knossos.

Nigel was managing Lolomarik Farm at Timau at the time. As Nigel tells it:

We had had a Friesian dairy cow stolen, and so I set off with a tracking team including one of our new staff, a young Kikuyu fellow called Muthee Ngarengare, to follow it. We leapfrogged with the vehicles and soon got after it, going north through Borana into the Mukugodo Reserve. We got east of Doldol, and by now we had run out of leapfroggers. I was in the car with Muthee and a local Ndorobo named Lemangen, and we had to stop driving as the road disappeared. Lemangen was in front, followed by Muthee and me bringing up the rear, unarmed, when a buffalo charged straight at us out of a patch of bush. Lemangen took off and Muthee, wearing only flip-flops, turned and ran straight up, over and down the other side of me.

I naturally turned and ran as well, and hoping to get it to go by me I grabbed a young tree and swung round, only to be confronted by the thing right in front of me. I did the only thing possible. I grabbed its horns, pulled myself right up to it, and hung on with its chin against my hip. Luckily it was not full grown, and its horns went straight up, so I had something to hold onto on either side of me. As it ran forward my feet went under it and it tried to dip and grind me, but each time it stopped I was able to get my feet back again. Eventually it stopped with its hind feet lower than its front in a gully and Lemangen reappeared with his penknife open, calling "Nitachinja wapi?" *(Where shall I cut it?).* He later said that he had intended to hamstring it, but he'd have had a hard time with just a penknife. I then let go, ran off and promptly got a stick between my legs, which landed me flat on my face. The buffalo came after me, stopped, took one look, snorted and then took off at right angles. ✸

7

"BORN FREE" LIONS ON TV

In October 1974, I get an urgent call to go to Naivasha to work on a TV version of the George and Joy Adamson Born Free saga. I run into the less attractive side of Joy Adamson.

THE REQUEST came by telephone on October 7, 1974, late one evening at home.

"Hello, is that Dr. Jerry Haigh?" said a man with an American accent.

"Speaking. Who's calling?"

"Hubert Wells here. I'm with the *Born Free* TV production at Naivasha. Can you get down here tomorrow by 9:00 A.M. to do some lion immobilizing for us? We need to have a lion appear to be sick and then recover."

"I thought Dr. Duncanson did the work for you. I can't really butt in there."

"Graham is away. I called Dr. Sayer to see if he could help, and he recommended you."

It was time to do some quick thinking. I had never immobilized a healthy lion, only the sick one at Solio, but I did have a couple of articles in my files that described techniques and doses for the use of Sernylan—the drug that I had used on Jonjon the chimpanzee—in lions. The drawback was that its effects seemed to last several hours, so the "recover" part of Mr. Wells's requirements might be difficult to meet in any reasonable time. I had recently acquired a new drug named ketamine that might be worth a try as its effects were shorter acting, and in cats and the three lemurs in which I had tried it, signs of recovery started in well under an hour. The trouble was that a lion would likely weight at least twenty times as much as an adult cat or lemur.

In calculating the right amount of ketamine to inject, it was probably going to be a matter of scale. I could always call Paul Sayer if needs be, so I jumped in.

"Sure, I'll try to rearrange my schedule. How do I find you?

I had learned about ketamine when two visiting zoo vets from the USA told me about it after it came onto the market. They said they were using it to good effect with big cats. I had quickly ordered a supply and had three bottles of it in my office safe. The visiting vets had recommended it over anything else that we previously had available, especially the Sernylan. They did warn me that recoveries from ketamine were not always smooth. This had been pretty plain, when I watched one-and-a-half-kilogram kittens rolling about like recovering drunks in their pens. A lion doing that was going to be more interesting and worrying, but it might actually fit the script.

Graham Duncanson, who was a rugby teammate and colleague who had stayed in my Meru house during my bachelor days, and whose infectious laugh and riotous good humour was always guaranteed to cheer up a gathering, had told me about the lion film at Naivasha and the work he was doing there. Once, as we flew in his Cessna to a rugby match, he had shouted over the noise of the engine, "Someone in Hollywood has decided to make a TV series based on the famous *Born Free* film; the one that starred Virginia McKenna and Bill Travers. I can go in in this thing and do my calls and be back home by lunchtime. The only hairy bit is the airstrip. I had a close call a couple of months back when a telephone wire someone had strung up caught in the undercarriage. Luckily, it snapped."

The idea of working with the *Born Free* people was probably the main reason that I had made the reflex decision to go to Naivasha. The original *Born Free* story was all about George and Joy Adamson, who had been clients of mine in my Meru days. Its theme, based upon Joy's books, had been the need to introduce captive lions back into the wild by gradually weaning them off their dependence upon humans for their food supply—that's "for," not "as," of course.

I had downed many a cup of tea with George in his camp at Mugwhango, in Meru National Park, listening to him tell me stories of his early days as a game warden. As I drank tea, George sipped at his usual tipple of White Horse whisky. The evidence of his preference for this brand was there for all to see: a series of little white plastic horses hanging in a line on a wire under the palm-thatched shelter of his camp.

Visits to Joy's camp, a few miles from Mugwhango next to the Rojewero River, had been less enjoyable. She was thoroughly abrasive and treated her staff like dirt, shouting at her cook in abysmal Swahili for even the most trivial request. Our first encounter had been when I had visited the park with Paul and Elma Sayer. We were there just as tourists. We had ended up dealing with Joy's cheetah, Pippa, which she was feeding incorrectly, a practice that had led to weak bones and may have even contributed to the broken leg that ultimately led to the animal having to be put down. The reason that Joy was feeding Pippa was really quite simple. As she admitted in her autobiography, she did not really want to lose touch with the cheetah and her cubs, despite the fact that the task she had set herself, reintroducing the animal back to the wild, was a success. Pippa had been hunting effectively for some time and did not need the raw goat meat that Joy provided on a regular basis. As raw meat, without bone, sinew or the bits and pieces that accompany a killed carcass is more or less devoid of calcium, Pippa's weak bones were no surprise.

With thoughts of my previous encounters with the Adamsons at the front of my mind, I prepared to head to Naivasha. Early next morning, I packed up my kit at the office, making sure to remember to open the safe and get the immobilizing drugs.

I headed out across the Laikipia Plains, with Mount Kenya at my back and a wide flat horizon in front of me, the rounded hump of the Aberdare Mountains away to my left. An early morning mist soon gave way to clouds of red dust as another vehicle approached. This time I was lucky in that the southerly wind was blowing my dust plume across the road, and I could see the driver frantically closing his window to avoid the worst of the choking that the dust would bring. At Thomson's Falls (now Nyahururu) I stopped for a snack, admiring the tumbling water from my chair on the hotel verandah, which was obviously sited to give a good view of the cascade. Then it was down the gradual escarpment, past the towns whose Maa names are testament to Maasai occupation of the area in former days. First Ol Joro Orok, "the Place of Black Water" (as from a spring) and then Ol Kalou, "the Place of Harvester Ants."

After Kenya's Independence in 1963, most of the white farmers who had developed this part of the Kenya highlands from grasslands into large farms were bought out in government-sponsored schemes. Kikuyus occupy most of the land now, farming the area in smallholdings dotted with patches of vegetables mixed with white-flowered pyrethrum and a few dairy cattle, but the Maasai names remain.

As I drove I mused intermittently about the challenge to come. Until quite recently I would not have been able to take it on as my only method of anaesthetizing a cat had been to wrap it in a towel and then inject the drugs directly into the vein in the foreleg. Cats being cats, this procedure was not without risk, and it took some practise. Obviously this was not going to be the protocol with a lion. What was the dose going to be? How would I get the drug into the patient? What about safety? Those who have been bitten or scratched by a tabby know that it is unpleasant and can be painful. A lion? Not quite the same.

As I began the descent into the floor of the Rift Valley, I could see to my left the low bank of mist that hung over Lake Ol Bolossat ("the Flat Place Between Two Mountains Made by God"), where I had often enjoyed weekend duck- and goose-shooting forays. Past the small towns, as the road switchbacked down the escarpment, the trees changed from the imported gums to more and more native flat-topped acacias (*Acacia abyssinica*), with their dark bark. The acacias flanked the verges, and whydah birds bounced up and down in the long grass, the black males with their ridiculously long tails seemingly unable to get airborne. The drier climate showed itself as the drought-resistant flowers of red aloes began to appear and then Lake Naivasha caught my eye in the distance, a thin ribbon of silver at the foot of Mount Longonot, the volcano whose crater I had looked down into almost ten years earlier. I dropped into Gilgil ("the Windy Place"), one of the important railway stations and post offices in the early days of European settlement.

Then it was a left turn along the floor of the Rift Valley and onward across the Murera River. I had one of those instant flash-back moments crossing the bridge, and I was brought back almost ten years to my days as an intern and the urgent tug on the line and the bending of the rod tip as I caught my first Kenya trout a couple of kilometres up-stream from the bridge. My fly had been a simple concoction of black tying silk and thin silver tinsel wrapped in a spiral, aptly named the Kenya Bug.

Large groves of acacias, known to many English speakers as fever trees (*Acacia xanthophloea*), with their black-streaked, mustard-yellow-barked trunks, rising leafless to their crowns at least twenty or thirty metres above, flanked the road. They partially hid the productive farms, where I could see a herd of Friesian cows grazing, as I headed into the small town of Naivasha on the eastern side of the lake.

The fever tree was so named because of its association with malaria in the days before the disease was recognized for what it is. Of course the fact that the trees tend to grow in areas near water would explain why people linked the disease to the trees, as mosquitoes breed near water and their larvae live in water there before they emerge to carry on the deadly cycle of one of the world's major killers.

My instructions had been to skirt the lake and head to Crescent Island where the filming would be done. Leaving Longonot to my left, driving between giant euphorbias thrusting their many branches upward like overgrown menorahs, I turned right and drove to the small spit of land, which at times of high water does indeed become an island.

Things seemed to be pretty casual, and I had trouble finding anyone who was interested in my arrival, but after a while I saw, with surprise, someone I recognized. It was Markie Kenyon, the brunette daughter of

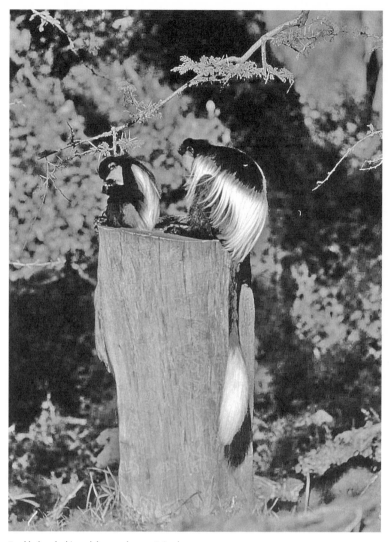

Two black-and-white colobus monkeys at Naivasha.

friends and beef-ranching clients, and I asked her what was what and who was the Hubert who had called me the previous evening.

She took me over to meet him and explained some of the situation.

As we walked across the grass toward another grove of fever trees, Markie introduced me to her partner, an entirely bald man named Eddie Steeples, gold earring in place.

"Eddie and I own these crowned cranes," she said, and then pointed to a beautiful black-and-white monkey with its long hair and white tail, "and that colobus. We raised all three from a young age."

The cranes, the national bird of Uganda, were mature, about one metre tall and resplendent in their grey and white plumage, brown wing tips and astonishing yellow top-knots. I had admired wild ones performing their elegant courting dances on a number of occasions.

"Tell me more about Hubert," I said.

"Hubert is the head lion trainer for the show," she said as we walked across the grass beneath yet more fever trees.

"He brought his animals from the USA, where they formed part of a company known as Animal Actors of Hollywood. He's got seven adult lions. There are five others here, as well, all immatures owned by other people, and there's also a leopard."

We approached Hubert, who was about the same height as me, at six feet (1.82 metres), fifteen pounds lighter than my 190, and had a full head of dark blonde hair, where I had virtually none, and what did ring my crown was mid-brown. After the introductions, Markie moved off while Hubert and I headed directly toward some lion enclosures. "What do you need me to do?" I asked him so as to have my task clear in my mind.

"Well, we need you to give her a shot to knock her out. She needs to appear sick."

The thread seemed to be that "Joy," the female star played by Diana Muldaur, would express grave concern to "George," her male counterpart played by Gary Collins. Apparently "Elsa," the lioness being played by one of Hubert's menagerie, was unwell, and Joy was worried about her. Their "houseboy" played by Kenyan Peter Lukoye, would overhear the conversation and cut in with his "traditional" remedy, a concoction of herbs and blood meal, to set things to rights.

We did not have a TV at home, so I did not realize that this (to me) unlikely or impossible scenario would be pretty tame stuff to audiences who could be lead to believe anything about nature. "Because it was on the box it must be real" was already in vogue at that time, and the mantra seems now to have become hard-wired in the psyches of many people.

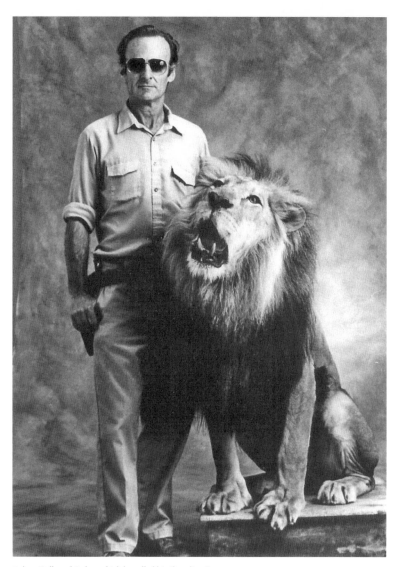

Hubert Wells and Sudan, which he called his "best lion."

During my two-hour drive I had mulled over my line of action, and I had eventually decided that I would do one lion with Sernylan, which I knew would work, and then see how things unfolded. If needs be I could try the ketamine. I ran this plan past Mr. Wells and he seemed fine with it.

"Should be no problem, Graham has used Sernylan on this fist one—named Lamu—before. In fact, she had some a month ago," he said.

Now it was time to do my thing, despite being somewhat nervous about it all. We walked together over to a series of cages where several lions were resting, and Hubert opened one of them up and called the lioness. There was no point in procrastinating, although the lion was no doubt seriously valuable, and I did not have any practice insurance.

"She weighs about two hundred and fifty pounds," said Hubert in reply to my enquiry. I converted that to its metric equivalent and figured out a dose that should work.

I had no idea how I was going to get the needle into her and still keep my various body parts intact. Hubert seemed quite blasé about the whole thing as he brought over one of his charges.

"Don't worry," he said, "I'll just slip this chain around her neck, cinch it up to the fender of that Land Rover, and you can go ahead."

The fact that he used the term "fender," instead of what I knew to be the bumper at the front of the vehicle, passed me by. I had other things to worry about.

With what seemed to be a pitifully small piece of chain, suitable for a miniature poodle's afternoon constitutional, he casually wandered over to the animal, slipped it around her neck and walked her over to the Land Rover, which was parked in the shade. Hubert didn't actually say "Heel" as he might have done to a well-trained dog, but the lioness did indeed walk with her head level with his left hip.

I approached, in a very gingerly fashion, and stood well back, more or less leaning round the side of the mudguard. At full stretch I held the needle between index finger and thumb and patted her on the rump with the back of my hand a couple of times. This patting technique is something that all horse vets use routinely to stick needles into their patients, and I had been able to fool many a horse into thinking that I was merely being sociable. The next move, again, just like that of a horse vet, was to turn my hand over and continue the patting, but with the business end of the needle entering the target area in the heavy muscles of the hind end at the first pat. The trick was not to stop for two or three more pats in order to hopefully fool the patient into thinking that nothing of consequence had happened.

I then connected the syringe and began to inject the drugs. It was no surprise when the big cat turned her head and looked at me with the typical supercilious stare used by so many cats of my acquaintance in such situations. She seemed only mildly curious, rather than angry, as if to say, "What is that silly man doing?" It was over in seconds and then we walked a short distance with the animal to a clearing where there were two cameras set up.

My medical records from that day show that she did almost nothing for seven minutes and then seemed a little groggy. At this point Hubert undid the leash and we stood back and waited.

By eight minutes the animal was obviously not seeing straight and did not respond. She walked groggily for a few metres and fell in a disjointed fashion eleven minutes after the injection. At thirteen minutes, she was hardly responding.

I let the cameras roll for a brief while, and then I stepped in, stethoscope in hand, and began to worry. My clinical instincts superseded all else as I went into a routine check of vital signs. Temperature check, pulse check, gum colour check, breathing, eye response. How was she doing?

Her fur was bristle rough, a complete contrast to our own long-haired blue-point Siamese at home. Without being conscious of it, I noted her massive teeth and clean gum line as I checked the pink colour of her membranes.

I need not have worried. For the next forty minutes she lay there, out cold. The only part of her that moved was her rib cage, up and down, up and down, twelve times a minute, as regular as clockwork. Even the head cameraman, whose name I never learned, got bored after about ten minutes. Some of the most monotonous footage ever to be filmed went into the can.

"Can you wake it up or make it move a bit?" asked the cameraman.

"I'll try," I replied.

So saying, I got out a stimulant from my drug box and injected a dose into the vein on the lion's foreleg. She responded by breathing more deeply, twitching an ear, and with little movements of her head for about one minute.

She lay, virtually immobile, but breathing steadily, for the next two and a half hours. Hubert told me, when I visited two weeks later, that she had still been groggy the next morning and did not fully recover for thirty-six hours.

"Can you try that new drug?" said Hubert. "I'd like to get more footage and it would be interesting to see how it works."

Making the dosage switch from a two-kilogram lemur or kitten to a one-hundred-kilogram lioness presented a challenge, but it seemed to be just a question of maths. The visiting vets' warning about the stormy recovery, and the potential for trouble with so large a patient, prompted me to think about trying something a little different. I had been using the sedative Stresnil in a cocktail for my work with rhino and other wild animals, and I decided to try it in the lioness to see if it would reduce some of the adverse effects.

My medical records show that the ketamine might have been designed for this particular scene. In two minutes the second lioness, named Tammy, had developed a strange gait. A minute later she made a staggering run of thirty metres, quite uncoordinated, her spine weaving, and then she sat down all in a heap. She was never as deeply anaesthetized as Lamu had been, and thirty-five minutes after the injection she was back in the truck, with her ears in the "alert" position. After an hour she was belly crawling in her pen, and she had fully recovered after two and a half hours.

The ketamine dose I had used would be inadequate for more detailed or close-up work with a lion, such as blood sampling or placement of a radio collar, but the drug is still in use by lion researchers in 2007, albeit in combination with different and more powerful sedatives.

As I had sat there watching Lamu doing almost nothing I had heard and seen some other action going on nearby. I was not sure whether it was rehearsal or material that would eventually be used in the episode, but a bowl of something dark red was being offered by a Kenyan, presumably Peter Lukoye, to a different lioness as she lay beside Diana Muldaur.

"This medicine will make her better, memsahib," he said.

"What is in it?" asked the blonde woman in a clear American accent about as far removed from the real Austrian Joy's fractured English as Mongolian is from Spanish.

The dialogue seemed no more realistic than the script I had heard during the rhino capture filming of two years before.

The handwritten medical record reads approximately:

TAMMY

for Elsa N. series

8.10.74 nearly adult female abt 100 kg.
Required as sick lion, getting up & down, known to be sick

Try Ketamine + Azaperone not for immobilizⁿ.
dose at 8mg/kg K. + 0.4 mg/kg Azaperone

dose 800mg Ketamine 40mg Azaperone by hand, separate syringes

2mins strange fore-leg gait exaggerated lift.
3mins 30 yard staggering run all 4 legs incoordinated + wearing off spine
  then sat down in a heap
4mins shouting etc by handlers, same run 20yds slow to pick up back end
-15mins lay on side looking over shoulder, some ear twitching & fairly
  bright look to stimuli, attempted to move but failed when tail
  stuck.
20mins inco-ordinated attempts to strike when handled, into truck
25mins sitting on basket in truck ears alert
1hr slight problem removing from pen, belly crawl with loss of
  coordination in pen.
2½hrs fully recovered.

The medical record of October 8, 1974, showing the effects of ketamine on the lioness named Tammy.

Mirella Ricciardi, whose superb photographic eye has captured so many images of Kenya and its people, was also on the film set at some time during the series, no doubt on a promotional shoot. She later published photographs in her book *African Vision: The Diary of an African Photographer* that say so much about the entire *Born Free* enterprise. I tried to obtain permission to use them in this book but had no luck. One black-and-white picture shows a young blonde woman, hair deliberately unkempt, kneeling behind and slightly over the top of a recumbent male lion whose mouth is fully stretched in a yawn. The woman is clad in very little of what seems to be some sort of animal skin. To accompany this and the other images on the double-page spread, Mirella wrote, "On several of the sets I worked on as a special photographer, the scripts had been conceived and written in countries that had no affinity with Africa, by people who had no understanding of the true nature of the land and their films invariably resulted in false superficially stilted portrayals that ignored its vibrant nature and true extravagance."

On the opposite side of this same double-page spread is a large colour photo of a pubescent girl wearing some sort of ultra-short skirt that shows a fair bit of her pantyless buttocks, with a single thin strand of the same material over one shoulder. She is walking hand-in-hand with a chimpanzee. Both pictures are steaming with only-just-latent sexuality, which was no doubt exactly what the producers were after for promotional material.

In another brief sentence of text on these pages Mirella states, "Kenya's ideal film location often made for corny films like the ghastly 'Born Free' series."

With exceptions, such as the evocative *Out of Africa*, these are my exact sentiments. What little I saw of this show, which I later learned did not run for very long, was very different from the original film and the books by the Adamsons, which have done a great deal to make people in many countries aware of conservation issues.

In later years I heard of a rather sad end to the black-and-white colobus monkeys I had met that day with Markie. Markie told me that Joy Adamson (the real one), who lived farther round Lake Naivasha at Elsamere, had decided that she wanted the monkeys for herself. Markie recalled the saga with some cynicism. "We had all the right permits and we'd worked bloody hard to make sure that the animals had a diet as near to natural as possible." Black-and-white colobus are highly specialized feeders and need the right food, especially as youngsters, in order to thrive.

The game department had contacted Markie and Eddie to let them know that they were taking the colobus monkeys from them.

Markie told me, "We took a folder full of paperwork to the game department offices several times. We went higher up the chain of political command. The response was the same each time: 'I am sorry Madam, but we have to take your monkeys.'"

When told that the monkeys were to be taken directly to Elsamere, Markie balked, but she reluctantly accepted that they would go to the so-called Animal Orphanage in Nairobi, knowing full well that this would be only a staging post en route to Lake Naivasha again. Markie and Eddie were not permitted to visit them.

Joy did indeed wield huge political clout. She took over the monkeys, which were dead within a few months. The cranes had a happier end. Markie and Eddie left them at Sanctuary Farm on Crescent Island, where they lived for many years.

Joy's work was a study in contrasts. Her marvelous paintings of Kenya's flowers, and especially her unique historical record of Kenya's peoples before modern influences changed them, are testament enough to her talents. That she raised the profile of the conservation movement worldwide, though her books about the lions, cannot be denied. She was instrumental in getting the fascinating Hell's Gate area of the Rift Valley floor declared a park, and she ensured, through generous donations for the Elsa Trust, that park wardens throughout Kenya had the opportunity to obtain pilot's licenses, which enormously increased their efficiency. I also benefitted directly from funds that she raised. My work with the sick White rhino in Meru was paid for by the Elsa Wild Animal Appeal through its Veterinary Aid Fund, which she had started for the specific purpose of paying veterinary expenses for wildlife conservation.

Other aspects of her life were less attractive. I, like others, found her difficult and abrasive. Like her third and final husband, George, she simply failed to grasp the risks associated with the taming of big cats. Her feud with George, toward the end of her life over royalties to his books, was an ugly chapter that has not been well publicized, although Adrian House, in his extensive and well-written biography of the couple, *The Great Safari*, gives it a mention. In the biography House quotes *The Oxford Textbook of Psychiatry* and appears to conclude that Joy suffered from a condition known as Histrionic Personality Disorder, stating that this diagnosis is "tragically accurate." Even in the brief dealings I had with her, the definition fits.

I am not quite sure when the *Born Free* TV project was abandoned, but I have a series of certificates, all dated October 24, 1974, not long after my visit, that cover the health examinations of lions Hatari, Mooshie, Blake, Arusha, Lamu and Asali, as well as a leopard named Lolita that I was asked to carry out so that the animals could be exported back to the USA.

I suppose that the best thing about the show, for me, was the chance to find out how to immobilize a large dangerous carnivore, something that would stand me in good stead for many years to come when I moved to Canada and started to work with bears and wolves. ✳

8

WHITE RHINO IN MERU

The White rhino in Meru Park become my intermittent patients between 1968 and 1975. A visit to the park almost forty years later brings a sense of déjà vu as Jo and I meet the new warden and learn about the roller coaster ride that the park has undergone since we left Kenya in 1975.

SEVERAL WELL-RESPECTED EX-GAME WARDENS, including Ian Parker and the late Peter Jenkins, have made it clear that the only way of preserving rhino in today's world is to maintain them in small heavily guarded refugia. It would be vastly overstating the case to suggest that the first six White rhino introduced into Meru in 1966 were placed in a well-guarded refugium designed to deter poachers. A boma about one hundred metres on a side was built for them, with two woven wire cables stretched between posts all round, except for a gap that could be closed with a couple of logs. Two Meru park rangers were issued ancient Lee-Enfield .303 rifles, which they carried as they watched the animals that were initially held inside the boma and fed alfalfa hay.

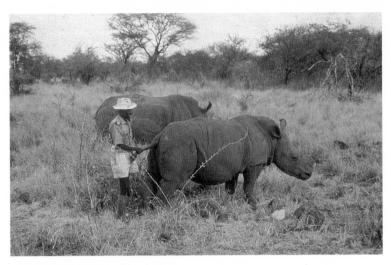

White rhino in Meru with one of the askaris, c. 1970.

Gradually the rhino were allowed to wander outside the fence but were brought back in every night, as much to allow for health checks as for any other reason, such as poaching.

The animals had come north from what was euphemistically called Lesotho—this was the time of Apartheid—but had actually been brought from Natal, captured in the Umfulozi National Park by Ian Player's team and brought up by game warden Ken Russell, who bore an uncanny resemblance to me, with exactly the same hair style and head shape. In Meru they had initially been looked after by warden Ted Goss, who gave me his meticulous notes when I started to take over their medical care in 1968. For a while, their main problem had been trypanosomiasis, the animal form of sleeping sickness transmitted by tsetse flies, and Ted had instituted a program of regular injections to deal with this.

After Ted was severely injured during an attempt-gone-wrong to immobilize an elephant bull—it stepped on him and crushed his thigh—game department veterinarian Dr. John King paid regular visits to the park to look after the rhino. As John tells it, "The regular Berenil treatments had become a major source of problems in themselves. Every rhino had an abscess caused by the treatments, and none of them seemed to be getting trypanosomiasis any more. Rather than continue to subject them to frequent treatments I decided to stop all injections and wait to see what would happen. It was the right choice as the animals had obviously been exposed to the parasites often enough and must have had sufficient mild infections that they had developed immunity. No further cases occurred so it looked as if the tsetse fly was no longer a problem."

I had had several dealings with these rhino between 1968 and 1970, all at the request of warden Peter Jenkins, and these did not cease when Jo and I moved from Meru to Nanyuki, although we were then living an extra two hours away, by car, from the park. We stayed in touch and of course made the occasional visit, just for the pleasure of going to this jewel of a place about which Joy Adamson wrote in *The Spotted Sphinx*: "The combination of its ecological conditions was excellent and with its varied fauna it could become a true 'Garden of Eden.' No other East African game park has so many permanent rivers and swamps, so great a variety of vegetation and scenery, such differing attitudes."

When Peter called me one evening on the radio phone at our home in Nanyuki and asked me to visit as soon as convenient, it was not the big surprise that had come when I had first been asked to go there from the old wooden house I lived in during my bachelor days in Meru. That house in Meru was prosaically name HG2, which was presumably the best that some bureaucrat with as much imagination as a sledgehammer could come up with when naming what must have been the second government-built house in the community.

Our cottage in Nanyuki had no name, but the murram road on which it lay made up for that deficit. It was known as Lunatic Lane, due to the fact that a retired couple who had moved there before the Second World War had had a somewhat discordant marriage. Every week or so the wife would appear at the club at a dead run screaming "Get that lunatic away from me!" as her husband chased her while brandishing something lethal, perhaps an axe or cleaver.

Those first two calls I had made to Meru had been to deal with rhino victims of overly vigorous foreplay, one female having been picked up and slammed into a large pepper tree, and another so severely injured that she had been constipated for three days.

In the first of these, my penicillin injections had not saved her life, which was no real surprise when I learned that a broken rib had punctured her liver. In the second rhino case, an hour spent with my arm up her rear end, followed by a four-gallon enema, had been a success, both in terms of the animal's rapid recovery and the huge pile of processed grass that she deposited on the ground behind her not long after the treatment was completed.

The new radio call to Nanyuki came in over a clear line, which was a nice change. "Good evening Jerry," Peter had said. "Can you come down and see one of our rhino females. She's another one with one of those huge *kidondas* on her side, and it seems to be getting bigger every day. It's about the size of a dinner plate. Over."

Like most bilingual Swahili-English speakers, me included, Peter freely mixed words from both languages, using the best words to fit the situation at hand (*kidonda* is a Swahili word meaning sore or wound), and I processed the sentence as a whole, without having to think about it. Of course the addition of an "s" to turn *kidonda* (singular) into an Anglicized plural also seemed natural. Today it comes as no surprise to hear educated Africans mixing three languages—English, Swahili and a native tongue such as Kimeru or Kikuyu—in exactly the same fashion.

"Hello, Peter. I can get down in the next day or two, but how are the roads with all the rain? It's been very wet over this side. Over."

"Yeah, the roads are pretty bad, especially the road down from Maua. Have you got a four-wheel drive? Or can you get a ride by plane? Over."

We had recently sold our Toyota Land Cruiser, so the four-wheel drive option was not open, but as we spoke I had a glimmer of an idea.

"Let me get back to you. If I can't get you tonight is this time tomorrow a good time for you? Over."

"Sure, I'll look forward to hearing from you. Over and out."

Our friend Buster Cook had maintained a strong interest in my rhino work ever since he had helped design my robust darting needles, and I knew that he had not only just purchased a brand-new twin-engine Baron Beechcraft but also that he was keen to use it. When, as soon as I had hung up after the radio call, I put the idea of a trip to Meru to him, he was only too pleased to join in, and it was then just a case of confirming things with Peter. I called him back within ten minutes and arranged to be at the park by mid-morning next day. He said he would keep the animal in the boma.

We took off from the Nanyuki airstrip at 9:30 the next morning, skirting the low clouds that obscured the shoulder of the mountain. I got a new perspective on the many farms in the Timau area and my old stamping grounds in Meru as we flew more or less due east toward the Nyambeni Hills. Although Buster was Instrument Flight Rated, he had no desire to fly into the heavy weather that was all around us but particularly ominous over the mountain.

We slipped over the shoulder of the Nyambenis, flying above Mikinduri market, where, as District Veterinary Officer Meru, I had vaccinated dogs for rabies and sprayed hides and skins with Magadi soda to kill any residual foot-and-mouth virus before the skins were shipped to Nairobi.

Peter met us at the park airstrip in his Land Rover, and we were soon looking at the rhino.

He had not been exaggerating. On the side of the beast, about halfway up its body, was an almost round suppurating sore, exactly as he had described it, thirty centimetres across and no more than two centimetres deep.

As Peter was talking to Buster, I confirmed with the wizened *askari* (guard) who was on duty that day that the sore had been there for less than a week and was growing day by day. As with the previous half-dozen cases of it that I had seen, it was obvious that I could not simply leave it alone. I needed to take a closer look.

Having dealt with those previous cases related to foreplay and this skin condition—we still did not know its cause—I had by now figured out drug immobilizing doses with this group of rhino to a point where I was confident of being able to stop her in her tracks so that I could do a variety of things, but at the same time not have her go down.

"*Lete kifaru kwa munanda,*" ("bring the rhino to the crush") I said to the askari, as I picked up a nice green swath of hay from beside the fence and passed it to him. He walked over to the rhino and waved the bundle under her nose, at which she promptly followed him into the robust wooden crush that was wide enough for an adult rhino to stand in. He dropped the hay at the front end and slipped between the three heavy cross rails that had already been inserted there, as his companion slid a horizontal bar behind her. As long as she had enough of her favourite food in front of her, she would not bother with

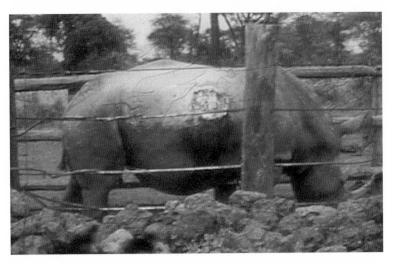

Every now and again these large eroding ulcers would occur on the rhino skins. No cause has ever been established. Photo enlarged from Super8 movie.

the restraint, although of course she could easily have broken out had she had a mind to.

Using a small needle, I slipped her sedating dose into the soft skin beside her tail and stepped back to await results. Within five minutes she had stopped eating and a half mouthful of hay hung from her lips.

To deal with the mess on her side, I simply went back to first principles. It was a case of cutting all around the suppurating material and excising a circular strip about two centimetres wide. Then I scraped the surface with the edge of my scalpel, until I could see healthy tissue underneath. After cleaning it all up with copious quantities of a warm salt solution, I turned to a tried and true remedy that came in the form of a proprietary drug called Cooper's Healing Oil. The ingredients were not indicated on the four-litre tin, but there would not have been a farmer or a large-animal vet in Kenya who did not swear by the stuff. To cover my bases, and to try and prevent a backwards progression if flies came to the wound, which they surely would, I also applied a blue powder called Negasunt, which claimed to have not only a sulfonamide but also an insecticide and maggot-killing component. A large dose of antibiotics in her rear end completed the treatment, so I then gave her the antidote and instructed the askaris to remove the rails.

"That should do the trick," I said to Peter, handing him the rest of the healing oil tin, as well as the blue powder puffer. "Get the askaris to put these on morning and afternoon and with any luck she should be fine."

Buster and I were soon on our way back to Nanyuki, arriving ahead of a huge thundercloud that would have made my somewhat queasy stomach turn somersaults had we had to fly through it. It was a pleasure to offer him some lunch, as our cottage was more or less on his way home, and I knew that Abuyeka could be relied upon to come up with something appropriate. I also knew that we would not be able to match the hedonistic feed that we had had with Buster a couple of months previously, when he had invited Jo and me out to share a bottle of claret and a stunning Swiss cheese that practically poured itself off the plate onto our biscuits. Even the smell of it at ten paces set my saliva running.

As Buster already owned a single-engine Cessna 180, the Beechcraft seemed a bit of an unnecessary luxury, but we soon learned what lay behind the purchase. Within a couple of months of our trip together to Meru, he flew the new plane to Australia, taking the long route via Aden, Pakistan, India, Malaysia and Indonesia, and returned by scheduled airline. A year later he immigrated to Western Australia after selling Endarasha to an African Cooperative, so I lost my ready, and cheap, way to get to the park.

Our last visit to see Peter and his wife, Sarah, before we left for Canada, occurred in late May 1975, when Jo was heavily pregnant with our son. It was during that visit, after dealing with yet another rhino skin case, that a really weird coincidence took place. Biology professor Dick Neal was in Meru, studying kangaroo rats. He was there with his wife, Jenny, and children, Mark and Christine, four and two years old respectively. The Neals were from Saskatoon, Saskatchewan. While they were there, I was able to ask them about the city and the university, as I had been offered a job there, to start in the September of that year. We have been firm friends ever since.

In 1978 Peter was posted out of the park and in the following few months fifty-six black rhino were killed there by poachers, including all the ones that I had had a hand in translocating with Tony Parkinson.

Peter officially retired form the Kenya parks service in 1985, but the Duke of Edinburgh persuaded the British government to support him, because of his well-recognized work with rhino conservation. Between 1985 and 1989 he returned twice to the park, only to find it pretty much of a shambles. In one of these intervals, the deterioration had reached the point at which only one road was passable; not surprisingly, it was the road between the park headquarters and the tourist lodge, which had the only bar within miles. It was not unusual to meet the new warden there. Peter finally did retire—sort of—in 1991, but he continued with conservation work after that. One of these projects was his work with the Lewa Conservancy, of which more in the next chapter. He died on September 17, 2001.

If you leave the Bwatherongi campsite in the park and turn left you will come to a gravel road called the Chuma track. *Chuma* is Swahili for steel and Peter was given this name by his African staff because of his uncompromising attitude. Peter's ashes are scattered in a ridge up the track, almost a private family site.

The entire history of Meru National Park has been a real roller coaster since we left Kenya. Poachers killed all the last eight White rhino in a single night in 1988. Before that ugly event, one of them, named Mkora ("rascal" in Swahili), which had not fitted well into the group, had been transferred to the Lewa Downs Sanctuary.

To begin with, the park's effective conservation area was expanded by the inclusion of several neighbouring reserves, the whole being named the Meru Conservation Area (MCA) complex. After Tsavo East and West National Parks, the MCA, which encompasses Meru and Kora National Parks, Mwingi and Bisandi National Reserves, and Ngaya Forest, is the largest conservation area in Kenya—over five thousand square kilometres in area. It would be nice to think that this expanded conservation area was of benefit to the animals within its boundaries, but it would be wishful thinking.

Between 1997 and 1999 the populations of all mammals in the park itself took a huge nose dive, as poaching became a daily activity. Surveys taken at either end of this period tell the tale. A comparison of aerial game counts done in February 1997 and repeated in July 1999 show that all species except buffalo had declined by something between

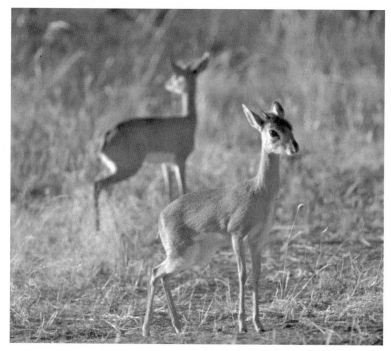

Two dik-dik under the canopy of wait-a-bit thorn.

80 and 100 per cent. That means that animals like impala, waterbuck, giraffe and both species of zebra had virtually disappeared. How much this had to do with the fact that a member of the Kenya Wildlife Service (KWS) staff owned a butchery in Meru town is unclear.

One species that did not seem to have taken a hit was one of the smallest antelopes of all, the dik-dik, perhaps because the amount of flesh available would be little more than that on a large rabbit. In some parts of the park, especially where masses of wait-a-bit thorn is common, one comes across pairs of these delicate creatures every few hundred metres.

In 1999 another Jenkins—Mark, who had been mauled by George Adamson's lion and survived, and whom I had last seen in his father's house at park headquarters as a ten-year-old boy in 1975—returned to Kenya after two years at Cirencester, the agricultural college in England, and stints working with wildlife in Kenya, Zimbabwe (where he learned to fly), South Africa, Uganda, Mozambique and Malawi. He had heard of the chance to return to Meru when Richard Leakey, back as director of the Kenya Wildlife Service for a second term, had offered him a role.

Things were a trifle desperate. As Mark put it to me, "The place was finished. The entire budget for everything was enough to supply diesel for one vehicle for about six months"

The challenges that Mark Jenkins and his staff of three hundred faced in Meru boiled down to four basic categories. As he wrote in his 2002–2003 Annual Report the challenges were: attracting more tourists, improving KWS–community relations, extending education initiatives and guaranteeing security.

Tourism in general took a huge hit after 9-11, and the targeted bombing in Nairobi and at the coast did further damage. Visitor numbers plummeted to less than two thousand people in 1997 and 1998. The new program, as run by Mark, sought to involve more local communities and especially to involve schoolchildren. In 2001 over ten thousand people came in, a rise of 61 per cent from the preceding year.

Our own visit in 2005 was highlighted by a stay in comfortable cottages, swims in the pool at Bwatherongi and then a real commotion when a hippo decided that she, too, wanted to go for a swim, smashed the fence around the pool and left behind a considerable volume of vegetable material as a challenge to the filtering system.

An education and public affairs outreach program has been started and will hopefully grow as more people use the new education centre. It will not be easy. Locals have been involved in fence building to reduce human-wildlife conflicts and have been employed in road clearance efforts. Water remains a major issue.

The thirteen rivers that flow through the park are a huge draw for many purposes. Therein lies the rub. The local residents know about the water as well as anyone. The Bwatherongi River in the park was bone dry when Mark arrived in 1999. It had been dammed upstream and had become a source of drinking and irrigation water for local families. The soil is rich, and although the climate is probably too hot for maize growing, millet grows well. If the rivers were tapped, there could be widespread cultivation, supporting hundreds of families. With modern approaches to tsetse control, cattle could do extremely well in the rich grazing areas. In 2005 I heard the wife of a (white) Kenyan businessman say, "Ach, Meru, the place should never be a park, the land is much too good."

Poaching also continues to be a major issue in the park. In the introduction to that 2002–2003 report, Mark wrote: "Then disaster struck. Between 1980 and the late 1990s poachers slaughtered 90% of the Park's elephants. Rhino were completely wiped out. Disease took a terrible toll on wildlife. Lawlessness and land use conflicts between humans and wildlife devastated the area. The Park's infrastructure decayed. The blow to conservation was extensive. As a result, tourism plummeted."

Security was another major issue. It had two components, the first to control cattle incursion into the park, the second to control poaching. As Mark put it to me, "The livestock issue is huge, and getting worse. Cattle, mainly stock from Somalia, are dumped at the boundary and naturally find their way in. Since 1999 with regular helicopter surveillance and expenditure of about $400,000 the cattle numbers in the area were reduced from 150,000 to 4,000. Now the helicopter has gone after crashing in the Aberdares and cattle numbers are back up to 120,000." Mark expressed the wish that the Tanzanian solution could be adopted, but was not overly hopeful. If cattle in Tanzania are caught inside their parks, up to 50 per cent of the herd can be confiscated. As far as Mark is concerned, a tax is needed on the huge herds owned by the small number of people, all very powerful individuals, who come into Meru.

On top of cattle incursion, there were several outbreaks of Rinderpest or cattle plague in the 1990s. This is the same the deadly virus disease that killed an estimated 90 per cent of all hoofed animals in Africa in the late 1800s.

The almost three hundred people who had been charged with illegal grazing or trespass and were found guilty between 1999 and 2005 were fined from 8,000 to 16,000 shillings, which is about half the value of a good cow (eighty shillings to the US dollar). Most of the owners had brokers in the nearby town of Maua who paid the fine in about four days. Mark was unimpressed.

Security was not straightforward, of course, and carried risks to personnel. Since Mark has returned to the park, nine rangers have been attacked with knives or with the main weapon of murder in Rwanda's genocidal war, the ubiquitous *panga* (machete). In today's litigious society, the askaris have had to be very careful about how they conduct themselves. Mark cited one example in which a Somali man stabbed a ranger after taking his rifle. The ranger was charged with the use of excess force because he defended himself.

On a more upbeat note, Mark has been able to attract major funding to deal with the problems and has received support from Kenya Wildlife Service HQ. From the report again: "Most of the 250,000 USD provided for the FY 02/03 went to a combination of revival of basic operations, security equipment and training and community relations. The biggest single expenditure (almost 65,000 USD) was for capture and transloca-tion of animals."

The funding for all this came from several sources, but the main off-shore ones were through the International Fund for Animal Welfare (IFAW) whose US$1.25 million helped lever a combined ten million Euros from two French donors, Agence Française de Développement and French Global Environment Fund.

The translocated animals came from three main sources. Elephants, fifty-eight of them, came from Laikipia, where they had become a serious nuisance. A total of over six hundred zebra (both Grevy's and Burchell's) came from Laikipia and the Lewa Wildlife Conservancy, and 411 impala and fifty reticulated giraffe arrived. Even cheetah and leopards were brought in. Several White rhino were brought in from Nakuru National Park, with more to come. Mkora returned from Lewa and has already sired new calves.

The management approach that Mark took with the new rhino owed much to the development of effective tsetse traps in southern Africa as to anything else. The traps are quite simple. Blue flags, about a metre tall and twice as long, are erected on frames and sprayed with fly-killing chemicals. A can of cow's urine is suspended near the flag and that's all there is to it. The combination of colour and scent draws in the flies, which come to rest on the flag, and the chemical does the rest. While the attraction of urine is easy to understand, the blue is less so. There are no blue-coloured animals in Africa, and the blue wildebeest, or gnu, is in fact mostly dark grey. What is not grey is black. Why blue works I have no idea. Perhaps tsetse are colour blind in this spectrum.

Mark did not confine the newcomers to the park in a small boma, as Ted and then Peter had had to do in order to be able to take daily temperatures and frequent blood samples. Instead he took the calculated risk of releasing them into a forty-hectare area in which he placed the recommended number of traps. Of course tsetse traps are effective only if they are properly serviced, and an area of that size needs considerable surveillance in order to deter poachers.

When we spoke in 2005, Mark recognized the divide between so-called scientific and practical sides of management, and he was rather skeptical of the former. He felt that not enough of the available money had been spent on the management side of the park and too much on research. Despite this, his report included the information that "the MCA has recently attracted eminent, reputable researchers, students and institutions to partner in research, including Princeton, Tufts and Nairobi Universities."

THE LODGES, Leopard Rock and Mulika, that we knew in the days when we lived in Kenya fell into disrepair and have gone. A new and very special place has been built at Mughwango, in fact right on top of the rocks that used to overlook George Adamson's camp. It is called Elsa's Kopje and is obviously designed to cater to a very specific sector of the tourist trade. Virtually all guests arrive by air. They can lounge in the pool that has been cleverly built into the rocks, relax on comfortable chairs under the thatched roof of the lounge, or stay in rooms that are designed so that none overlooks another. Apart from the mammals that have been reintroduced and that can be seen around the park, there is the added bonus of a chance to see the delicate, grey-coloured lesser kudu, with its white vertical stripes, the males with long spiral horns (we saw a dozen in April 2005), and the marvelous variety of bird life that abounds. The rivers, the swamps, the dry thorn bush and the open glades make Meru National Park a special place. As the sun sets and frames a grove of doum palms against the Nyambeni Hills, it is like a slice of paradise.

The upbeat introduction to the park's 2002–2003 report states: "Despite decades of wanton poaching and the collapse of Meru's management, 'Elsa's country,' as Meru national park is popularly referred to, is once again an explorer's paradise and a showpiece of Kenya's unique wilderness. The Park's pristine natural features and alluring biodiversity are unequalled anywhere in Kenya."

Then in late 2006 things came off the rails for Mark. He and his family received ugly death and rape threats conditional to his remaining in the park. He was able to find out who had sent them but decided that he would take it no further. As he said to me over the phone, "We have closed that chapter of our lives. It is time to move on."

There were a couple of problems that Mark had to deal with. One was the fact that despite years of great practical experience, he has no diploma or degree; another is that he is not a Kenyan citizen. With young degree-holding Kenyans chomping at the bit for a job, he was under constant pressure that even reached the national newspapers. Then there was his uncompromising attitude, much the same as that of his late father, seen by his critics as arrogance.

A Jenkins man has become warden of this beautiful park on four different occasions. On two of Peter's returns he found the place much degraded, and he worked hard to resurrect things. The same happened to Mark.

Based on its history, I am skeptical that Meru will remain a game park. It is much more likely that it will become a mix of cultivation along the rivers and a large grazing area for cattle. It is wonderful country for both. ✻

9

RHINO REFUGES

A trip to Solio Ranch in 2006 takes me back to days of rhino captures in the 1960s and 1970s, and a meeting with Court Parfet gives me the chance to catch up on the history and tribulations of rhino conservation in his park, the first rhino refuge in East Africa. Another former client and rugby teammate runs a successful conservancy that also acts as a rhino sanctuary.

THE FIRST AREA IN EAST AFRICA heavily fenced enough to hold rhinoceros was at Solio, on the Laikipia Plains between Mount Kenya and the Aberdare Mountains. In 1968 ranch owner Court Parfet put up a game-proof fence and started to stock the area with both Black and White rhino, and it was to Solio that some of the rhino that we caught in the Isiolo area in the early 1970s were trucked. I also helped catch several rhino on surrounding farms and put them inside the Solio fence. Between 1968 and 1978 a total of twenty-three Black rhino and sixteen White rhino came into the park, the latter arriving after we had left Kenya to take up residence in Canada. Two of the earliest

Black rhino came from the neighbouring ranch, and it was a delight, over thirty years later, to learn that they were still alive.

In fact, Joseph Muna, a Meru, who had been a junior clerk at the ranch in the early 1970s, when reminiscing with me in January 2005, remembered the capture of this particular cow and her calf very well. We had been told that she spent most of her time with her half-grown calf in a thorn bush thicket not far from the house of a neighbouring ranch, and so Mr. Parfet had arranged for a small helicopter to come and help with the work of moving them. At first it had been proposed that I dart the animal from a very small light aircraft, known as a Super Cub, but I had vetoed this idea, as darting from a helicopter is difficult enough. A fixed-wing aircraft would be an impossible platform from which to shoot a moving object that can jink in any direction. I had had no intention of being found in the wreckage tangled up in acacia thorns.

We had had good luck and I had been able to get two darts away within about fifteen seconds, one into the rump of each animal, and they had run only a short distance, sticking close together, before becoming immobilized at the edge of a dry luggah. Joseph told me that the animal, known as L1, has the longest horn of any rhino in the park. Even when we caught her, as the accompanying photo shows, her horn was impressive.

Another capture for Solio that I remember from this era had a Chaplinesque element. I had just arrived to work on some monkeys at the Mount Kenya Game Ranch orphanage when John Kariuki, the manager, passed a message to me. The note was cryptic. "Please call Rose Caldwell at the Sports Club." The old crank-handle phone was working, and I was soon through to Rose, whose husband, Jimmy, was the Solio Ranch general manager.

"Jerry," she said, "can you take your dart gun and get out on the plains road toward Solio where Mr. Parfet and Jimmy are having trouble with a rhino? I was driving past on the way into Nanyuki to get some groceries when Jimmy saw me and simply asked me to get you if I could."

This sounded like something that needed dealing with promptly, so excusing myself with John I headed down the hill to the house and grabbed my dart gun from the safe, as well as a bun, which I smeared with generous dollops of peanut butter and jam. I headed out again,

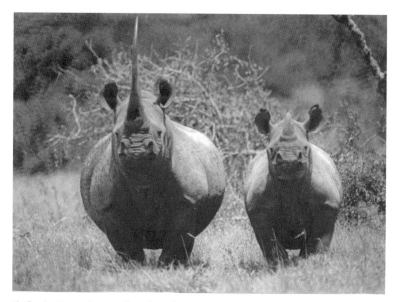

The female rhino number L1 and her calf at Solio. I caught her in 1973 and she was still alive thirty years later. (Courtesy Mr. Court Parfet)

past the office to pick up the potent immobilizing drugs that were safely locked in the big wall safe. Luckily, Mutua and I had had enough experience catching rhino to be able to put our kit together very quickly. The darts, syringes and other bits and pieces were already in the Styrofoam-lined box. The drug vials each had their assigned slot in the cushioning material designed to prevent breakage as we drove on the rough roads.

We turned right at Naro Moru, crossed the tracks and forked left toward the Aberdares. About ten kilometres across the plains we were astonished to see a fully grown rhino staggering around like a Glasgow Gorbals Saturday-night drunk. He was going round in circles, at the closest point not more than twenty metres from us, and turning at the fence, which was merely three strands of barbed wire that he would normally have barged straight through. It was obvious that he had some sort of drug in him, but I had no idea what. It was also obvious that we could not get over to Mr. Parfet and the others, as they were on the other side of the animal. The gate at the roadside was locked and I was not going to risk walking over. I really didn't know how the huge animal would react.

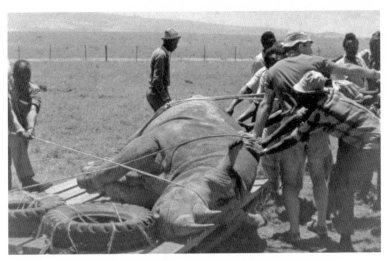

Rhino capture on the Laikipia Plains. Starting to tie down. (Courtesy Jimmy Caldwell)

We looked things over as I considered my options. I decided to make up a dose at about three-quarter strength and managed to get it into the rhino's backside with my first shot. Mutua and I waited for him to fall over, and when he did Jimmy drove over and opened the gate, and we went in and got to work. We loaded him onto a sled that Jimmy had made beforehand, and we took him into the park to release him.

I asked Jimmy why and with what he had already been drugged. He replied, "Mr. Parfet has some Immobilon, and he fired several times into it. He took one of the shots from much too close, about three metres, and the dart burst and sprayed all over us."

"Ye gods," I said, "that stuff's very dangerous! A few drops injected would probably have killed you, and it can even be absorbed through mucus membranes in the eye or mouth. What did you do?"

"Och," said Jimmy, a fellow Scot, "we had lots of water in those chargals on the bumpers and wing mirrors, so we just poured it all over ourselves."

"So you didn't have to use any antidote?"

"No, none of that blue stuff, what's it called?"

"Revivon," I said, smiling inwardly at the name.

"Anyway," Jimmy went on, "soon after that I saw Rose driving by on the road, and we were able to attract her attention."

One surprise was the six needles that we pulled out of the rhino's hide. They were all little short ones meant for cattle, all quite useless for rhino. None had fully penetrated the thick hide. The partial drugging must have been due to the accumulated effects of very small doses.

It was quite a surprise to discover that a drug like Immobilon, about ten thousand times as potent as morphine, could be purchased and used by someone with absolutely no training in its use, no anaesthesia experience and no veterinary degree, but the acquisition was easily explained. Mr. Parfet had been helping out with some studies conducted by scientists from the East African Veterinary Research Organization at Muguga who had been immobilizing buffalo in order to work on the scourge of East Coast Fever. They were trying to develop a vaccine that would be effective in cattle, which contract the disease from buffalo via the ticks. The people who left the Immobilon behind for Mr. Parfet would seem to me to have been overly cavalier with it. People have died after accidentally injecting themselves with it.

Although Solio was not a heavily guarded refuge in the early years, the very fact that Mr. Parfet had the vision to start it up needs to be acknowledged. By any standards the park has to be considered to have been a success, particularly where rhino conservation is concerned.

The rhino translocations have been spectacularly successful and by 1992 sixty-four Black and twenty-four White rhino had been moved from Solio to various refuges, both public and private. An important move was the shipment of White rhino to Lake Nakuru National Park in 1987, and Meru National Park has also received animals from Solio. In 2001 two White rhino were shipped to Uganda, where all trace of any sort of rhino had been removed during the Amin regime. When I was with students in Uganda in 2007 we saw these first two and more that had come after them.

In April 2005 Jo and I visited both Edward Parfet, who now lives on the ranch, and his father, Court, who has moved to the Muthaiga suburb of Nairobi, amongst numerous embassies and the tightly guarded and highly priced homes of the wealthy. Parfet senior gave me as much information as he could about the records of the game ranch part of the operation. Unfortunately a vengeful ex-employee who had been caught stealing ranch property had returned with a can of petrol, poured it over the office buildings and set the whole lot on fire, destroying all written records, but Mr. Parfet's excellent memory, with its information since transferred to paper, tells the story of the successes.

After meeting Edward, Jo and I drove around the park, which was still as beautiful as ever in 2005. We saw plenty of evidence of the success of the conservation effort. Every one hundred metres or so, we came across a rhino midden, where animals had repeatedly marked out their territory by scattering their dung.

Not everything connected with the Solio game park has been plain sailing, of course. In the early years the poachers did not come onto Solio, but in 1997 and 1998, when I was writing my first book, a few rhino were poached. Mr. Parfet gave us a graphic description of the type of activity engaged in by the early poachers. An animal was found in a snare that had been placed between two stout trees. The cable, about two centimetres in diameter, lay around her head behind the back horn and over her eyes. She had been fighting the thing for about two days, but had had no success, as the makers had cunningly constructed it so that it would only move in only one direction, tightening with every pull. The ranch team was able to free the animal, not without risk to themselves, but she was found drowned in a pond two days later. She may have been blinded by the snare, or perhaps she succumbed to the stress of her prolonged struggle.

Mr. Parfet reckons that he and his staff removed at least twenty snares from rhino during those years.

Another interesting consequence of the poaching pressure at Solio has been that the Black rhino there are thought to have stopped breeding altogether in about 1997. The constant harassment had been too much of a disturbance.

In 2004 at least twelve rhino were poached at Solio, despite the high-voltage electric game-proof fence. The poachers used more than an AK-47 to kill and a saw to cut off the horns. By this time they had polished their methods and taken shovels with them. Working at what must have been a feverish rate, by the middle of the night they had dug a hole beside each dead rhino that was big enough to roll the body into. The carcasses were then covered in dirt and brush so that telltale vultures would not spot them and begin their give-away circling and descent. This is why I say there were at least twelve rhino poached in the park. It is certainly possible that more were taken and were simply too well concealed to make the count.

Very positive action was taken in January 2005, however, when a crack anti-poaching squad was posted to the ranch. Soon afterwards it was widely reported in the local press that the newly adopted policing at Solio had yielded an interesting result. One poacher had been shot inside the park fence. The belongings found on his body identified him as an off-duty Kenya Wildlife Service employee who was stationed in Mount Kenya National Park. Another poacher was tracked by bloodhounds several kilometres to the nearby town of Naro Moru and arrested. Most people involved in the investigation seem to think that the manager of the poaching operation is someone highly placed in the nearby town of Nyeri.

Mr. Parfet told us that it is very hard to stop the poaching when fines imposed in court are only about 40,000 shillings (about US$500), although for those who cannot pay, ten years imprisonment is also a potential sentence. With the value of rhino horn as high as it is, $500 is no sort of deterrent. The most recent prices (2002) for horn in the Yemeni capital of Sanaa were $1,200 per kilogram, so twelve rhino with a roughly estimated average weight of three kilograms of horn each would have a potential market value of over $43,000. Even at the export price of $750 per kilogram, the fine would be about the value of one quarter of one horn.

Despite the problems, it must be noted that the 1993 Kenya Wildlife Service report titled *Conservation Strategy and Management Plan for the Black Rhinoceros in Kenya* has one important acknowledgement. It states "Solio Ranch has been the most successful of any rhino sanctuary in Kenya by a substantial margin, this success achieved entirely at the owner's expense. As a result it has served as a model of a fenced rhino sanctuary followed successfully by other areas."

The heightened security must have been a great success because by early 2007 the ranch had once again become overpopulated, especially with Black rhino, and a further thirty-one head were moved a short distance to a newly created refuge on the neighbouring Ol Pejeta Ranch, which had recently been expanded to 31,000 hectares and become an important conservancy. This move was accomplished in fifteen days with great efficiency by two teams led by Kenya Wildlife Service vets, both on foot, who were guided in from the air by spotters flying light aircraft. The rhino were not held in any kind of quarantine but simply loaded into crates and trucked over for quick release, probably spending less than two hours in confinement. Every rhino had a radio transmitter placed in its horn so that it could be monitored.

The Ol Pejeta website states that in one case the free release of a mother-calf combination took place. Batian Craig, the wildlife and security manager, told me via e-mail that although the calf took off on its own when released, the pair were back together within three days. Black rhino are highly territorial and pretty intolerant of intruders, so there must have been some real ding-dong battles among them as they began to try to establish new home ranges in strange surroundings.

There are now several rhino sanctuaries around the country. A major one lies to the north of Mount Kenya at Lewa Downs and backs onto what was once the Isiolo Quarantine Area, where I frequently had to check cattle that were being brought from the NFD before they could proceed to the slaughter plants farther south.

In 1983 Anna Mertz started the construction of a rhino sanctuary at Lewa, which had once been a cattle ranch. The owners, David and Delia Craig, had run beef cattle there and were regular clients as I went there to pregnancy check cattle or issue health certificates for sold animals. Their eldest son, Ian (father of Batian at Ol Pejeta), had played rugby as an aggressive wing forward alongside me in the pack for the Mount Kenya rugby team. After leaving school in England, he made his first purchase of a vehicle, a second-hand Toyota Land Cruiser, with the proceeds from an elephant he had shot under license.

Anna had come to Kenya with her husband to retire after a successful career as an engineer in West Africa, where she had witnessed the wholesale destruction of wildlife for the bushmeat trade. She was determined to stop the same thing happening to Kenya's rhino and so approached the Craig family, who wholeheartedly embraced the concept. My old friend Peter Jenkins, now retired from Meru, had been the game department liaison officer assigned to the project. It was he who designed the first fence at what became the Ngare Sergoi sanctuary. They initially fenced two thousand hectares, and within five years they had expanded the area to four thousand.

The first rhino to come to the sanctuary was captured by a team led by my old friend and colleague Paul Sayer, no doubt using the darts and needles that I had designed myself and had left him when we headed for Canada. Anna named this animal Godot because, as she wrote in her book about the whole experience, she had waited for him for so long. At least he arrived, unlike Beckett's famous absentee.

More rhino followed, these darted by another friend, Dieter Rottcher, who had been an intern at the veterinary school at Kabete at the same time as Paul and me.

Anna then proceeded to make the most detailed long-term study of rhino behaviour ever and documented many things that had never been previously recorded, including their various calls, most of which consisted of tonal variations on what she described in her book *Rhino at the Brink of Extinction* as "eeeak."

The entire sanctuary, now called the Lewa Wildlife Conservancy (LWC), today covers 25,000 hectares as fundraising has become ever more sophisticated. The ranch not only supports rhino, but it is also home to a variety of species, including fifty reticulated giraffe, five hundred Grevy's and Burchell's zebra and four hundred impala. Elephants have also taken up residence, but they can come and go through special gaps in the fence on the sanctuary's northern boundary. The success of the program can be measured in various ways, one of which is the fact that many of these animals have bred very successfully and Ian has had to move many of them off the conservancy to places like Meru National Park. He and his team have become so proficient at the capture methods for each species that they are frequently employed to undertake similar exercises in other parts of Africa.

A major part of the US$2 million annual budget at the LWC goes toward security, which includes highly trained, well-armed askaris, trackers and dog handlers. The LWC also has three tourist lodges on it, as well as a tented camp, and it can offer six thousand bed nights per year. Ian's brother, Will, runs a business called Wilderness Trails that offers experiences varying from walks to horseback and camel safaris and is based upon the ranch, as well.

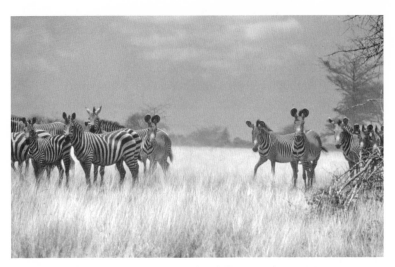

Grevy's and Burchell's zebra in a mixed herd. Grevy's have the large ears and narrow stripes. Once abundant throughout much of northeastern Kenya, southern Ethiopia and Somalia, there are now fewer Grevy's zebra left than there are Black rhino. Much of the loss is due to hunting pressure and the international market for the beautiful striped hides. (Photo by Dick Neal)

There are now over three hundred staff on site, many of them well educated, some with university degrees, and a full-time research team studies many aspects of the ecology of the area. One of the most important of the current research efforts is centred on the Grevy's zebra. These striking members of the horse family have undergone a massive decline—over 85 per cent—in the last twenty years, and there are now fewer of them in the world than there are Black rhino. There were named after Jules Grevy, a nineteenth-century French president who received one as a gift from Ethiopia's Emperor Menelik in 1882. Fewer that two thousand are believed to live in the wild, with a further 220 or so in zoos. They are confined to northern Kenya and Ethiopia. Populations in neighbouring countries having been decimated by hunting.

The Grevy's zebra's situation was not made any better by a 2007 outbreak of anthrax in the Samburu region, north of Lewa. The disease affected many species, including both Grevy's and plains zebra. The Kenya Wildlife Service took action and report that they vaccinated at least sixty of the animals, which would have been far from easy.

The other big step that the LWC has made is to embrace the concept of community conservation. To his end they have linked with and helped the development of Il Ngwesi Group Ranch, which has a tourist lodge owned and run by the Mukugodo Maasai.

THE FUTURE FOR RHINO, as I stated at the start of this chapter, is delicate. In the LWC newsletter of October 2004 appears the following phrase: "never in our lifetime will rhino within East Africa be safe from the threat of poaching; this threat is current, real and pertains to every single rhino area in the region." It has been estimated that there were no more than three hundred Black rhino in Kenya in the 1980s, a huge decline from the estimated twenty thousand present when I began to work with them, usually translocating them out of areas intended for settlement, in the late 1960s. The numbers appear to be creeping back up, though; in 2005 the figure was put at about four hundred. In late April 2007 the precise number of 539 was given on the Ol Pejeta website.

However, when heavily armed guards are not available, things can quickly come unstuck as was illustrated in a BBC website story filed by John Kay under the November 23, 2007, headline "Shootings threaten black rhino project."

The story is about Charles Hamilton, whom Jo and I met in 1992 at Imire, his family's safari park one hundred kilometres (sixty miles) southeast of Harare. Hamilton broke into tears when he showed the reporter images of the three adult female Black rhino, one of them only days away from calving, which had been shot by an armed gang who came to Imire in the dead of night, killed the animals and cut off their horns. ✳

1995–2007

FORESTED AFRICA AND THE BUSHMEAT CRISIS

Mwenye njaa hana miiko.
A hungry man observes no taboos.

—SWAHILI PROVERB

Until you have crossed the river,
don't insult the crocodile's mouth.

—FROM *The Ewe*,
IN *An African Treasury*,
SELECTED BY LANGSTON HUGHES

10

FOREST ELEPHANTS

My family and I move to Saskatchewan, Canada, where I join the faculty at the Western College of Veterinary Medicine. A trip to Cameroon gives me my first taste of West Africa as I work on forest elephants in less than comfortable conditions and meet people whose beliefs systems have little to do with Western values.

THE WEEKEND BEFORE I MOVED TO CANADA with Jo and our two children, Karen and six-week-old Charles, in September 1975, I had to turn down a request for more rhino work from my client Court Parfet. Had Prince Bernhard, the president of the World Wildlife Fund, made his trip to Kenya a week earlier, my last rhino capture in Kenya could have been at Solio. Mr. Parfet had called me up and asked if I was free on the 15th to give the prince a demonstration of immobilization. I had to tell him that we would be on the plane for Europe and then Canada that day, and that I could not oblige.

We had made the decision to move to Canada after I had received an offer to join the faculty of the Western College of Veterinary Medicine in Saskatoon as a zoo and wildlife vet. I knew that the change would be dramatic but had not really reckoned with the winters or the management of captive wild animals. We dealt with the winters easily enough—warm clothes, a well-insulated house and, most peculiar to us, a block heater for the car. We had never encountered this gadget, which allowed us to plug the engine into a power outlet to ensure that the oil would not freeze at any temperature below about-15°C. Not exactly equatorial!

The captive wild animal issue was, in some ways, harder to accommodate than the weather. I went straight from the Pleistocene freedom of Kenya to the sight of two lions in a wire mesh cage no more than five metres in diameter. There was plenty to occupy my mind as I initiated a herd health program for the zoo's collection and began to try and learn the business of teaching. Most exciting, however, was the arrival in my office, within about six weeks of starting the job, of a stocky bearded man named Bob Stewart, who would become a good friend. Bob was with the provincial Department of Natural Resources and was looking for drugs to use on a long-term moose ecology study that would involve placing radio-collars on a large number of animals. It did not take me long to convince him that I had the right experience and could get the right drugs for the study. Better yet, the drugs would come free as I could readily get them as a research tool from the Janssens Pharmaceutical Company in Belgium, which had supported my work with rhino, elephant and several other species in Africa.

This opportunity, which was soon dubbed by a colleague as my "having a horseshoe in the right place," led to a continued career with free-ranging wildlife that took me all over Canada. I have worked with species as diverse as polar bears, seals, elk and wolves. It also led me to active involvement with veterinary associations concerned with wildlife and zoo animal medicine and ultimately to my next opportunity to work in Africa.

It's funny how casual conversations round the coffee urn can lead to new opportunities.

"Morning, Billy," I said to dynamic dark-bearded Billy Karesh as we stood in line for a cup. "I've just gone half-time at the university, so if you have any field work with which you need a hand, let me know."

It was August 1995, on the first morning of the annual meeting of zoo and wildlife veterinarians in East Lansing, Michigan, and Billy and I had met at many such conferences before. Of course my statement had been 90 per cent hope and 10 per cent maybe. I didn't think any more about it until the next morning, when I saw Billy, who is the Director of the Field Veterinary Program for New York's Wildlife Conservation Society (WCS), talking to his boss, Bob Cook, the senior vet at the Bronx Zoo.

As I walked over to greet Bob, whom I also knew, he turned to me and said, "Morning Jerry, were you serious about the offer of some help?"

"Sure, what's up?"

"Would you be able to get to Cameroon next spring? We've had a project there on forest elephants going for a couple of years and Billy has a conflict in commitments. Could you get there in March or April?

"How long for?" I asked.

"About a month."

It sounded too good to be true, but I was soon chatting to Jo about it, and within a few days of getting back to Saskatoon and my university duties, I was trading phone calls with Bob and Billy and getting things like vaccinations and other paperwork organized.

One task was to take a heavy elephant radio collar as part of my luggage, something that would cause quite a delay at customs in Cameroon's main port and commercial centre, Douala, and needed a bit of tricky explanation at the airport in Saskatoon. Although this was well before 9/11, large bits of electronic gear tend to make check-in people inquisitive.

Before leaving, I did some reading and found out that Cameroon is a pie-shaped country about the size of Spain or Britain, stuck between the giants of Nigeria and the Congo Basin. The population of about 12 million has at least 130 ethnic groups, each speaking its own language. As I would soon find out, sometimes villagers in the forest regions, living only a few kilometres apart, had to converse in pidgin, the *lingua franca* of West Africa, because they could not understand one another's mother tongues.

Before long I found myself walking through a dripping rain forest. I soon came to realize that if it wasn't raining, it had either just rained or was about to rain. The Korup Forest of western Cameroon must be about the wettest and rainiest one anywhere. It gets about six hundred inches (15,000 millimetres, which sounds much more impressive) a year: that's over forty millimetres a day.

The rain forest was something entirely new to me. The undergrowth was so thick, and the canopy so dense, that I felt as if I were walking in the middle of a wet green sponge. The giant trees, reaching limblessly up through the greenery until they found a spot high up to catch the sun and branch out, were another new sight. Many of them lacked the traditional shape I had become used to in Canada. Two or three metres above the ground the trunks started to spread down and out in a fan-like series of solid buttresses or an amazing interwoven mass of root-like stems. Their shapes of course, have evolved to increase the trees' stability in the thin soil and improve their access to nutrients.

I had flown into Douala from Saskatoon, via Montreal and Paris, and had been met by Paul Elkan, the slim dark-stubbled Peace Corps volunteer acting as team leader while Buddy Powell, the project director, was away on family business in the USA. After a night's stay in the city, we had set out in a battered Toyota Land Cruiser on the five-hour trip to Nguti, in the west central part of the country, where the project was based.

At first the road had been a reasonable quality tarmac, bounded on both sides by date palm, rubber and banana plantations that had replaced the native rainforest many years since. As we got farther away from the city, the tarmac ran out and the road deteriorated. Red dirt, either seen as a dust cloud behind the vehicle, or worse yet, enveloping it when traffic came the other way, brought back memories of many years of driving in East Africa. Spring-breaking potholes had to be avoided at all costs. Large trucks, carrying either fuel or huge hardwood logs, would come against one's flow and take no mind of one's presence. It was best to pull to the side when one saw them coming.

"That's about the fifth truck loaded with hardwood logs this morning," I said to Paul. "I wonder what each one is worth."

"Each load would be worth at least $100,000 in foreign exchange," he told me.

We passed six of those trucks that day. I was only just beginning to learn about the impact of logging on Cameroon's forests.

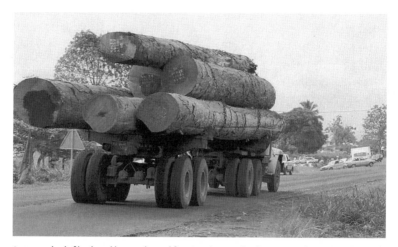

A $100,000-load of hardwood logs on the road from Nguti to Douala. This was one of six such loads I saw during a five-hour drive.

As we progressed, we entered areas of native forest, with small plots dug along the roadside where individuals had tried to eke out enough tillable ground to grow some food. Then, inevitably, came larger agricultural areas, stretching back several hundred metres, completely cleared of trees. Some tree stumps stood still smoking from the fires that had been lit to help in their felling, and straggly cassava and maize plants grew in the open spaces.

Suddenly, we came upon an amazing sight. A huge set of pillars held up a giant causeway above our heads. We twisted up a narrow escarpment and then the road changed. From the dusty pot-holed red ribbon, we drove down a ramp onto a wide stretch of tarmac. We were at least two hundred kilometres from Douala, and here was a road as good as any you would see in Europe or North America.

"What on earth?" I exclaimed.

"It's an example of a European Aid program that has become completely disorganized," Paul explained.

"The whole road was supposed to have been built in concert by a group of contractors from different countries. This one had been finished first, but the others were abandoned, as contractors weren't being paid."

The new road led us all the way to Nguti, where the first thing I saw at the main road junction was the concrete shell of a two-story building containing about ten rooms on each floor. Rebar rods stuck out into the sky, and the whole thing seemed to have been abandoned during construction.

I spent the night trying to get over my jet lag, and then we got down to the business of preparing the gear for our trip into the Korup Forest. This is one of Cameroon's national parks, and the Wildlife Conservation Society team was studying many aspects of the area, including the ecology of the elephants.

The park was strangely chosen. Inside its boundaries are three villages. That in itself might not be unusual for a park, but in this case the men folk of all three are traditional hunters. Even though the villages are small—one of them has only eight homes in it—there is a steady drain on the wildlife in the park because of them. It is impossible to go anywhere along forest tracks without coming across shotgun cartridges about once an hour. On one day of elephant searching we heard shots six times. The main targets for the hunters are a variety of birds and small antelopes. There have been elephant hunters in the region, although their activities had been somewhat curtailed at the time that we were there because of the wcs project and its attendant publicity. The villages were in the area long before the park was gazetted (legally declared a National Park in the official document known as the *Government Gazette*), and the villagers naturally do not want to move unless suitable amenities and locations are found for them. The situation, at the time, was at a stalemate.

One of the species that lives in the area is the forest elephant. They are far less well known or studied than their much larger and more familiar cousins, the bush, or savannah, elephant. They stand only about two metres at the shoulder, have smaller and rounder ears and lighter narrower tusks. Even the number of toes on the feet is usually less, being only four, as opposed to five. However, the two races can interbreed, and intermediate forms of elephant are known. In 2001, reporting in the journal *Science*, Alfred Roca and his colleagues showed that there was sufficient genetic evidence to consider forest and savannah elephants as separate species. However, they are closely enough related to be able to interbreed.

My role was to provide veterinary care during the capture of some of these animals and to assist in the placement of satellite collars so that the folks in New York could get some idea of how the animals make their living. Buddy was doing his doctoral work, a fascinating study of the means by which these elephants act as architects of their own environment by breaking trees and dispersing seeds.

As Buddy explained it to me later, "The elephants roam through the forest in search of food because the trees come into fruit at different times of year, so they are constantly searching. Of course many of these fruits are a real draw. A good example is the wild mango, which they love. Inevitably, some seeds and nuts are swallowed whole. Then they reach their ultimate end point and exit from the elephant."

"I wonder if any of the seeds are like those from the tambalacoque tree that allegedly needed to pass through a dodo in Madagascar in order to propagate," I mused.

"We don't know yet, but the seeds take root in their new spot and so the elephant acts as an unknowing free ride for many plants, thus maintaining the diversity of the forest," he replied.

Paul took me to see the tree nursery that Buddy had started up, planting seeds that he and the team had found in elephant dung. There were about seventy species, carefully tended by a local gardener. Part of Buddy's study involved complex radio tracking, using signals sent via satellite, so that daily movements could be followed in New York. Eventually a map could be built up that would show each specific tracked animal's entire home range.

The gear, apart from the camping equipment that had been prepared by the field team, consisted of the radio collars, crossbow and other drug immobilizing equipment. I knew that we would be using the crossbow because Billy Karesh, who had darted the first elephant collared, had told me an interesting story.

"We got one elephant," he said, "but we were using a dart rifle with a powder charge and the animal scented it and came straight upwind toward me. I dived behind a big buttress tree, and he began to chase me. It was ring-around-the-buttress-tree for a few moments."

It was funny when he told the story, but it must surely have been terrifying at the time. Hence the shift to the crossbow, which would not leave a powder scent trail and in addition would be silent.

Paul and I sighted in the crossbow on a target next to the tree nursery. Using the laser sight, we found that we could both shoot a bolt, adapted to carry an immobilizing dart, about twenty metres with good results. One of the confounding factors was that each dart had to be attached to the bow by a piece of strong braided nylon, known as a tracking string, that would fly out of its container like a fishing line and keep the shooter and the dart in contact. The intent of this system was to enhance our chances of tracking an animal, should we be lucky enough to find and dart one.

Buddy's team had been trying to find and capture elephants in the Korup region for almost two years, but it was difficult work, as the elephants were not only well hidden by the masses of green but also were thoroughly alert, having been persecuted by hunters for many years. The local villagers have another explanation. They know that at night, usually after drinking alcohol, some of the village elders transform themselves, leave their human bodies and enter the elephants, which explains the animals' foreknowledge of attempts to catch them. Billy and Buddy had had to undergo a ceremony with the elders in order to have their dart guns blessed. In his entertaining 1999 book *Appointments at the End of the World*, Billy also relates how, at the ceremony, their minds were addled by potent brew made from palm wine.

During the two years before my arrival, the team had only succeeded in catching two females, whom they had named Angelina and Isabella. This was not going to be a picnic.

Before leaving for Cameroon, I had phoned Buddy, who was in Florida, for advice on clothing and work conditions.

"Bring a minimum of clothes for the actual hunting trip, some in a waterproof bag. Don't take a good camera, as it will get covered in mould in the rain forest," he told me.

"What about footwear?" I asked.

"We all wear locally made plastic sandals."

"Are you serious? I wear a size twelve. Can you get them there? What about running shoes, or maybe hiking boots? Surely they'd be more comfortable."

"Sure, come in your boots, but don't wear them in the forest. You will get so damp that your feet will turn to mashed potatoes. Size twelve will be no problem," he said.

The day we set out to dart elephants, we drove for an hour to the park edge at the village of Baro, where a really strange sight met my eye. Every twenty metres or so down the single central street of this typical mud and sticks village, the only concession to modern technology being the corrugated roofs of the houses, there was an electric street light!

When I asked about this bizarre sight Paul explained, "A team of Exxon staff arrived to build a high-tech suspension bridge to replace the traditional one made of natural materials. During their stay they installed a generator and these lights. Within a week of their departure the generator packed up and the lights are as you see them, nothing more than decoration."

We loaded our gear and set out across the suspension bridge into the bush. Now the serious walking began. The trail was well defined at this stage. In fact, Felix, a slight wiry man about 1.7 metres tall, who was one of the team, described it as a road. At the time, I presumed this was because he regularly travelled the trail on weekends to visit his wife and son, who lived in one of the three villages in the park. The trail varied in width from 1.5 to 0.5 metres. About every five minutes one had either to crawl under or climb over a fallen log.

Despite the fact that I was wearing only a pair of light cotton coveralls over my boxers, within ten minutes I was soaking wet with a mixture of sweat and water dripping off the vegetation. I kept stopping to marvel at the greenery and the life forms on the forest floor. One of the most intriguing things was the termite hills, each built up with its own mud umbrella on top. The looked like overgrown bowling pins covered by a hat of the sort worn by people in Thailand. The termites obviously knew a thing or two about living in a rain forest.

After about a three-hour walk, by which time I was exhausted, we arrived at the research camp. Three porters hired at Baro had gone ahead, carrying with them our food supplies and some of the other gear. Upon arrival, I was immediately plunged into a medical situation. One of the porters had fallen and gashed his foot on a sharp stick. The triangular flap of skin and muscle, about four centimetres at the base, was laying back, exposing a bone in the top of his foot. We boiled some water and I added a teaspoon of salt as a disinfectant. Once the water had cooled, we used a syringe intended for elephant work to flush out the wound. We did have some suture material in the first aid kit, but no instruments. I broke open an antibiotic capsule and poured the powder into the wound and then made do with the pliers of my Swiss Army knife as a needle holder while stitching the wound. We had no anti-tetanus serum with us, but in that sort of environment it would be an absolute must, so I told him to get himself to hospital next day and seek help from the doctors. He was in no condition to walk home, but that was the only way out, and so, with a foot that must have been hurting horribly, he set off for his village. I just hoped that the stitches would hold together. I saw him a few days later, and, happily, things were on the mend.

Supper consisted of rice and curried sardines mixed with onions, followed by a single cup of hot chocolate. Not what I would call haute cuisine, but Paul explained that with limited availability of preserved foodstuffs, and no possibility of keeping anything safe from mould, mice or overheating, there was little choice. He also said that the other team members, all men from the local villages, would not have eaten so well at home.

After a fitful night, still trying to get over my jet lag, we got going at dawn. First came breakfast. I discovered what is meant by a limited diet. The meal consisted of rice or *gari* (a cooked form of cassava that has had the cyanide boiled out of it) and the remains of last night's curried sardines: a thin sauce. Plus, of course, a cup of tea. Luckily, I checked about lunch at this time. My choices were still limited. Cold rice or nothing. As I am one of those folks who has to eat fairly regularly in order to avoid headaches and stomach cramps, the future did not look bright. We were planning to be in camp for up to a week, that is, if we did not get an elephant before then.

I also discovered why Felix had called the trail into camp a road. Within about ten minutes of leaving camp, we were on really narrow tracks, hemmed in by a mass of green leaves of every imaginable size and shape, not to mention the intriguing variations in shade. Visibility varied from about one metre, if one looked sideways off the trail, to a maximum fifteen metres, if one looked straight down it. James, just as slim as Felix but four centimetres taller, was the head tracker and took the lead. He soon stopped and lopped off some branches, trimmed

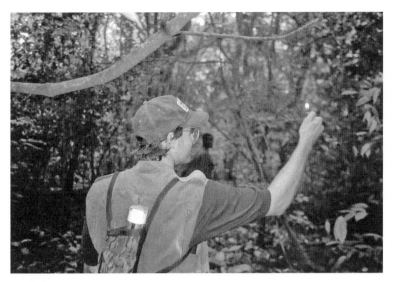

Paul checking the wind in the Korup Forest.

the leaves and passed around short stems. Everyone at once started to chew on them, and James told me that they were called chewing sticks. The plant has been used since early times as a toothbrush. Analysis has shown that the juice of the plant (*Salvadora persica* commonly known as Muswak) contains the antibiotic triclosan, which is known to be effective against gingivitis

This is but one of the many plants in the forest known to have medicinal properties. In other parts of Africa, researchers have described sick chimpanzees knowingly selecting and eating plants that contain medicinal compounds. In the case of one research effort with chimps, an antibiotic new to human science was found. Cameroon has a thriving traditional medicine industry, catering not only to its own citizens through practitioners of the art, but even exporting some compounds to the West.

We had been walking in single file, and in total silence for about ninety minutes along a sort of trail, with visibility down to a maximum of about five metres when something finally happened. Every now and again, Paul had stopped and tested the wind. This involved lighting a standard Bic lighter and observing the flame. The action was silent, essential in the forest when tracking animals. With the winds swirling in the underbrush, it was important to know that we were not walking downwind.

Suddenly, James held up his hand. All of us promptly found the largest tree available, hid behind the buttresses, and waited, not knowing what was going on. We could now hear branches cracking and other quiet noises associated with feeding elephants. Paul went forward with the crossbow and darts. He told me later that he got within about three metres of the animals but could not tell, because of the vegetation, whether he was looking at a rump, shoulder or side. The elephant group spooked and moved off, but not very far, and about two hours later we had a mature bull collared and standing up wondering what had happened.

If the elephant felt caught in a Salvador Dali painting, the actual capture also had elements of the surreal. We tried to follow the group when they spooked but had lost track of them in the underbrush. Paul, James and I had moved ahead, leaving the team safe behind a large buttress tree, and had spread out on a front of about thirty metres. Suddenly James came past me almost at a dead run, looking for Paul and telling me to get behind some large roots as he had seen a single bull elephant standing quietly by a tree. James soon came back to wait with me, and we soon heard a loud "thwack!" as a dart hit. However, no call came from Paul, and so we waited.

Paul, who had been able to get up to within twelve metres of the bull and lie behind a bush, related the rest of the events.

"I waited for a suitable moment and was finally able to get off a shot at the side of the animal's shoulder. Unfortunately, he chose this precise moment to flap his ears, and my dart went right into the middle of the left one and emptied its contents on the other side of it, into thin air."

"What happened next? Didn't he take off?" I asked.

"No, that was the weird thing. He took very little notice of the dart but started almost at once to play with the tracker string. He reeled in several metres of it before I was able to cut it with my Leatherman. I loaded my back-up dart, which was tricky, as I couldn't stand up and had to be very quiet. It took me almost twenty minutes to get off another shot. I tried to work my way around him to get a side shot, but he must have known I was there, as he turned each time I moved."

"You were lucky he didn't simply shove off," I said.

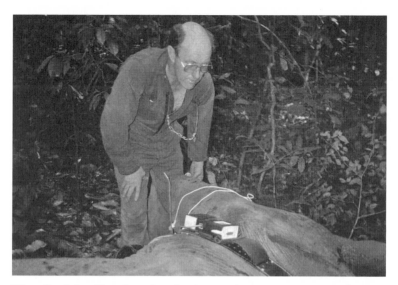

Billy, our first elephant. The equipment is a pulse oximeter, used to measure oxygen concentration as an aid in monitoring anaesthesia.

"I know. Eventually, in desperation, I fired a shot into the front part of the shoulder. This time the dart went home and the elephant took off."

The first dart had been equipped with a miniature radio transmitter, and so we were able to get a good idea of the direction in which he had gone. We also picked up a blood spoor that came from the ear that had been pierced. This turned out to be a stroke of luck, as the radio dart had either fallen or been pulled out after about twenty-five metres.

We now knew that we had an elephant with a dart in him. While most darts work well, there is always a question and a worry that some-thing mechanical may have gone wrong, even when you can see the animal you've darted. The worry was amplified considerably by the working conditions, especially the very limited visibility. As the radio dart had come out, and the tracker string was not in play, we had to rely on James and Felix to find our elephant. Luckily, they never lost his tracks, and within about five minutes we found him lying on his side and with enough clear ground around him that we did not even have to use the machetes to cut back any foliage.

There is an extra layer of worry when working with elephants. El-ephants, different from all other mammals, cannot lie upright on their chests for any length of time. Early on in the days of elephant immobilization, workers discovered that elephants that fall into this position, called sternal recumbency, will die after about twenty minutes. It is likely that when in this position, the tremendous weight of the animal, combined with the enormous pressure from the huge volume of intestines, prevents the lungs from moving. The animal can suffocate. I had queried Billy Karesh about the difficulties of darting elephants in such an environment, and we had agreed that the risks, although recognizable, were acceptable. Elephants usually do fall on their sides when they are immobilized, and we felt that we would be able to topple a patient onto its side if we needed to.

Perhaps, as had been suggested at Billy's meeting with the elders, the villagers had forgotten why the White folks were in the forest and had stopped warning the elephants. Anyway, we had been in luck. I had been in the Korup for less than twenty-four hours, quite a contrast from the amount of time and effort that others had put into the captures of Angelina and Isabella.

Now, we got down to work, which consisted of the collection of a considerable range of samples. We took blood, feces, hair, a tiny biopsy and a small piece of the tip of one tusk. Using these samples we would be able to identify the DNA makeup of this animal and also identify his ivory for all time from its chemical makeup, as each elephant's tusks have their own unique characteristics. We measured everything we could think of. Body, leg and tusk length, girth, foot diameter, tail length and so on. The interesting thing about this animal was that he was probably a cross between the forest and the bush variety of the species. He was 2.12 metres tall and had intermediate type tusks, both thicker and more curved than those of a true forest elephant might be. In addition, his ears did not have the characteristic rounded shape of the forest species. One forefoot had four toes while the other had five, again an intermediate characteristic.

Our most important task was to place his heavy collar that had two radio transmitters on it and weighed over forty kilograms. The radio on the top was designed to communicate with a series of satellites and was geared to go on every other day for the short period that these would be overhead. The lower radio was a VHF type that could only be

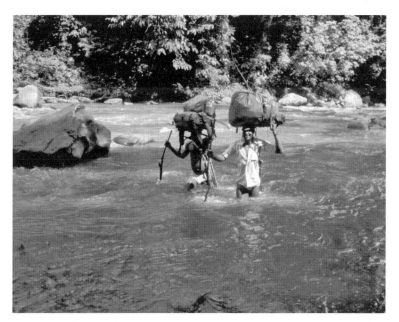
A river crossing in the Korup Forest.

read from a maximum of twenty kilometres, and even then only if the weather allowed and there was a more or less direct line, without hills in the way, between the elephant and the receiver.

All this time I was checking his breathing, pulse and the hue of the pink interior membranes of his mouth, which was telling me how his circulation was doing. Finally, we collected as many ticks as possible off his body, and then it was time to give him the antidote and watch him walk away.

Now it was decision time. By the time we had finished, it was past three o'clock in the afternoon. Some team members had to go back to camp and clear up. Could others of us get out to the car before dark and so keep the blood samples in good condition? For me, there was another excellent reason to get out. Another supper of curried sardines and rice did not appeal, and the thought of a breakfast similar to that morning's was a complete deterrent to a return to camp.

Anyway, there was no point in returning to camp if we did not have to, as there were no more radio collars available and so no more work could be done on this particular trip. Paul and I decided to have a go at getting out. Felix volunteered to go with us. It would mean a stiff walk straight through the forest. No set paths, just a compass bearing and a rough idea of where we were at the moment and where the river was. Once we got to the river, Felix, being a local, would have no trouble in guiding us to the bridge.

When we first started, I thought I was tired from the enervating heat and the lack of sleep. I had not realized the half of it. We crossed two small rivers on the way out, and I had absolutely no hesitation in simply diving in and giving myself a good soak. I was already dripping wet from sweat and high humidity, so it made little difference to my clothes. The walk seemed to go on for ever, with Paul and I checking our compasses at regular intervals while Felix just marched on. It was really a case of his being entirely at home, as I would be leading someone through the streets of Saskatoon. Once back at Nguti, I indulged in a meal of pancakes, syrup, fried eggs and a tin of fruit. I certainly had no trouble with insomnia due to jet lag that night!

When we phoned New York the next day with the good news, we had considerable trouble convincing anyone that we were not doing a big leg-pull. We had failed to realize that we were calling on April 1st! I don't think that they really believed us until the satellite radio began its transmissions and showed that the collar was moving around the Korup.

Now began a period of frustration for me. There were no more collars in Cameroon. The company that had contracted to make them had been slow to deliver, despite plenty of warning, so I could do nothing. Paul and Felix were able to go back into Korup and follow Billy's movements on the VHF radio. (The elephant had been nicknamed Billy in honour of two of the senior scientists at the New York Zoological Society).

While I was waiting for collars, however, we embarked on a checking trip in another part of the forest. It turned out that Angelina's satellite collar had not been working as well as it should, and so we set out to see if we could find her on the VHF. This trip was more relaxed, and I had had time to make some minor adjustments to the menu: less Spartan. I have always had a philosophy about camping. Anyone can be uncomfortable in the bush, wherever they are. However, with a minimum of forethought, one can ameliorate some of the discomfort. So, I purchased a couple of loaves of bread, some peanut butter and some jam for myself.

These extra food items provided me with a lunch and a welcome change of diet. The peanut butter also provided me with a vehicle for the horse de-worming medicine that I had brought along to prevent myself from contracting river blindness, a nasty parasitic disease that one can simply not avoid, spread by black flies. The medication came in a toothpasty-looking tube, and I simply calculated the right amount to spread on my sandwich. It had no taste but the consistency of mayonnaise, so it was ideal in a sandwich.

My experiences with the first two-day trip into the forest had also made me wiser about clothing. I still wore just coveralls and boxers, but I washed and changed them daily. The accumulated salt from sweat in the waistband and between the legs had made a raw mess of my back and inner thighs before I learned the importance of this piece of laundry management.

Because we had no collar, the entire four-day trip to check on Angelina was more relaxed. There was no pressure to find new elephants or to worry about the risks associated with collaring them. It also gave me a good chance to get to know the rest of the team members. They were an impressive unit.

James was the son of a well-known chief and famous hunter. As a young lad, he had surreptitiously borrowed his father's shotgun. In trying it, he had inevitably been knocked flat on his back, but he persisted, becoming a hunter himself. He said that he had been an elephant hunter for many years, killing animals on contract when they became problem animals around the many villages scattered through the forest. He claimed numbers that seemed to be beyond possibility, saying that he had killed over two hundred elephants in his life. Certainly there was good evidence that he had taken out about twenty in the last three years before joining the capture team. He used one of two borrowed heavy rifles and had been with the team for about a year. By the time I met him, he was being paid a substantial bounty by Buddy or Paul if he brought in a rifle confiscated from another hunter. His skills were another clear example of the old adage "set a thief to catch a thief." Many of the best members of anti-poaching units in Kenya were made up of reformed poachers.

Elias, a stockier round-headed version of Felix, was the best educated of the local crew. Since he seemed to know much about the history of the area, I asked Elias about the abandoned building that I had seen on my first day in Nguti. He said, "It was built by a local businessman, intended for a hotel, but not completed, because when he went to check with the witchdoctor he was told that it could not be finished as it had evil spirits inside it." By the time I saw it, the jungle was beginning to take over, and several plants were staking their claims, both inside and around the edges.

Gregory, taller than all the others, and sporting a bright multicoloured shirt, was another team member. He knew this part of the forest better than James and was also a marvelous tracker. He spoke less English than any of the others, so I had to rely on translations and an embryonic understanding of pidgin.

There was a real camaraderie and a healthy amount of leg-pulling and joking, as well as discussion of serious subjects, in camp. We used hunters' huts in the forest as our night stops. These were simple structures, roofed with palm leaves, that provided a focal point for the cooking fire. The huts were located close to a small river, and it was a real delight to strip off and go for a warm dip at the end of an exhausting day's walking in virtual silence.

"Murphy" had obviously gone for a walk elsewhere, and his "anything will go wrong" rule had gone with him. We woke up the first morning, and just for practise Felix turned on the vhf receiver. Angelina's signal came in loud and clear!

It took us no more than two hours to catch up with her group. They were as difficult as ever to see, but there seemed to be about five of them, and there was at least one small calf. We decided to sit on a nearby hillside and watch events. After about an hour, during which time we had not seen the animals, Felix mounted the antenna again and discovered that the animals had moved off. He estimated that they were probably at least two kilometres away. It seems ridiculous, writing from a comfortable office in Canada, and recalling the thousands of elephants that I have seen in East and southern Africa, to state that these huge animals had simply melted out of sight, but that is precisely what happened, despite the watchful eyes and listening ears of five bush-experienced humans.

We spent another day exploring the forest, and I was particularly enchanted by a salt lick and open grove in a stream bed where elephants obviously came regularly. I spent over an hour down on my belly next to the stream as a host of multicoloured butterflies came to feed on the copious amounts of processed vegetation (partly decayed elephant dung) scattered on the banks. With the pressure off, James and Gregory were able to help me identify some of the sounds that they heard in the forest. They identified chimpanzees, which they said are extraordinarily difficult to see, as they are so shy, as well as a couple of species of monkey and several kinds of bird. The shyness of the chimps was no real surprise, as they are a favourite prey of bushmeat hunters. We heard some squirrels chattering, and James darted off the track to show us a tortoise that these characters were scolding. He said that the squirrels would continue to abuse it all day. He also said that a hunter should not kill this kind of tortoise, as it would bring bad luck.

HAVING FOUND ANGELINA there was no point in staying, so we headed out of the forest and back to Nguti. There was still a period of ten days before Buddy would return with the new collars, so there was plenty of time to relax. I wandered down to the village to pick up a beer and watch a soccer game on the pitch beside the mission.

Next day Paul and I headed for the bright lights of Douala, where he was to pick up his girlfriend, and I started a brief holiday and exploration of some other parts of Cameroon. ✳

11

AN
INQUISITIVE
MATRON

*I take a holiday on Cameroon's coast. My
introduction to the bushmeat trade, more work
with elephants and an interesting taxi ride. I
meet with the survivor of an elephant attack. I
reflect on the impact of logging in West Africa.*

TO START MY HOLIDAY, I headed down the coast to the town of Limbe,
where Paul had recommended an inexpensive but reasonably appointed hotel. I had brought my fishing gear with me—I seldom travel far
without it—and tried my hand, with some success, on the coast, as well
as in some of the rivers.

For the purposes of my holiday I had been lucky enough to be grant-
ed the use of a Toyota Land Cruiser. After staying down the coast for
a while, I decided to make a trip up into the Fulani country north of
the rain forest. Here the culture was quite different. The fiercely independent peoples there did not tolerate interference from the south,
and "city slicker" criminals from the south seemed to disappear quite

quickly if they wandered into the Fulani region. I thought it better not to ask for too many details of how this happened, but the implication was clear. Relations between North and South seemed like a variation on those between gangs during the Prohibition Era in Chicago, complete with cement shoes.

As I headed back toward the coast after several days of exploring, a wheel bearing on the Toyota seized up right on the highway, near the headquarters of a huge banana plantation, bringing me to a grinding halt and destroying one brand-new tire. I walked up to the offices and soon found a charming manager who had spent time at England's Cambridge University and willingly helped me out. He found a guard to stay on duty with the vehicle and waited with me for no more than ten minutes until I grabbed a ride with the third bush taxi—a Toyota van—that came past, the previous two having been full. There was one seat left, in the middle row, although it was really only half a seat, as the rest of the bench was taken up by two very solidly built matrons.

It was a good thing for me that I was in the English-speaking, western part of the country as before the driver had shifted up into third gear the opening gambit from my immediate neighbour, the nearer, and larger, of these ladies, was, "And what church do you belong to?"

The conversation in the taxi shifted over many subjects in the next three hours, as every ten kilometres or so we had to slalom through upturned nails on boards at dozens of barriers set by one of the three arms of the police. The driver had had the good fortune or foresight to have as his front-seat passenger a retired policeman who had dressed in his uniform for the trip. The policeman knew that he would have a free ride to the capital to collect his pension because his presence allowed the driver to avoid paying bribes at any checkpoint.

One passenger sat quietly at the very back and was one of the last to alight, at a local market, just before my stop. He hobbled to the roadside, and I asked my large neighbour why he had a bandage on his leg.

"Oh, he was in a crash at the road junction just before you got on. His taxi hit another one head-on. He was the only one to survive," she said then added, "Twenty-seven people died."

After returning next day with a mechanic to fix the Toyota, I headed back to Nguti via Douala where I picked up supplies, especially more peanut butter and jam for lunches, some tins of fruit and the where-withal to make pancakes or bannock, the egg-free flour-based bread made famous in the story of the burned cakes of Robert the Bruce of Scotland.

At Nguti, where Buddy and his petite wife, Maureen, had now arrived, together with two new elephant collars, we soon prepared another ex-pedition. I headed into the small market to see if I could pick up any other supplies to augment the meagre diet.

While walking down the main street I was surprised to see three young women whose back-carried, milk-coffee-coloured babies had obviously been sired by Oriental fathers. I later asked Buddy about this, and he said, "There is a steady stream of foreigners coming through here. Last year there was a Korean construction crew working on log-ging roads—they were stationed in a camp at the other end of the town. The rest is easy to understand."

Sometimes fiction can be used with great strength to make points that are missed or ignored in other media. Cameroonian writer Juli-ana Makuchi Nfah-Abbenyi, known simply as Makuchi, has crafted a short story that gives yet other angles to foreign invasion of Camer-oon's forests and culture. Makuchi uses the term "Timber babies" to describe infants like the ones I saw in Nguti in her moving short story "The Forest Will Claim You Too." The timber baby element is a minor thread in her story. The main emotional impact comes when she de-scribes in gruesome detail the death under a fallen log of a young man who defies the village council and starts to work for a logging com-pany after being recruited by a Frenchman and a Korean. She goes on, in the words of her radio broadcaster narrator, to say, "how can we let the French, the Thais, the Italians, the Germans, the Koreans...crush us with our own?" Whether writing fact or fiction, Makuchi is pas-sionate about the forests in which we were working.

When we were ready to set out, we returned to the area of the for-est where we had seen Angelina and set up camp in the same bush hut as before. Buddy explained that this was one of the oldest for-ests in Africa, and there were signs of human activity that dated back many thousands of years, predating the last glaciation. Occasionally one would come across a palm tree in amongst the hardwood giants.

Palm trees are not native to the area and must originally have been brought up from the coast.

Even walking through the heavy underbrush, I found it difficult to comprehend the number of plant varieties.

"How many species of plant do you think there would be if one drew a circle ten metres in diameter and counted all the plants within the circle?" I asked Buddy as I pointed into the underbrush.

"At least two hundred," he replied without skipping a beat.

It took me a moment to digest that, not really having a clue if he was right.

The part of the forest we were walking through was laced with wide tracks that were partly overgrown. They are the legacy of logging companies that have surveyed deep into the interior and selected specific hardwood species, such as teak, and taken them out with giant skidders.

We had all waded across one of the many rivers in the forest and were resting for a moment before proceeding, when Buddy, with a strangled squawk, said, "I've got a tick up my urethra." This was not good. If the tick decided to quit moving and instead seek a blood meal, it could swell and cause a blockage, which would be very serious.

What to do? Paul, Buddy and I all carried knives in our belts. The other two had Leatherman tools, while I was firmly and emotionally attached to my Swiss Army knife, which had been given me by my mother-in-law. Leatherman knives do not carry tweezers, but all of the more fully equipped Swiss Army ones have exactly what Buddy needed in this situation.

I did not volunteer to do the minor surgery, but simply passed the little tweezers across. Only a couple of minutes later Buddy heaved a sigh of relief and passed them back, remarking, "Score one for the Swiss Army knife." Of course the red handle and white cross of this tool has been well known for many years, and at its public peak was the silent star of the television series *MacGyver*. I have a feeling that our Cameroon solution to a problem, while being challenging enough for the television writers, might not have been considered quite appropriate for family viewing when MacGyver was on the tube. However, with the splurge of so-called "reality TV" that now crops up at every turn, on just about every channel, a tick in the tip might not be considered too far out.

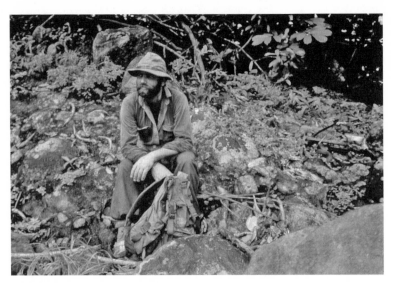
Buddy Powell resting after a river crossing.

The first night I was able to provide the whole camp with some new culinary experiences. Apparently only Paul, Buddy and I had ever eaten pancakes before, and Paul had never eaten an upside-down pudding made with bannock and tinned fruit. The all-round comments of approval made the effort worthwhile.

On the third morning, the crew moved our gear to the next hut left before first light, and as we ate our breakfast—rice and sardines for the crew, bread and peanut butter for me—they came back into camp in a hurry.

Almost out of breath, and obviously excited, Felix said. "We have seen very fresh tracks near the river, only a few hundred metres from here. Three elephants, probably bulls by the size."

We were soon on the trail, and even I could plainly see the overlapping footprints of three animals that had crossed a stream bed and walked on the sandy banks for a while.

Again, the tension mounted as Paul and James went forward with the darts and the rest of us waited behind a buttress tree. This time it was about forty minutes until we heard a thump as the dart hit home, followed by a tremendous commotion as the elephants moved off at a run.

We were on their tracks within two or three minutes. The underbrush was much thicker than it had been when we darted Billy. Indeed, we had to use machetes to get through some of it, despite the fact that a couple of tonnes of bull elephant had just gone through. This was where the radio dart paid off. Each of the three elephants had charged off in a different direction, and we would have had a desperate time sorting them out without the antenna that Felix was carrying and the blip-blip-blip in his earphones when he turned it on. We found the dart after about ten minutes, and I began to worry about the time lapse since the dart had been fired.

Suddenly Felix dived back through a particularly heavy bunch of lianas and said that the animal was down on the other side of them. I checked my watch. It was thirty-two minutes since darting. I was next through the gap in the creepers and immediately saw that we were in trouble. The elephant was quite dead. Heroic measures, including an injection of stimulant, and an effort to roll him on his side and perform artificial respiration by jumping on his chest, were to no avail.

It was plain that he had started to fall backwards and to one side, as they normally do, but the drugs had overcome him at the worst possible site. He was leaning up against a tree, unable to fall to his side, and worse yet his sternum was on top of an old termite mound, adding even more pressure to his chest.

It is difficult to tell how long he had been dead, but the drugs we were using, and with which hundreds, if not thousands of elephants have been immobilized, normally start to show signs of working in about five minutes, and would be expected to immobilize an animal in something from seven to ten minutes. Even if this animal had been lying down as long as twelve or fifteen minutes after darting, he would have been lying on his sternum for twenty minutes, unable to breathe because of the weight of his abdominal contents pressing forward onto his lungs.

The mood of the crew that had been so upbeat just a few moments previously, took a nose-dive. It was now that I gained new respect for the team. Despite the huge letdown they began the tedious task of data collection, and we conducted a post-mortem examination.

After a brief discussion Buddy decided that the capture component of the project would be closed down, at least temporarily. There were several potentially important political decisions to be made, both in Cameroon and in New York, before there could be any thought of continuing.

As I look back years later, I can view the trip and the experience with what I hope is a balanced perspective. In the report of this death, and the rest of the exercise, written for the decision makers in New York, I concluded that the very presence of the Wildlife Conservation Society in Cameroon, and the continuation of the radio tracking and work on other species, was likely to exert a positive influence on conservation. Buddy had gathered an excellent team of about ten people who were all funded from overseas sources. If the project were to be shut down, what would a man like James do for a living? Elephants had been an integral part of his life for many years. He had achieved a certain status in the community. If he could not maintain that status as a tracker and team member, I am fairly sure that he would return to his former craft. If he had been able to shoot elephants before the WCS entered his life, what would stop him from reverting? His success rate was known to consist of several elephants killed per year. The one bull that we had lost was a serious emotional blow to all of us. However, in terms of the overall population of forest elephants in the Korup region it would have nothing like the impact of even one elephant hunter working for a couple of months.

I can also reflect that stalking elephants in almost impenetrable rain forest for hours on end, never knowing when you might come across one within a few metres, and then trying to get a dart into it without being sure what part of it you are looking at because of the thick vegetation, is about the most adrenal-squeezing work I have ever done.

There are two postscripts to this story.

About six months after I had left and returned to the "normal" life of Saskatoon, Paul had an escape that makes him a member of a very small club. He, Elias and another guide, whom I never met, were following a collared elephant in a different part of the forest. Unbeknownst to them a lone bull had caught their scent and charged. He caught Paul from behind, ruptured his hamstring and threw him in the air. He then proceeded to drive a tusk through the front of Paul's chest, penetrating far enough to break his shoulder blade. Inexplicably, the elephant then took off. Paul's companions split up. One stayed with him, nursing him through the night, while the other ran back to the village (about four hours away) and brought help. Paul has described his feelings and the subsequent events in an article in *Wildlife Conservation* magazine. He lay all night wondering why he had not bled to death, and in the morning he was hoisted onto an improvised litter upon which he was taken first to the village, and then a further eight hours to the roadside. From there he was picked up by helicopter and flown to Douala, thence to Paris, and finally to New York. The surgeons there rebuilt his leg, and eight months later he walked back into the village to thank them for their help. I can only imagine their amazement at seeing him alive.

It would take an intimate knowledge of anatomy, and a good deal of bravery or sheer stupidity, for anyone to deliberately drive a stake through a man's chest and avoid hitting the esophagus, heart, lungs, or any major blood vessels or nerves. Paul was very lucky.

Attacks by elephants have no doubt been a fact of life for Africans for millennia, and in recent years newspaper headlines have highlighted the conflicts as elephant range shrinks in the face of continuous human expansion. No doubt many human deaths during these confrontations go unreported, although they are known well enough in the local communities.

There have been a few recorded survivals after elephant attacks, and no doubt there are some unreported ones, but in most cases a human is not going to survive such an uneven contest. Other survivors of elephant attacks whom I know include wildlife photographer Peter Beard, park warden Ted Goss and Muraya Kiai of the Mount Kenya Game Ranch, whom we met in 2005.

I asked Muraya about his experience, and he was only too willing to share it, as it has given him considerable notoriety in his village. He is a tall (1.92-metre) forty-year-old Kikuyu from Nyeri, whose maternal grandfather was a Maasai, and his imposing figure lends to the drama of the story, which he has fine-tuned over numerous retellings.

He and other ranch employees had been building a fence on the ranch when a herd of seven elephants broke in. The team had made three failed attempts to drive them out when Muraya turned and saw a bull that he had not noticed coming after him. He ran but unfortunately tripped. The elephant was on him and drove a tusk through his back, down through his diaphragm and liver and then tossed him into a tree. He fell from the tree and the elephant again speared him, opening up his belly, and once more flipped him six metres into a tree.

Holding his stomach, which had spilled out, more or less in place with his blood-stained jacket, he scrambled through the branches and was able to get to ground and hide under and behind a large log. He had somehow hung onto his walkie-talkie radio all this time.

"I used the radio, which I had kept through God's grace, and told the others to stay away, as the elephants were now all around me. I did not want anyone else to be killed."

Eventually the elephants left, and the crew called Don Hunt who drove Muraya to the Nanyuki Cottage Hospital. As Don put it, "We took him there to die."

They had not reckoned with the skills of the resident doctor, Jo's successor Abid Butt, or with Muraya's innate toughness, or with the kind of luck that so often seems to play a part (Muraya's eldest son turned out to be a suitable blood donor).

Three weeks later he walked out of hospital, and a year later he was fully fit and willing enough to show not only his impressive scars for the camera but also the unrepaired hole in the back of his jacket where the first tusk drove into him. He keeps this jacket as a kind of trophy in the office. It is a good example of the hazards of working with elephants.

The other postscript to this chapter is that wcs have given up their work in the Korup Forest, probably due to the continued hunting activity and declines in wildlife populations. Elephants are now more readily found in the adjacent Banyak Mbo Reserve. wcs has not left Cameroon and has a very large and active program there, but the logging issue has not gone away.

As Billy Karesh put it in his 1999 book *Appointments at the End of the World*:

> The logging industry has wreaked considerable havoc on the rain forest. The rate of destruction is approximately half that of Brazil—about 0.8 per cent per year, far surpassing other countries in Central Africa. The French government recently relieved Cameroon of a large part of its foreign debt burden in exchange for exclusive logging rights for French-owned companies...The French deal with Cameroon reduces their debt burden in exchange for destroying their environment. ❋

12

BUSHMEAT

Bushmeat has supplied people with food for millennia, and it has gradually evolved into a major commercial enterprise. I see how the system works in Cameroon.

MY FIRST EXPERIENCE WITH BUSHMEAT in an African forest came soon after the start of my first elephant-collaring effort in Cameroon in 1996. On the second night out of town, when I was getting a bit worried about the limited rice and curried sardine diet we were facing, Gregory, our most skilled tracker, stood and picked up his shotgun, a crudely made, single-barrelled concoction, the stock bound with copper wire just behind the trigger guard. He had an old and somewhat battered brass dish about twenty centimetres across mounted on his forehead and held in place by a band made from a piece of inner tube.

He said something in pidgin of which I got enough to understand "bushmeat" and "hunt."

"What have you got here?" I asked, gesturing to the headpiece. Gregory's English was limited, and he said something more in pidgin that I did not understand at all. I turned to Buddy with a raised eyebrow and a query in my face.

"It's an old carbide lamp. The sort coal miners used to wear; they are sometimes used by spelunkers—cavers," he said. "He will add some calcium carbide when it gets dark, and light it with his Bic so as to create a sort of spotlight for hunting."

Gregory quickly disappeared along the overgrown path, gun in hand.

An hour later he was back carrying a small crocodile, no more than a metre and a half long. I understood enough of his pidgin to realize that he had not fired the gun but had used his machete to dispatch our supper near a stream. It was a welcome addition to the meal, although it had the consistency of very tough chicken and tasted distinctly fishy.

The term bushmeat means different things to different people. For those who study the subject, the term bushmeat covers meat from all wild animals, whether obtained legally or illegally. Bushmeat includes animals that are ranched, like those held behind fences in any of South Africa's six-thousand-plus game farms, as well as free-ranging animals. Others are more restrictive in their definition of the term, choosing not to include ranched animals. The range of species that can become bushmeat covers the gamut, from insects, reptiles and birds to small mammals, from rodents and bats to antelopes, such as duikers, and all the way to elephants. I think of it as meat obtained from free-ranging animals.

The bushmeat trade has become the "concern du jour" among conservationists in Africa, not without good reason. When I searched the word bushmeat (or the separated term "bush meat") on the Internet in May 2007, I got over 3 million hits. It has a long history and its use has increased steadily in synchrony with the rise in human numbers. As *New York Times* columnist Raymond Bonner so aptly put it in 1993 in his important book *At the Hand of Man*, "People were once an island in a sea of wildlife. Now wildlife survive in parks that are islands in an ocean of people."

Traditionally, forest dwellers have always hunted for their food near home and then preserved what was not eaten right away by smoking it. When cattle are not available—lack of grazing and tsetse flies see to that—the only animal protein around is living in the forest, so it has been natural to take advantage of it. Bushmeat hunting has probably gone on since humans first moved into forest environments.

As forested areas became more populated with people, small-scale hunting developed as a form of commerce. Billy Karesh recorded how he found pangolin (a small anteater covered in scales) and porcupine on a menu in Yaoundé, Cameroon's capital city, and articles in local African newspapers discuss the need for bushmeat in the absence of beef.

Bushmeat hunting has always had some impact on wild animal numbers, and it is logically a major element in the decline of many species that has been going on for at least a hundred years. This decline has been thoroughly documented by Tanganyika- (as it was then) born and University of Oxford-affiliated biologist, author and artist Jonathan Kingdon, in his seven volume *magnum opus* on African mammals *East African Mammals*. Ian Parker and Alasdair Graham, ex-Kenya game wardens and authors, then collated Kingdon's data and tabulated the declines of thirty of the species Kingdon lists to make the message quite clear.

My first encounter with the bushmeat trade occurred when I had some days off while awaiting a new elephant radio collar. I had headed west and then north through the palm-nut and rubber plantations from Douala toward the Fulani country lying between the belt of tropical forest that runs east-west across the continent and the southern edge of the Sahara Desert. While still driving through forest, I came across roadside stalls that offered a variety of animals for sale, and so I stopped to talk to one group as I went north and then again on my return journey. The first time they were reluctant to talk to me, but I did at least establish some credibility, especially once I had demonstrated my credentials in talking about hunting, which included a discussion about guns and cartridges. We talked prices for the various commodities, the fluctuating prices of shotgun shells—depending upon the openness of the border with Nigeria—and the suitability of particular shells for a given species. When I mentioned the English brand of Eley, there was general agreement that that was the best, if only one could get them.

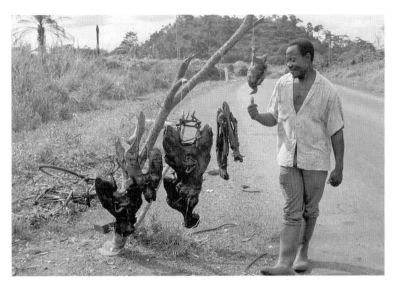

A bushmeat vendor. At the top is a fresh francolin. Beneath it are two smoked cane rats and three unidentifiable smoked monkeys.

On the way back, late in the afternoon, I had a much longer and more interesting stop. This time there were several different types of animals on show, about ten specimens of seven species. The most expensive was a two-metre-long crocodile, still very much alive, its jaw tied shut and its tail pulled round and tied to its snout with string while its hind legs were firmly bound to its body. It was on sale for 80,000 CFA, the local currency. This translated to about Can$400 at the time. The reason for the high price was that both the meat and hide were of value.

Other meats that were on display had a fascinating price structure. The next most expensive was a cane rat (also known as grasscutter or, in pidgin, cutting grass) of about four kilograms.

"How much is that?" I asked.

"Twenty-thousand for the cutting grass," was the abrupt reply.

"And that?" I asked, pointing to a freshly killed duiker antelope, about the size of my black Labrador dog at home.

"Ten thousand."

There was a very fresh bird, about the size of a small chicken, hanging on a thread by its neck at the tip of the dead forked branch that the hunter was using as his eye-catcher, right by the road. It looked very much like the Scaly Francolin of the East African highlands but I could not be sure.

"And that?" I said, pointing again.

"Fifteen hundred." This translated into about $7.50, about as much as a supermarket chicken double its size in Saskatoon. At these prices the meat was obviously available only for relatively wealthy people.

There were three carcasses on display under the palm-leafed shaded counter behind the branch. One, a monkey I did not recognize, looked a bit puffy. The other two were dried up, uniformly dark-brown. After taking a second look, I realized that the two dried ones were animals that had been smoked, one a monkey, the other a duiker, but I could in no way identify them, as all the hair had been singed off them.

"How much do they cost, and when did you get them?" I asked.

He pointed to the unsinged monkey. "Six thousand CFA, shot last night. If you had come this morning it would have been ten thousand."

He obviously realized that I wanted to know the other prices, as well, so he simply continued down the line, saying, as he moved, "I got these the night before last. Didn't sell yesterday so I smoked them overnight, while I was out hunting. Cost you four thousand each."

I internally shook my head at the meat hygiene implications of the whole price structure, especially as none of the carcasses had been disembowelled.

Although technically illegal, bushmeat supplies were openly discussed in the English language newspapers in Douala, where the point was made that in the southern half of the country there is no cattle ranching and that bushmeat forms an important part of the diet for many people. No doubt poorer people continue to gather what they can to feed their families.

In 1958, before she came to Kenya, Anna Mertz, who had been the driving force behind the rhino refuge discussed on pages 112–115, had witnessed the trade in Ghana and wrote "lorry loads of antelope arrived (at the local market) every morning. Many were carried alive with their legs broken, others arrived already smoked and salted." That must have been a grim sight.

Historically, using history in its broadest sense, which includes oral history predating the written records of the last two thousand years or

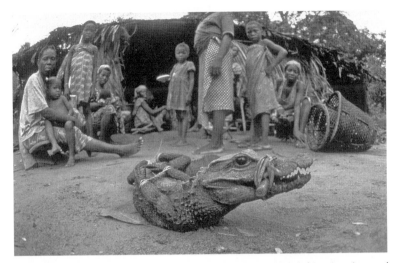

Many hungry mouths to feed and some welcome cash income from the crocodile hide. (Photo by Karl Ammann)

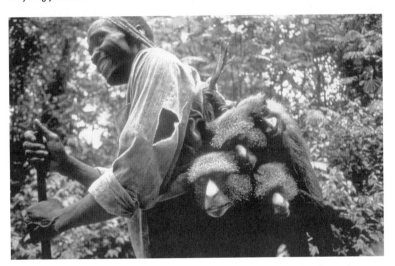

A successful hunt. A moustached guenon (top) and three Martin's putty-nosed monkeys being taken to market. (Photo by Karl Ammann)

so, humans have hunted for food worldwide. They had to in order to survive. Being omnivores, we have hunted for roots, leaves, fruit and of course for a wide variety of animals. The Inuit waiting for a seal to surface at an air hole, or joining his companions in a whale hunt was, and is, engaged in a form of bushmeat hunting, just as is the fisherman casting his net into a shoal of sardine-sized fish inside the reefs off Fiji. So also the Orang Asli hunter with his blowpipe in Malaysia and the Baka pygmy deep in the forests of the Congo Basin. In modern Western cultures, there are still people who rely upon wild meat for their protein intake. Some have to, as they lack financial resources to buy meat in stores. Others, like the Aboriginal peoples of Canada, including the Cree and other First Nations peoples of my adopted province of Saskatchewan, are entitled to hunt wildlife (a.k.a. bushmeat) on a year-round basis, and do so.

Technically I am a bushmeat hunter, although I certainly do not have to be so to survive. I buy hunting licenses every year, and our deep-freeze is packed with venison and a variety of species of waterfowl that are so abundant in Saskatchewan. We have not purchased meat, other than bacon, in thirty years. I hunt because I enjoy it, and also because we like the flavour of wild meat and choose it as a healthy alternative. Hunting is healthy both because it gets me out and about, with plenty of walking, and because of the meat's dietary properties, especially the low-fat content.

Rob Barnett, working for the wildlife trade monitoring network TRAFFIC, an arm of the World Wildlife Fund for Nature (WWF) and the International Union for the Conservation of Nature (IUCN), put together a detailed report on bushmeat in seven African countries ranging from Kenya southward to Botswana. The bushmeat trade in western and central Africa is well recognized as an important element in consideration of gross domestic product and national revenues. On the other hand, most people have generally considered that in the countries Barnett studied, Kenya, Tanzania, Malawi, Zambia, Zimbabwe, Mozambique and Botswana, bushmeat acquisition has been viewed as a subsistence activity. He concluded that the perception was misguided. For instance in Tanzania, he reported that the bushmeat trade exceeded the value of wildlife in the tourist industry, trophy hunting or legalized hunting. Much of the trade is informal and secretive, but in Botswana it is recognized as a cultural right, and the supply of wild meat has been legalized through a comprehensive licensed resident hunting sector. In Zambia and among the WaKamba people in the Kitui area of Kenya, bushmeat makes up the bulk of all meat protein consumed by the people, especially as meat from domestic animals in this area is often much more expensive than bushmeat. Some of Barnett's overall conclusions were that demand for bushmeat is increasing, supply is dwindling and prices are rising. They rise even more in festive seasons.

Other figures quoted confirm that the trade is anything but trivial. Writing in the *New Scientist* in August 2004, science writer Amitabh Avasthi reported that annually from one to five million tonnes of bushmeat is consumed in the Congo Basin alone. The higher figure almost exactly matches a study published in the journal *Conservation Biology* by John Fa, who is director of Conservation Science at the Durrell Wildlife Conservation Trust in Jersey, and his co-author Carlos Peres, who is a tropical ecologist at the University of East Anglia in England. Fa and Peres calculated an annual consumption figure of 4.9 million tonnes for the same area. They collated data on fourteen hunting profiles from Cameroon, east and south throughout the Congo Basin, and estimated that 579 million animals are consumed every year. Fa and Peres are certain that this number is an underestimate because it does not deal with local consumption in households. Wildlife expert Douglas Williamson of the United Nations Food and Agriculture Organization, and his colleagues, in a summary of the trade as it affects forest conservation, relayed an even more specific figure. In Ivory Coast alone, 120,000 tonnes of wild meat were harvested by over a million hunters in 1996.

Any way you cut it, these numbers are huge, but what they tell us, because of the ranges quoted by some authors, is that nobody knows the true size of the trade.

In terms of weight, the duikers, small forest antelopes that lead mostly solitary lives, make up about 75 per cent of the catch. Other favourites are cane rats and any primate. Almost all of the scientists studying the subject agree that the harvest is unsustainable. We already know what is happening to the animal populations. What will happen to the people who have relied upon the animals in the forest for their protein through the centuries? What happens when the meat runs out?

It is not just the scientists who are reporting on the crisis. In October 2001 Ghanaian journalist Vivian Baah wrote a series of articles under the title *Guess What's Cooking for Dinner?* in the *Evening News* of Accra in which she not only stated her love of bushmeat, particu-

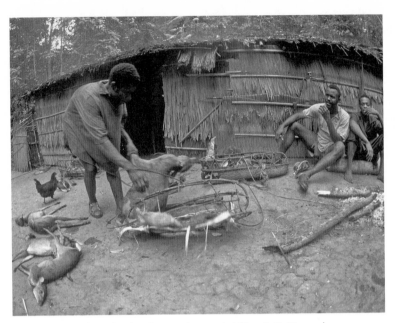

Several species of duiker ready to be taken to market or cooked. (Photo by Karl Ammann)

larly grasscutter, but also described in detail how, for her article, she joined a group of hunters who were finding it increasingly difficult to obtain meat for market and who were resorting to the burning of forests in order to improve their success rates. Ms. Baah speculated that the long-term effects of all these activities and the likely effects on the plants used in traditional medicine and the environment in general could not be anything but decline and disappearance.

There are other factors that govern which species may, or may not, end up as bushmeat. Some are, or have been, taboo: witness the tortoise I was told about by James Ako when I worked in Cameroon. In Zambia hippo and zebra were long considered taboo, but that is no longer cast in stone. Vivian Baah, in that same article, relates how in parts of Ghana "among the Ekona clan of the Ashanti's, it is a taboo to kill the Ekuo [buffalo]. But these days, the members of this clan themselves are the worst offenders. Having turned their backs on the taboo, they now butcher the Ekuo with cheeky ease."

I have chatted with Ian Parker about the subject of what may or may not be eaten by members of various Kenya tribes. He told me that "in

Kenya's Kitui District the North African Crested Porcupine was once off-limits. Not any more."

The hunting of primates was once largely confined to West and central Africa, but that, too, is changing. The subject of taboo and totem alone, relative to the bushmeat trade, would make a fascinating, if grim, study.

Other factors effecting wildlife populations in Africa and the need for people to eat, which cannot be ignored, are the massive growth in human populations and the increased ability of people to move freely about the continent.

There is little doubt that the huge increase in human population has been the underlying cause for the increased demand for bushmeat. Several authors have pointed out that the rapid rate of human population growth has its roots in improved medical services, which have led to a decline in infant mortality and an overall improved survival rate. Contraception is actively discouraged by the Roman Catholic Church, and in some areas veterinary and livestock services have led to an increase in the numbers of cattle, sheep and goats to levels at which the land cannot sustain the numbers.

In the rain forests, there is no doubt that the ability of increasing numbers of hunters to get to their quarry has been enormously enhanced by the development of the network of access roads built by logging companies. The straight lines that mark the logging concessions transect vast tracts and can readily be seen from the air. I return to the effect of this activity in the next chapter, particularly how it affects primates.

It is not just the logging industry that is having an effect on access to animals, however. Justin Brashares of the University of Califronia, Berkley, and his colleagues have reported on almost thirty years of data about the relationship between fishing and bushmeat hunting in Ghana. The study was intense and detailed, the team having conducted seven hundred wildlife counts per year in six nature reserves. During the period 1970-98 the biomass of forty-one large mammal species declined by 76 per cent, and of these species 16 to 45 per cent were locally extirpated.

With a slightly later start, in 1977, fish trawl surveys began off the West African coast and the numbers also showed a marked decline, by at least 50 per cent in the same period. Brashares and his colleagues show clearly that declines in fish catch are closely correlated with increased hunting in nature reserves and declines in numbers of those forty-one species. The human population in the region has of course grown, in this case three-fold, and as people need protein to survive, when fish numbers drop, the hunters turn to the only other obvious source. While this makes eminent sense in a nation where fish make up an important part of the diet, there is a sinister side to it that points the finger at the European Union and its subsidy programs. The authors state: "Declines of fish stocks in nearshore and offshore waters of West Africa have coincided with more than a 10-fold increases in regional fish harvests by foreign and domestic fleets since 1950." They go on to write that "EU financial support of its foreign fleet increased from about $6 million in 1981 to more than $350 million in 2001."

With few exceptions the techniques used by hunters to capture their quarry involve guns, nets, pit traps, poisons and cable snares. Of these, snares may be the most effective and are certainly cheaper and easier to use than guns. Snare densities as high as thirteen per square kilometre have been reported, and they are indiscriminate, being effective against some birds and reptiles and virtually all mammals, except hippo and elephant. Even if they are not captured, hippos and elephants often suffer severe and ultimately fatal damage due to snares, something I witnessed in Rwanda in 1975 and wrote about in *Wrestling With Rhinos*. In this case we saw 37 per cent of elephants in the country with partially or totally severed trunks. The most dramatic of these was an adult cow that had had her trunk almost complete cut through by a snare within thirty centimetres of its base, just below her eyes. There was a gaping hole in the front of it, and it hung down, completely flaccid, like a two-metre lump of grey sausage.

One exception to above methods is a highly effective hunting technique used in the Taita–Taveta region of Kenya, just inland from the coast. Dubbed "panic and slash" by Ian Parker it involves the use of torches, klaxons and whistles to totally disorient herds of animals at night during dark phases of the moon. The animals do not flee but simply freeze. The men then use razor-sharp grass-cutting slashers across the Achilles tendons of the victims. Two men can immobilize

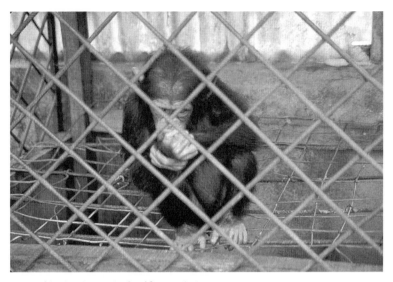

A young chimp in a tiny cage in a hotel forecourt in Cameroon.

at least eighty animals in a single night and then return at leisure to dispatch them. The best thing about this technique, from the point of view of the hunters, is that the random and chance elements of snares are redundant.

Four of the hotels I stopped at in Cameroon during my time there in 1996 showed another horrifying side of the bushmeat story. The most dramatic example of this was at a lunchtime stop on the way south from Nguti toward the coast. In a hotel forecourt there were two wooden cages, no more than a cubic metre each in size. Each had a wire mesh front and floor, and inside the one nearest the hotel gate was a mangy-looking white-nosed monkey, no more than three kilograms in weight, its hair all patchy where it had been pulling at itself in frustration. The neighbouring cage held a skinny juvenile chimpanzee, sitting with arms folded, staring into nothing.

I saw two more chimps with that same vacant look at another hotel I stopped at. One of the apes also looked hopeless, the other was screaming defiance at a human family group who were standing a metre or so back, the little boy laughing nervously as he clung to his mother's skirt. It is chilling to think that these monkeys and apes were a by-product of the bushmeat trade. A chimp infant becomes available only if the entire family, which may comprise several individuals, has been killed. Chimps are much too aggressive for it to be any other way. If a hunter were foolish enough to try to capture an infant ape without killing the entire group he would be torn limb from limb.

Karl Ammann is a noted wildlife photographer who devotes his life to stopping the slaughter of protected species for bushmeat. On his website he bemoans the fact that what sells to documentary makers and other media, and what has supposedly persuaded people to want to preserve wildlife is its "beauty and diversity." In an e-mail of May 2007 he told me how he had just completed an interview with *Associated Press* in which he stated that forest elephants in central Africa are now hunted for meat, and that their ivory is just a by-product. He wondered if any of the AP outlets would pick it up.

One paragraph on his website is a biting condemnation of some aspects of how getting the situation out to the viewing public is such a problem.

> *While the print media and its editors were generally more open minded, the world's documentary outlets were mostly interested in success stories, happy endings and heroes. Packaging the three was pretty much an outright sale. Destruction, finger pointing, eco criminals, conservation failure was and is not considered to be 'entertainment' plus it brings into the picture the real editors: the network lawyers which have no problem with the happy ending and success stories.*

Ammann has concluded that we need to go beyond the "feel good" and "happy-ending" approach and tell the real story behind complacency, and he has taken up his camera and used it as a cudgel to shock and horrify with images of bushmeat items, particularly primates, and especially gorilla and chimp, for sale in markets.

Ammann's are not the first photos of hunted gorillas. Forty years ago, in his 1963 autobiography, Armand Denis published several remarkable photographs of gorillas that had been hunted by large gangs of Ituri hunters deep in the forests of the Congo Basin when he accompanied them on a well-orchestrated hunt. Denis and his wife, Michaela, were among the very first to recognize the potential of television for showing natural history stories. They were forerunners of today's David Suzuki and David Attenborough, but their photos did not have any major impact on conservation in the 1960s, which was well before the bushmeat issue became so widely studied and written about.

Of course bushmeat does not just involve apes. The roadside stall in Cameroon showed this clearly. A more upmarket version of such a stall could once be seen in some British butcher's shops in the winter months. Outside a butcher's shop in a covered market in England's Oxford I have seen pheasants hung by the neck in pairs, rows of European brown hares and the gutted, but not skinned, carcasses of deer on show for potential customers.

It is also important to realize that the eating of primates, including chimps and gorillas, is not a continent-wide activity, and it is certainly nothing new. However, it is equally important to realize that among some of those who do eat ape and monkey meat, it has become a delicacy, and that new converts to this "cuisine" occur because of the fad. Bushmeat, especially that of primates, is more expensive than beef in some markets, but still preferred when available. It may be a supply and demand situation.

Not everyone eats primates. Indeed, many are opposed to the idea, including most Kenyan and Ugandan peoples. The differences in opinion are no doubt similar to those held about other species in other countries. An Englishman or American would be horrified to think that humans eat dogs, but in China and parts of Nigeria no such restriction applies. The French consider horsemeat a delicacy, but ask the average Englishman about this and you may get a look of disgust, at the very least.

Another element of cultural, and hence dietary changes, relative to bushmeat is occurring near Fort Portal in Uganda, only a short distance from Kibale National Park, which holds thirteen primate species in its 776 square kilometres. Refugees from the carnage of many years of war in the Congo, now the Democratic Republic of the Congo (DRC), have not unreasonably drifted eastward. Many have settled in the area, and of course formed relationships with locals. Children have been born. The spouses and offspring have been introduced to the completely new (to them) practice of monkey eating. Senior scientists at the park will admit, privately, that there are an increasing number of hunters taking bushmeat, especially monkeys and apes, out of the park. It is a real worry for them.

Of course, the bushmeat culture has not remained confined to West and central Africa, as I have discussed with Ian Parker over tea and cake in his Langata home on several occasions.

"Kenya's Kikuyu are poaching on a wide scale throughout the Aberdare Mountains for their own benefit," he told me. "They are overcoming their traditional aversion to the eating of game meat and will now eat antelope and elephant quite readily."

"And what about primates?" I asked. "As I recall they have never eaten them. They have a strong aversion to the idea."

"An interesting thing has happened there," he replied. "Successful Africans, most of them of the Kikuyu tribe, now own farms in upper Kiambu, where their tea estates lie along the fringes of the Aberdare Forest. As these folks want their children to be well educated, the youngsters are not available in the labour pool, so they hire migrant workers as tea pickers. Most come from Uganda and even further west, bringing with them their hunting culture, taking time off to hunt anything for food, including primates. There has been a marked decline in the populations of Syke's monkey in the southern Aberdares, and most people put this down to hunting activities."

Beyond the food element there are other long-held beliefs about some wild animals. While people used bushmeat to survive for thousands of years, not all of it ends up on the table. Some species, or their specific parts, have played, or still play, an important role in cultural activities, and for medicinal purposes. Ostrich plumes and lion manes decorate ceremonial dress in several cultures. The Acholi of Uganda use the hides of kob for their dance costumes. An unstated element that runs throughout Joy Adamson's book, *The Peoples Of Kenya*, is the use of wildlife parts in traditional costumes. Hardly a photo or painting of a warrior or witch doctor in traditional dress lacks some hide or feather, particularly those of leopards or ostrich.

Evolutionary biologist Francesco Angelici and his colleagues, based in Rome, studied the use of mammals in the rain forests of southeastern Nigeria. Twelve of the thirty-seven species he listed were used in some way for religious purposes, for native medicine or in sexual rituals.

For example, hyaena parts are widely used in many countries for medicinal purposes. This practice has a long tradition. An English translation of the writings of Pliny the Elder, who lived almost two thousand years ago, devotes five pages to the pharmacological properties of the hyaena. These range from alleged aphrodisiac properties of the genitals taken in honey to the use of the gall for cure of ophthalmia. Uganda veterinarian, Margaret Driciru's recent survey in and around Uganda's Murchison Falls National Park revealed that over 6 per cent of the people reported using a hyaena's nose to help blind people. The nose is even called "blind man's eye" because when dried, ground and sniffed, or given to a blind man as a whole piece, it is believed that it will "lead him to any destination he wants to go, and would make him recognize people coming ahead of him by smell and without seeing them."

Hyaena liver is widely considered to be poisonous when fed to an intended victim. So much so that the chief warden of one of Uganda's parks was recently offered a large cash inducement to allow a hyaena to be killed so that the liver could be extracted. I was told of a horrific example of hyaena use in 2005. It involved a live hyaena that had been trapped and released after its nose and foot pads had been sliced off for medicinal purposes.

Osei Adow, a political scientist from Ghana, writing about bushmeat use in her country in 2002, catalogued several species and their parts that play a role in traditional medicine. She stated "the meat of the elephant is combined with other items as cure against undue flirting. The faeces is used for various medicines. The vein of the buffalo is also used to treat mental disorders, while the skin is used to check witchcraft." The skins of various animals are obviously an important element in traditional medicine, as she mentions the skin of leopard (used with other ingredients to defeat opponents in wrestling matches), chimpanzee (as a talisman against miscarriage), waterbuck and giant rat (the former for treatment of smallpox, the latter as part of a mixture for use as an antibiotic bath for children). Bones also play a role. Porcupine spine bone is used to prevent premature death in children while "the bone of the bush buck is ground and mixed with other ingredients to prepare concoction for children to develop strong bones. Pregnant women also depend on the concoction to enhance foetus bone formation." The use of these bone remedies has an interesting parallel in the way that Westerners use calcium tablets.

Adow also mentions python teeth and liver and the liver, intestines, feathers and skin of the guinea fowl, which are mixed with alligator pepper—a tropical perennial used as a medicinal plant—to cure dizziness. Finally, "the skull of the green monkey is used for the cure of stomach problems in children. The tail of the flying squirrel when mixed with other ingredients is used to avert abortion."

David Kahwa is a fisheries specialist at Makerere University in Uganda. He is a member of the Banyoro people of Uganda, a small group whose ancestral lands lie near the town of Masindi. As we chatted about traditional beliefs and enjoyed an evening drink around the campfire together in 2007, he told me of an ancient belief among his people.

"There is a ground-nesting wasp—I don't know the species—which has the ability to always find its nest. It has very accurate homing instincts. If you can kill it with your bare foot, which is a bit risky, and then feed it to your hunting dog you will ensure his skill and create a *muhigi takanda* which means a hunter who does not get tired." He concluded, "Of course, our hunting traditions are gone, and I don't suppose any of the young people even know about this matter."

With the decline in wild sources of bushmeat there has been an interest in the possibilities of domesticating some species and so supply the market. In a 2006 article on the BBC website, Oria Ryan describes how some farmers have taken advantage of the lust for bushmeat, especially cane rat, by turning to their production as farm animals, an activity that has been going on for many years but may be growing as the demand continues and the supply from the wild continues to dwindle. Cane rats breed at the age of one year and can produce from two to six young twice a year. They can attain a weight of as much as seven or eight kilograms and mature quickly. This has some potential to make them profitable for the small holder supplying a popular niche market. French veterinarian Phillipe Chardonnet, who has worked with international development and wildlife for over twenty years, and his co-authors have summarized the value of wildlife worldwide and concluded that cane rats and guinea fowl both have good potential in Africa for rural farmers.

However, a detailed analysis conducted in 2005 by wcs scientist Miranda Motkin and her colleagues of the potential for wildlife farming in tropical forests raises a number of serious concerns. The authors pointed out that cane rats are not easy to raise and are subject to stresses that reduce their productivity when they are held in captivity. One stark conclusion they give is that "until wildlife numbers in the wild become so low that it is no longer worthwhile hunting them, wildlife farming is unlikely to reduce hunting, due to high costs of farming compared to hunting, lack of appropriate technical skills and funds, and cultural constraints."

THERE ARE SMALL GLIMMERS OF HOPE that people are waking up to the problem of the bushmeat trade. Vivian Baah's article won her the Biodiversity Reporting Award, hosted by Conservation International for print media, and a nine-minute documentary film, *Say No to Bushmeat*, made as a result of its publication was selected as a finalist at the 2003 Jackson Hole Wildlife Film Festival in the USA. Chosen from a field of 550 international entries, the film was nominated in the Best Non-Broadcast category at the festival.

In the same press release that announced the nomination of the film came a telling quote: "Since the release of the video and the awareness campaign we launched in Ghana in August 2002, the bushmeat trade has been reduced considerably," said Okyeame Ampadu-Agei, executive director of Conservation International (CI) Ghana. "The campaign has helped dramatically change people's attitudes about bushmeat consumption. Of the 300 restaurants in Accra that were selling bushmeat before the campaign, 92 percent no longer participate in the trade."

I wonder how many had to go out of business.

On his website Karl Ammannn ends on a slightly optimistic note. He comments that interviews with the iconic National Geographic Society and a YAHOO news video illustrates that his efforts "are getting through on some level."

It would be nice to think that actions of the kind Ammann and Baah are talking about could take hold in other parts of Africa, and indeed worldwide, but burgeoning populations, added to the very long-standing cultural role of bushmeat, will make it an uphill struggle. Alternatives to bushmeat are hard to imagine, as cattle, sheep and goats are difficult to keep in most of the forested areas across the continent, and the masses of people need to eat. ✻

13

A ONE-WOMAN CRUSADE

Jo and I pay a visit to a chimp sanctuary and meet a human dynamo. A tug at the heart-strings for us both. The bushmeat issue and the political posturing around it are part of our discussions.

OL PEJETA CONSERVANCY, which lies to the west of the town of Nanyuki, is one of the largest ranches on the Laikipia Plains that stretch for many kilometres to the west of Mount Kenya. When we lived and worked in Nanyuki, it was a cattle ranch, but it was also home to large herds of zebra and several species of cloven-hoofed mammals like giraffe, impala and buffalo. It was owned by a succession of wealthy individuals, first Court Parfet who sold it to the arms dealer Adnan Khashoggi. The ranch now incorporates the neighbouring property of Sweetwaters, formerly owned by my tennis partner Seager Bastard, then passed on to Lonrho's Tiny Rowland. The scuttlebutt around Nanyuki was that he had acquired the land from Khashoggi in settlement of a gambling debt. The latest change in ownership of the ranch came in mid-September 2004, when an American philanthropist who likes to keep a very low profile, and does not wish to be named, acting through Fauna and Flora International, took over and dedicated himself to continuing and expanding the conservation component of the joint ranches.

Within Ol Pejeta is the Sweetwaters Chimpanzee Sanctuary, a small series of pens surrounded by many strands of high-voltage electric fence that stretch up over three metres. Inside the pens is an unlikely collection of orphan chimpanzees that have been brought here from many parts of Africa. The site is just one of over a dozen across the continent at which confiscated orphan primates end up. They stretch from The Gambia in the west to Johannesburg in the south and include Ngamba Island in Lake Victoria (see pages 407-08). All of these orphanages are members of PASA, the Pan African Sanctuary Alliance, and are dedicated to the keeping of animals that have been rescued from a variety of unsavoury situations just like the grim hotel cages that I saw in Cameroon, or worse.

Ann (Annie) Olivecrona is a larger-than-life Swedish extrovert who spent nine years of her life at Ol Pejeta managing the chimp sanctuary and dedicating herself to the cause of conservation, particularly the conservation of Africa's tropical forests, which would of course protect the primates that live in them. She poured heart and soul into her work. When Jo and I first met her in her small bungalow in late 2004, she was caring for thirty-four rescued chimps of various ages. More animals were arriving with alarming frequency.

In late January 2005 six infant chimps, aged between about seven months and two years, were seized at Nairobi's Jomo Kenyatta airport. They had been loaded as part of the luggage of a woman reputed to carry both Egyptian and Nigerian passports. The luggage was routed from Lagos to Cairo, via Khartoum, and because the contents of her luggage were obviously not the dogs that the paperwork stated, the baggage had ended up in Kenya on their way back to Nigeria. An alert baggage handler had noted that the sounds emanating from the small crate in a corner of the warehouse did not sound like the dogs listed on the manifest, and he had seen a tiny black finger poking up between the slats. After some considerable discussion with officials of the Kenya Wildlife Service, five of the animals had been shipped to Ol Pejeta. The sixth had died while with the KWS officials, probably from pneumonia, no doubt exacerbated by dehydration or malnutrition, or both, as they had all been cooped up in tiny compartments without food or water for goodness knows how long, certainly for three days over a weekend at Nairobi. It is perhaps a wonder that the five survived. If Annie is right, the woman who was attempting to transport the chimps is the same one who drowned two ape infants, a chimp and a gorilla, in acid when she could not get them through the system and into the marketplace, no doubt to be kept as pets.

The "owner" of the chimps had long since departed for Nigeria when Annie received them at the orphanage, although she later had the gall to demand the return of "her" chimps. Ongoing investigations that involve Interpol and other police agencies may bring the culprit to book. The findings of their investigations may even inculpate a high-profile medical specialist in Cairo, who is alleged to have been involved as the intended importer. Unfortunately, bigger fish may have escaped the net, and one has to ask what proportion of the overall smuggling effort of chimps does this one investigation actually involve? Probably a minute one, if the statistics on the illegal animal trade are anything to go by.

There seems to be some debate about which illegal trade worldwide generates the most income, but the top four are drugs, arms, people smuggling (including women as sex workers) and animals. All are worth billions of dollars a year, and the animal trade involves the death of a vast proportion of its victims even while in transit.

One problem that Annie identifies with the investigation specific to the chimp case is that the officials at CITES (The Convention on International Trade in Endangered Species) had, when we met in 2005, so far chosen not to do anything about the chimps involved in the case. She and Ian Parker are both pretty skeptical about CITES. Parker considers them to have become a top-heavy bureaucracy that is held up by its own inertia; he describes it as "an orgy of silliness" in a chapter titled "CITES—The Unworkable Treaty" in his book *What I Tell You Three Times Is True.*

On our return to Sweetwaters in March 2005 it was impossible not to feel an immediate tug at the heart-strings when we saw the five pairs of doleful eyes staring out from under the table on Annie's verandah, or when one or two of the slightly bolder ones came and reached up to be cuddled. None of the chimps weighed more than about eight kilograms, although all were beginning to recover from the undernourishment that they had been subjected to during their captivity in various places. Two were attached to one another like limpets and Annie speculated that they might have been together in captivity for some time, having only one another to bond with.

As if these five chimps, all under twenty-four-hour watch from the team of helpers (nursemaids) that Annie has had to take on, were not enough, she was waiting for the arrival of more animals following confiscations in Rwanda, the DRC, Ghana and South Africa. Julia Wanjiku, the matronly Kikuyu woman whose own children have grown up and left home, does duty as cook and housemaid for Annie and doubles as expert chimp surrogate mother. She must be the only person in Kenya whose duties cover such a wide range, and she certainly has more experience in the care of infant chimps than anyone should ever need.

When we visited again a month later, one of the orphans that had graduated four months previously from the verandah of Annie's house to the main compound, rushed out and latched on to Julia as soon as she saw her. The chimp, named Saidia (Swahili for "help") was one of the youngest ever rescued, possibly as a little as a month old. She could not crawl, had severe burns on her head and back when she arrived and was so dehydrated that she looked as if she was near death. Julia spent many hours with her and brought her back to life. There can be no doubt that Saidia knew exactly who she wanted to hug. In fact, we had a hard time getting away until the little creature joined the other chimps in a game of tag in the trees, and we were able to slip into the Land Rover.

From time to time, Annie has to get some veterinary assistance, which is no surprise. She has a network of medically trained folks who are ready to help at short notice. Our old friends and colleagues Paul Sayer and Dieter Rottcher, with whom I worked in our intern days at the veterinary school in Kabete, just outside Nairobi, are two of them. Dr. Bengt Ole-Roken, from the Kolmarden Zoo in Sweden, is another. Locally, Dr. Abid Butt, the physician who currently does the

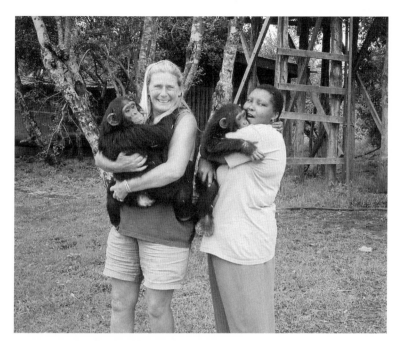

Annie and Julia at Sweetwaters with two orphan chimps.

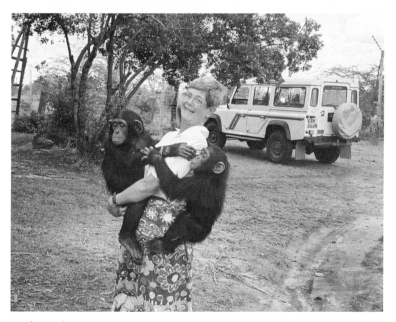

Jo and two orphans at Sweetwaters.

human work at the Cottage Hospital in Nanyuki, where Jo spent five years, also helps out with the chimps when they need medical intervention. It was he who examined the five young chimps that arrived at Sweetwaters just a few days before our return visit and removed homemade shotgun pellets from two of them. For dental problems in the chimps, Annie is able to call on Dr. Anders Glimberg, who travels up from Nairobi at his own expense to help out.

While we were with her in 2005, I was able to help her out with advice on a suitable dose of anaesthetic for one of her charges whose teeth needed to be dealt with.

The directors of the Max Planck Institute in Germany have generously donated their expertise and time to laboratory work, especially the evaluation of the DNA of these and previously acquired animals. Each population of chimps has a slightly different DNA fingerprint so that the precise origins of the chimps can be pinpointed.

One of the most important medical interventions is to control breeding in the group, and this is accomplished in all the various sanctuaries by borrowing from human medical technology and using commercial contraceptive implants that have to be replaced every now and again.

While it may seem utterly bizarre to the average reader to prevent breeding in an endangered animal, there really is no option. First, these chimps, every one of them, are emotionally scarred and will never be able to live a normal chimp life. They may develop natural-looking social groups in the enclosures where they are released after being cared for by Annie, Julia and their helpers, but they have no idea of how to forage for their normal food items, and even if they did know there are none available, so they require daily feeding by humans. Their natural habitat in the forests of the continent is being destroyed at a phenomenal rate, and there really can never be any thought of returning them to the wild.

In an ideal world, one would wish that they could indeed be returned to a forest environment. Even if a suitable unlogged forest could be found, it is highly likely that it would already be occupied by other chimps. If it were already occupied, the newly translocated group, or groups, would have no idea where the individual fruit trees might be, which would limit their access to food. A much bigger issue would be that the resident chimpanzees would simply not tolerate newcomers, and fierce fighting, with certain loss of life, would be inevitable.

As we sat on the verandah of Annie's home, looking out across Laikipia to the slopes of Mount Kenya—sometimes shrouded in cloud, but in the early morning standing stark and backlit by the rising sun—it became clear that Annie was passionate about the cause of the chimpanzee problem with which she dealt. And the problem finds its source in the bushmeat trade. ✻

14

BUSHMEAT AND BUREAUCRATS

Annie and Karl Ammann manage to get the bushmeat issue front and centre at the EU parliament, although the outcome is not exactly riveting. An important part of the bushmeat story is the potential of disease transmission, not only among wild species, but directly to humans. This transmission has had devastating consequences.

WHILE BUSHMEAT, as I have pointed out, has a long and perfectly reasonable tradition in all parts of the world, in the central and western African forests it is closely linked with the logging industry and has become a major commercial enterprise. According to research conducted by several people, including Annie and Swiss author and photographer Karl Ammann, the link is clear and unarguable. Dale Peterson's book *Eating Apes* and Anthony Rose's *Consuming Nature*, both full of photos by Karl Ammann, document the sorry tale. An ever-increasing demand for hardwood lumber from Africa's forests is met by the supply cut from the giant trees across the continent. In order to get to the trees, and to get the lumber out, roads have to be hacked out with heavy machinery. Once the roads are built, the machines can drive deep into the forest and whole communities quickly become established. The people in them need food and hunters can go in on foot, carrying the inevitable weapons, which may be anything from a homemade shotgun or rifle to the ubiquitous, and now very cheap, Kalashnikov, or a facsimile thereof. A panga acts as a butcher's knife, and as Karl's remarkable photographs show, the trucks taking out the logs can readily accommodate the partly butchered carcasses of many species, from duiker to gorilla and everything in between. In David Western's fascinating *In the Dust of Kilimanjaro*, an account of his work in Kenya's Amboseli and other areas, he quotes a colleague talking about the disappearance of large mammals in the West African country of Gabon: "Poachers are killing anything within a day's walk of settlements, roads, and rivers."

Annie tells how in May 2004 she witnessed an amazing interchange involving bushmeat at London's Heathrow airport. Her plane happened to arrive at more or less the same time as a flight from Lagos. During the time that she watched the procession, customs officials stopped every one of the Nigerian passengers and asked for the huge suitcases to be opened. Almost all were packed with smoked bushmeat. What shook her was that the customs staff simply passed the passengers on, without making any attempt to confiscate product or arrest anyone. Naturally, being afraid of no one, she approached the officials and remonstrated with them. The reply she got shook her to the core. She was told that there was not enough capacity at Heathrow to incinerate the smuggled meat, which is what should have been done, and so they were simply letting it go.

No doubt the inaction of the customs officials would have delighted the large expatriate Nigerian contingent based across Britain, to whom the gifts of bushmeat would be a most welcome reminder of home. The meat would possibly also have found its way into any homes or restaurants where there is a community of folks from central or West Africa, amongst whom the meat is so favoured. One such area is Belgium, where there were, at the time, reportedly over a hundred restaurants serving bushmeat in Brussels alone. In Britain there have been at least three convictions involving the owners of unlicensed restaurants

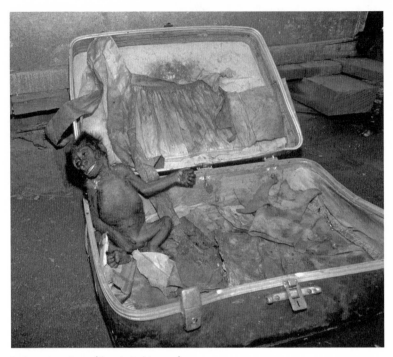

Bushmeat in a suitcase. (Photo by Karl Ammann)

where bushmeat, found to include chimp, was being served. Sadly, according to Annie, the fines were paltry.

The consumption of imported bushmeat also occurs in North America, and I found several reports on the subject when I searched on Google.

In an article dated August 20, 2007, David Pomerantz, writing for the *New York Sun*, described a court case in which an immigrant woman from Liberia has been prosecuted for smuggling monkey parts into the USA. Her defence appears to be based upon religious practices.

Pomerantz wrote she "took the stand for the first time this month, where she testified that she was baptized as a Christian, but that she eats the monkey meat at religious ceremonies like Easter 'because monkey from the wildlife is a very smart animal,' according to a court transcript. Her testimony suggests that she practices a hybridized religion that borrows both from Christian concepts and indigenous African religious beliefs...Seventeen congregants of [her] church in Staten Island, the First Christian Church at 54 Thompson St., filed an affidavit in July testifying to the importance of bushmeat for their religious beliefs."

When we met Annie in 2005, the appearance of African bushmeat in North America had not yet been documented, but it was certainly well known in Europe. The incident that Annie saw at Heathrow may have been early in the game, before British authorities began to get serious.

In a 125-page report titled *Assessment of the Solution-Orientated Research Needed to Promote a More Sustainable Bushmeat Trade in Central and West Africa* produced for Britain's Department for Environment Food and Rural Affairs in 2002, author Evan Bowen-Jones and his colleagues recognized that "much of the importation of bushmeat into the UK is commercial, organised and clandestine. While the conservation implications are often uncertain (because of the difficulty of identifying meat), CITES rules are being flouted with some regularity." In a footnote they gave a couple of startling figures: "200 seizures were made at Heathrow airport in one five-week period earlier this year, and 1.4 metric tonnes were seized from a single flight."

The annual report for 2004 states that there were almost 16,000 seizures of illegally imported meat, involving 185 tonnes, but that this may be as little as 1 per cent of the actual annual trade. If these figures really are only 1 per cent of the trade, then the numbers of animals coming out of the forests is truly mind-boggling.

All this occurred at a time when Britain was still recovering from the effects of the foot-and-mouth disease outbreak of 2001 and was dealing with the continued destruction of their beef industry due to Bovine Spongiform Encephalopathy (Mad Cow Disease) and its reported link to new variant Creutzfeldt-Jakob's Disease in humans. This brings us to another of many problematic layers in the subject of bushmeat.

There is increasing evidence of the risks of diseases of humans or their livestock being spread to wild animals and the zoonotic—diseases spread from animals to humans—part of the equation has become a major medical concern. Recent reports by Mark Woolhouse and colleagues, of the Centre for Tropical Veterinary Medicine at the University of Edinburgh, have shown that a staggering 868 (61 per cent) of the 1,415 human pathogens known are zoonotic. Many of these are seen in wild animals, as Dr. Bill Karesh and his colleagues at the New

York-based Wildlife Conservation Society have reported. Bill is the director of the Field Veterinary Program at wcs and also co-chair of the World Conservation Union's Veterinary Specialist Group.

One wonders if the customs staff Annie reproached at Heathrow, or their superiors, had ever heard of little problems like Severe Acute Respiratory Syndrome (sars), Ebola or hiv. sars spread to humans from wildlife in China, and both hiv and Ebola have been linked to the butchering and consumption of primate meat.

Simian Immunodeficiency Virus (siv), the primate version of the human virus that causes aids, has been reported in twenty-six species of ape and monkey and has many genetically different forms. Beatrice Hahn, a professor in the department of medicine at the University of Alabama, reporting in the journal *Science* in 2000, showed that chimpanzees, particularly the central subspecies, are considered to be the primary reservoir for the human aids virus, hiv-1, while hiv-2 came from the sooty mangabey, a small, almost uniformly grey monkey whose range is restricted to upper Guinea in West Africa. In humans these two viruses are genetically less closely related to one another than they are to their original primate sources. The siv counterparts of these two forms of hiv have been introduced into humans on at least seven different occasions.

Ebola, the deadly fever that kills humans and great apes so efficiently, has been found in central African primates and is easily spread to people when they handle the meat of infected animals. Infected humans develop severe internal and external hemorrhaging and up to 90 per cent of victims die. The virus also infects gorillas, chimpanzees and monkeys. As Billy Karesh and Bob Cook wrote in 2005 in the journal *Foreign Affairs*, "lowland gorillas and chimpanzees in Gabon and Congo and chimpanzees in western equatorial Africa have been decimated by the sickness. Since the disease first appeared, successive human outbreaks have been recorded in Côte d'Ivoire, Gabon, Sudan and Uganda. Each of the human outbreaks in central Africa during the late 1990s and the first years of this century was traced to humans handling infected great apes."

Jane Goodall told me about a friend of hers who has been studying gorillas in the drc and is now working on her third habituated group after the first two were wiped out by Ebola.

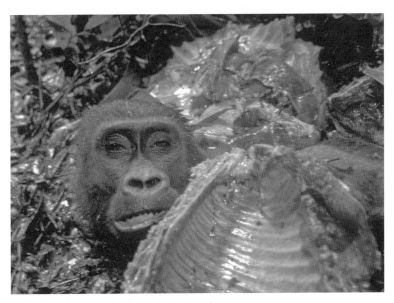

The butchers have been at work. (Photo by Karl Ammann)

It may not just be primates that are involved in the Ebola story. Suspicion has been cast on duikers, which are such an important part of the bushmeat catch. And the finding of both Ebola antibodies and portions of viral DNA were reported in December 2005 in thirteen specimens of three species of fruit bat by Eric Leroy and a big team working in Gabon and the Democratic Republic of Congo. It is not known if this was a chance finding, or if the bats are a virus reservoir, but Leroy and his colleagues speculated about the bats being carriers of the disease. Dr. Karesh told me in an e-mail that he thinks it is "highly likely that bats play a role, but to date we do not know when, how, how long or how often the virus may infect bats."

As reported on the international listserv *Promed* in August 2007, another deadly disease that has crossed the monkey to human barrier (if there is such a thing) is Marburg hemorrhagic fever, which killed a miner in Western Uganda after he consumed a colobus monkey. This was not the first case of the disease linked to monkey consumption. According to the World Health Organization (WHO), the last two recent outbreaks of Marburg hemorrhagic fever in the Democratic Republic of Congo during 1998–2000 and in Angola during 2004–2005 have claimed 128 and 323 lives, respectively. Rather than thinking of these diseases as being of monkey, ape or human origin, it is probably better to lump them all together as primate diseases.

Many viruses and bacteria can survive in carcasses for long periods, even if the meat has been smoked, and especially if it has been inadequately smoked. The classic Canadian example of this was the 1952 outbreak of foot-and-mouth disease that occurred in Saskatchewan. The outbreak was traced back to the importation of smoked sausage from Poland.

In May 2000 Karl Ammann initiated a correspondence with Koen Brouwer, the executive director of the European Association of Zoos and Aquariums (EAZA), an organization that has a direct impact upon the very segment of the public that has a real interest in wildlife. He had been trying to get the bushmeat issue, particularly as it relates to the great apes, into the consciousness of several influential groups since 1995, with little success. Karl suggested to Brouwer that a campaign aimed at the 120 million people who visit zoos annually in Europe might be effective, writing that "most of them would visit the ape exhibit, most of them could at that point be confronted with a bush meat display and a signature stand, featuring the standard petition letter addressed to the various heads of states with the signature list next to it."

In that same letter, Karl stated that the failure of his 1998 efforts, including a suggested signature campaign, with the Association of Zoos and Aquariums in the USA had been considered "too risky" (his quotes) in political terms. He further pointed out that at two major conservation meetings, one in Cameroon, the other in Gabon, the senior bureaucrats organizing the meetings had served bushmeat to the delegates (eleven species at the Cameroon gathering).

Karl also told Brouwer that he had spoken to Jane Goodall, and that she, too, felt that strong action was needed.

The campaign started, and then Annie, through her connections with several European zoos, was able to "marry," as she put it to me, EAZA with The International Fund For Animal Welfare (IFAW). Normally these two organizations would be highly unlikely allies, as they have very different views on animal issues.

Teamed up, the two organizations presented a proposal at the European parliament in November 2001 that was accepted, albeit in Annie's words a "washed out" version, in January 2004. The petition had been signed by a seriously heavyweight 1.9 million people, and had asked the politicians to ban hardwood lumbering. They showed a hard-hitting and brief—90 seconds—videotape about the logging-bushmeat link that would surely shock all but the dedicated logger who has no concern for wildlife.

Annie recounts, with a mixture of bottled rage and bitterness, how the video was sabotaged five times as the presenters tried to make their point. She saw the technician unplug the sound, and when she fixed that problem, he switched the machines from the PAL system of Europe and Africa to the VHS of North America so that the machines would not recognize the format. The chairman of the European Logging Association at the time was a Frenchman, and there were other very powerful German and French interests involved who wanted to make sure that their multimillion-dollar interests were not interfered with.

One more sabotage attempt was made with Karl's photographs that appeared in *Consuming Nature*. These had been on display at several European zoos and were to augment the presentation, but were, as Annie puts it, "suddenly were too horrible for the power [Annie's term] to see although all ordinary people had seen them for a year!" During the presentation, the photos were supposed to hang on screens that were mysteriously not delivered. In the end, Annie was delighted that every single one of the British Conservative members of the European Parliament supported the attempts, but she was sadly disappointed that not one of the British Labour members, or the seventy-six Swedish members backed up the petition.

Annie was also frustrated with the lack of action from major conservation bodies and her cynicism reached its apex when she stated that with Cameroon logged out, and the beginnings of similar destruction in Congo Brazzaville, the only thing keeping the loggers out of the Democratic Republic of Congo was the ongoing war. Although she recognized the horrors of the war, she also reckoned that it was saving the forests, and with them, the animals in them.

Grim though it sounded, Annie was not alone in this view, although the subject took a disturbing new twist in May 2007 with a news report about Virunga National Park. The rebel Mai Mai militia fighters attacked rangers in the park, killing one of them, and threatened to kill all the park's gorillas if the authorities came after them. By September the rebels had moved in and killed five members of one gorilla family, leaving the bodies where they lay.

Annie told us that she was planning, with help from others, to continue to bring pressure on the EU but that it was an uphill battle. The recent news that the Norwegian government was considering a ban on the importation of any African hardwood, and had moreover banned the use of any such wood in any new government building, cheered Annie considerably. As she put it, "Although Norway may not be a large importer of hardwoods, perhaps their approach may act as a beacon for others."

Annie and Julia left Sweetwaters in 2005, but they are still based in Nanyuki and Annie is trying to start up another sanctuary. Her efforts, and those of her colleagues, may not have been in vain. A postnote from the British Parliamentary Office of Science and Technology of February 2005 shows that the bushmeat subject has been taken seriously. The UK government has examined financial implications, as well as disease issues, including disease risks for UK agriculture and for transmission of zoonotic diseases. However, they admit to only £25 million in 2004 of funding for new initiatives on control, which included publicity and the training of ten meat-sniffer dogs for Heathrow Airport. This sum compares to ten times as much for the same task budgeted by the Australians.

The postnote authors use the term "bushmeat crisis" and have listed five components that are involved in its existence. They are:

- Uncontrolled development and population growth,
- Habitat loss and increased access to previously inaccessible areas (often a result of road construction for resource extraction such as logging or mining),
- Improvements in hunting technology (such as guns and wire snares),

- A lack of rural economic or nutritional alternatives; and
- A growing wealthy urban elite with a preference for bush-meat.

The British postnote also has a carefully worded paragraph that acknowledges how difficult control of the trade will be:

Weak governance is a problem in many of the countries where bushmeat is hunted. Where wildlife legislation does exist, the resources and political will to enforce it often do not. In corrupt administrations, officials can benefit from the trade in bushmeat through bribes. For those countries in a state of current, recent, or recurrent war, the conservation of wildlife is a very low priority. A sustainable bushmeat trade is theoretically possible given effective regulation to limit demand and protect vulnerable species. This will require multilateral political will, and some argue, political pressure or incentives.

In 2004, two years and two months after Annie's "married" EAZA-IFAW team made their presentation to them, the European Parliament also unanimously adopted a resolution on the subject, but it took almost four years to reach what is called a "Provisional Edition" of the text. Called in wordy fashion "European Parliament resolution on Petition 461/2000 concerning the protection and conservation of Great Apes and other species endangered by the illegal trade in bushmeat (2003/2078(INI))," the resolution covers the subject in recondite detail that could only have come from politicians and bureaucrats doing their thing to the 'nth' degree. It has ten "Having regards to" clauses, fifteen appearances of "Whereas," and twenty-one "Urges" and the like, a few with sub-clauses.

Three of the ones under the "Urges" category make interesting reading as they deal with the logging question. Numbers 11–13 read as follows:

11. *Urges the Commission to develop, together with the timber industry and the developing countries concerned, ways and means to control bushmeat hunting on concessions, e.g. by developing models for management standards, procedures and activities, criteria and indicators, to be financed by*

the timber companies themselves, as an integral part of their activities, and find ways and means of making these models mandatory;

12. *Urges the Commission to give special attention in this Strategy to the timber companies which allow, promote and facilitate the use of bushmeat, and to propose legislation to ban the import of products of companies which act illegally and aggravate the bushmeat problem by allowing their workers to hunt for bushmeat or use their transport facilities to transport poached bushmeat;*

13. *Urges the Commission to include bushmeat issues, criteria and indicators in the European FLEGT (Forest Law Enforcement, Governance and Trade) process to ensure that timber governance and certification systems support the regulation of bushmeat hunting and trapping in timber concessions; this will include taking account of the CITES Convention and the recommendations made by the NGO Forests and the European Union Resource Network (FERN) in its report of December 2002: 'Controlling imports of illegal timber, Options for Europe.'*

Maybe the "marriage" of IFAW and EAZA and the 1.9 million signatures did some good in terms of primate conservation and bushmeat in general, but in the EU pages there is nothing that offers any form of penalty for those who choose not to be "urged."

Another toothless resolution? Annie thinks so. She wrote to me that the EU is only saying it will "look into" the problem but that it has effectively done nothing and European companies today are logging more than ever in Africa.

Not mentioned in this resolution are other industries that have an impact on wildlife in the forests of central Africa. A local effect on wildlife in the east-central DRC has been created by the massive worldwide upsurge in the use of the electronic equipment, such as cell phones, DVD players and computers, over the last decade. In all such products a mineral called tantalum is used, and tantalum is extracted from coltan (columbite-tantalite). Eighty per cent of the world's known reserves of this ore are found in the DRC. Dr. Kerry Bowman, who is president and founder of the Canadian Ape Alliance based in Toronto, has been working in the Kahuzi-Biega National park in the DRC and has seen the truly terrible effects of the mining of coltan on the wildlife, during the height of the war. It sounded like a grim recall of Conrad's *Heart of Darkness* when Kerry told me that men, basically slaves, were being forced to mine at gunpoint and that the income from the mined coltan was being used to buy more weapons. Inevitably there was an increase in human encroachment into the forests, and the humans needed to eat. In this region of Africa the demand for coltan may have been a more important part of the bushmeat story than logging, but now that the war has simmered down, the full story is difficult to unravel.

THERE ARE OTHER COMPONENTS TO THE BUSHMEAT TRADE that have nothing to do with primates. In Kenya it has grown to a huge commercial activity that involves gangs of armed poachers, specially equipped refrigerator lorries or vans, and the shooting of anything that moves, often inside national parks. In Tsavo East National Park one lodge owner told us how he had counted one hundred giraffe snares in a single day, and as I described in Chapter Nine, Meru National Park, our favourite for many reasons, took a terrible hit in the late 1990s, losing virtually all specimens of some species in a two-year period. Mark Jenkins, chief warden in the park said to me in 2005, "The bushmeat trade is now vast."

Just before Christmas 2004, we learned of another example of what can be classed as bushmeat, although it involves fish. At Watamu, Kenya, a little coastal village with an amazing white sand beach, a local (white) resident told us how he had pulled up a net that was inside the reef that marks the boundary to the National Marine Park. As it was tangled in the coral he had to cut it in a few spots. The local ranger of the Kenya Wildlife Service would not act on the resident's complaint, and before long the resident was being advised by the local chief of police to pay reparations to the owner for not only the damage to the net, but "for loss of income." This, inside a national park where no fishing is allowed!

While this chapter, indeed this book, is about African wildlife, no one should forget the old saying about people in glass houses not throwing stones. Wealthy westerners and easterners have plundered the world's oceans and reduced many fish stocks to the point at which they can no longer be commercially harvested. The Japanese have recently stated that they will ignore the International Whaling Commission's votes and carry on killing whales. Millions of deer and birds are killed every year the world over. In an area like the rain-forest belt of central Africa, where tsetse fly or lack of suitable grazing entirely prevents the keeping of cattle, bushmeat may be the only source of protein.

The bushmeat issue (whether in Africa, Amazonia or anywhere else) is not going to go away because we want it to. The boatloads of Africans who flee the continent (and sometimes drown in the effort) are not taking the risks for the fun of it. Some of them are undoubtedly leaving to escape the wars that seem to wax and wane but never really cease, but a main reason for flight is the sheer driving force of hunger. Like the refugees stuck in limbo near the port of Calais and desperately trying to hitch an illicit ride on a truck heading across the channel to England, they are all trying to find a better life.

What is needed is a very strong political will from heads of government. They need not simply stop the hunting by making it illegal, which would of course fail completely, but they must find ways to cut off the supply chain from the sources to the mass markets, so that the hunters who are simply carrying on the activities of their ancestors can continue to feed their families. This will not happen unless alternative sources of food, particularly protein sources, can be found.

It will be a daunting task. Maybe it is impossible, at least until the numbers of animals decline so far that hunters' efforts are not rewarded.

As Armand Denis wrote in *On Safari* in 1963: "To the protein-starved forest dwellers, hunting is a necessity." ✳

1997

THE TROUBLE WITH LIONS

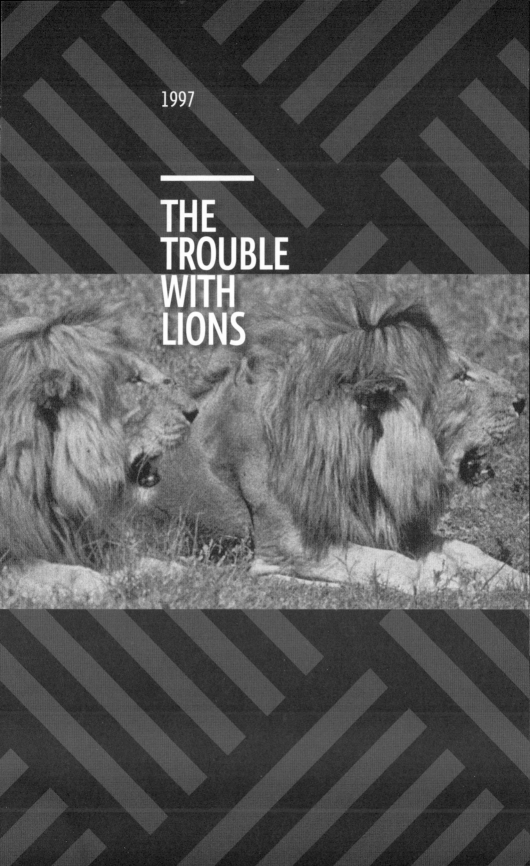

We must have sufficient humility
to approach local communities and
find out their needs and aspirations
before we start work. At all costs,
we must avoid planning upon
people, telling them what to do
without any form of consultation
whatever.

—JOHN HANKS, IN RAYMOND BONNER'S
At the Hand of Man

We can't run a ranch and a zoo.

—CHIEF LENGURO OF THE SAMBURU,
IN CHARLES CHEVENIX TRENCH'S
The Desert's Dusty Face

15

WHITE
WHITE
RHINO

Jo and I arrive in South Africa at the start of a sabbatical leave and land the luckiest chance imaginable as I am able to revisit old work and be involved in research on White rhino, the first species I worked with in a national park in Kenya almost thirty years previously.

"RIGHT! THAT'LL DO THE TRICK," SAID MARKUS.

The hot sun was already heading toward its noon position as we stood in South Africa's Borakalalo Park. It would soon dry the white-wash as it spread over the sleeping White rhino.

I had to agree with Markus. A grey rhino decorated with a large white splash, roughly the shape of Asia, all over its back, was not going to be difficult to identify from the air.

Markus and I walked with our gear to the two Land Cruisers parked about thirty metres away under the shade of a tree. We were just ahead of the rest of the team, five Africans whose names I had not yet learned, and wardens Ray Schaller and Rusty Hustler, who both about five-foot

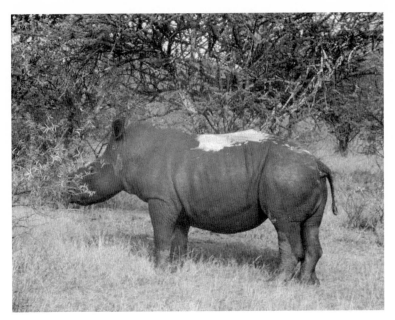
Up and ready to go. An immature rhino and his whitewash marker.

nine: Ray stocky and dark-haired, Rusty presumably nicknamed for his now thinning crop of light red hair. About an inch taller than me, at six-foot one, Markus's angular, shoulder-wide, slim-waisted figure, dressed like everyone else in more or less standard khaki shirt and shorts, showed the effects of a fit outdoor life. He flipped down the tailgate of the vehicle, leaned over and pulled the black plastic box, which looked just like a fishing tackle kit, toward him. Taking out a syringe and needle from the top tray, he reached in and removed a small bottle of antidote.

Markus returned alone to the sleeping rhino, injected some of the drug into his rump and then moved forward to his head, where he injected the rest into an ear vein. He turned and walked quickly back to the truck, stopping behind it as we all watched silently.

After about ninety seconds, the rhino's ears twitched once. Five seconds later they moved again, and then we saw the nearside eye open. It was if a light switch had been flipped. The animal lumbered to his feet and staggered around for fifteen metres like a Friday-night drunk before gradually regaining his balance. He looked back once and then moved smartly off into the bush, more or less disappearing within a hundred metres.

"He looks fine. Let's go back to camp for some lunch," said Markus, as he headed for the small helicopter parked fifty metres back from where our patient had lately been doing his induced Sleeping Giant act.

We were somewhere, I had no real idea precisely where, in the Borakalalo Game Reserve, which is only about 140 kilometres square and is administered by the North West Parks Board in South Africa. It lies about a ninety-minute drive northwest of the capital city, Pretoria. Like several other parks in South Africa, it has been developed from land that was once given over to agriculture and is completely surrounded by a game-proof fence. Bordered on every side by agricultural land, from a conservation standpoint, the park is an island. There are several standards of such fence in the country, the most complete of which will hold elephants, the major predators and just about anything else. In this case the fence was only good enough to hold antelopes, including gemsbok, the attractive curve-horned sable, giraffes and of course the White rhino we were working on. The park's game-viewing road network is about sixty kilometres in total, and like many of its counterparts it has a long list of recorded bird species; over 350. Another popular feature of the park is the fish-filled Klipvoor Dam, almost eight hundred hectares in surface area.

My being in the park on that particular day had all started with a telephone call.

"Hello, is that Markus?

"Ja, speaking."

Even with only those words, and the distinctive Afrikaans accent, there had been no doubt that it was our friend Markus Hofmeyr, who had stayed with us in Saskatoon for a few days when writing his qualification exams for licensing as a veterinarian in Canada. We had seen him from time to time as he also worked on several wildlife projects in the Rocky Mountains.

"Markus, this is Jerry Haigh. Jo and I are in Pretoria, starting our sabbatical, and I wondered if we could come and see you." Jo had taken unpaid leave from her clinic in Saskatoon to join me on our umpteenth visit to Africa.

"Ja, that would be great. When did you have in mind?"

"We can leave tomorrow, if that suits you."

"Oh...that's not very good. I'm leaving the day after to go to Borakalalo to catch rhino. Is there another time that suits?"

It was September 19, 1997, and we had a month or so to spare before heading to Namibia to work with Mike Briggs. We had started in South Africa, intending to spend time visiting several old friends before moving on to Namibia to meet up with Mike, but here was an unexpected chance to start to fulfill the mandate of my leave application, which had included wildlife research. Although some might call it work, I prefer to think of it in terms of J.M. Barrie's phrase, used at the 1922 convocation at Scotland's St. Andrew's University. He said, "It's not real work unless you'd rather be doing something else."

It was another case, like the delay in graduation that gave me the chance to go back to Africa in 1965, of the family motto, the "Tyde what may" willingness to take whatever chance arose.

It did not take too long to persuade Markus that my previous experience with large numbers of rhino captures might be of some value in the Borakalalo project, so he suggested that we come to his home in Madikwe right away and then follow him from there.

With the invitation to go with Markus in place, we promptly started to kit out the little Toyota sedan that we had rented for our two-month stay in South Africa. We headed off west and north, travelling through the towns of Rustenburg and Zeerust before checking the detailed instructions that Markus had given us to find the park in which he was currently acting as the field ecologist and veterinarian.

We soon found the park and Markus's home and met Michele, Markus's petite new wife, and a couple of students who were working in the park as part of the field experience in their diploma courses. After settling in and getting organized, it was time for a glass of beer for Markus and me and an orange juice for Michele and Jo.

Over dinner Markus told us that the main purpose of the Borakalalo exercise was to continue the conservation work begun by Ian Player about fifty-five years back, but updating the technology by ear-marking White rhino and placing small transponders in the base of each one's front horn. The ear notches were designed as a simple means of determining the sex and unique registration number of each animal when viewed from a distance, or even from the air. The males would have notches cut in a rectangular fashion, while females would have a V, about five centimetres wide at the top, cut into the edges of each ear.

"You'll no doubt be using a helicopter?" I had asked as we tucked into our steaks.

"Yes, I'll be shooting and we'll be working with Ray Schaller, the park warden, and Rusty Hustler, who used to be with the Rhodesian police and is now a warden in the park system. They've both got some experience, but I'm sure we'll find a job for you."

He knew that I had a track record with all of this, albeit experience that was from twenty-two years back. He also knew that I was still active in immobilizing lots of other species, from polar bear to moose.

"If you can take care of checking heart and respiratory rates, that'll ease some of my burden," he had said. The stethoscope that I had packed in Canada would be put to immediate use.

Early next morning we were off, following the dust plume created by Markus's Land Cruiser as we sped through dry thorn country. As long as we kept the window closed we did not have to deal with the flying grit, although vision was very limited if we did not stay well back. The only relief from the heat and dust came when Markus turned at one of the many junctions and the wind took the choking clouds off to one side. We occasionally passed through villages whose chief characteristics were masses of thorn bushes highlighted by what have been euphemistically called Natal Poppies. The real reason for the decoration on the bushes is the accumulation of plastic bags, mainly black, which have blown from the ground where they have been carelessly dropped and have caught in the thorns. As the bags are virtually indestructible, the number of "poppies" continues to increase; moreover they seem to multiply of their own accord, as they gradually shred, so that one large bag becomes several small strips, all caught up in the thorns. An ugly sight.

In an interesting example of parallel evolution, Natal Poppies have sprung up all over Africa, and have become a common sight wherever one goes. A more generic name might be African Wild Flowers, as we have seen them in every African country that we have visited in the last fifteen years. Eventually they either shred themselves so small that they cannot hang onto the trees, or they end up becoming the major visible form of garbage lining village streets. What a pity that they lack DNA and cannot propagate into useful bags every year or so. Since 1997, an attempt at control of this situation has been made by making the giving away of plastic bags illegal in South Africa, but Markus tells me that it has not had a noticeable effect on the flower crop.

The situation has hardly improved in the ten years since we learned the cynical nickname. Vast amounts of plastic clog up systems in most countries and recent reports indicate that even in Canada people are beginning to feel the grip of the man-made monster. In Uganda it is almost impossible to make a purchase without the item being stuffed into a small black plastic bag, called a *kavera*. The bags end up in roadside garbage heaps that may or may not be sporadically picked by an antiquated dump truck that drives off with its contents dribbling onto the road. The garbage piles are burnt from time to time, sending a plume of foul-smelling choking toxic fumes into the air. It is hard to know which is worse—the fumes or the garbage.

When, in February 2007, I took students to Uganda (of which more in the following section) there appeared to be an upsurge in the effort to pick up some of the messy piles, at least in and around the city centre, and I wondered what had led to this change. My host put it quite simply: "The Commonwealth leaders will meet in Kampala in November." He really did not need to expand, and when our bus made a detour through back streets to avoid some heavy traffic, we saw mass versions of the mess in spots where no foreign dignitary is ever likely to venture. Despite the clean-up effort, I saddened in November to learn from the BBC website that parts of Entebbe Road, the road between the airport and Kampala, had flooded because drains were blocked with plastic bags. The flood happened the Friday before the week of the Commonwealth meeting.

While the plastic intermittently occupied our attention near the villages, we had to concentrate on the numerous twists and turns in the road as Markus led us on our trip to Borakalalo. Without him as the leader the almost 150-kilometre trip would have had us lost in short order. We followed him into the park, stopping at the main gate where he identified himself, and drove along the gravel road, coloured creamy white by the pounded local stone. Suddenly we turned off the main track at a sign marked "No Entrance" and proceeded cautiously down a narrower and more rutted track, losing sight of Markus as he was able to move without concern about his clearance. We soon found ourselves at a campsite with dark green tents erected in a row alongside a river, thorn trees overhanging the far bank and on our side a clearing with a fire pit surrounded by large logs ready to be burnt.

The camp was well chosen, not a surprise when one realizes that park officials had, over time, had lots of opportunity to find the best spots. Ray greeted us warmly, and as we went to get our gear out of the car he said, "Don't worry about a tent. I've got a spare for you, that one at the end by the burnt stump."

We would be camping in luxury, with a wooden floor for the tent, a vestibule and mosquito nets provided.

"Be sure to use the wire twists when you close the zips," he said. "If you don't the baboons will get in without trouble, and you know what will happen if they do."

We needed no second warning, as we had seen the results of just such a raid during our days in East Africa. Everything had been opened, laid waste and wrecked. The monkeys are none too fastidious about their excretory habits, either. At one of our favourite spots, in Kenya's Meru National Park, a staff member had been employed to walk around the camp with a slingshot. He used it to great effect, and many a vervet monkey and baboon would have had a painful lesson from the golf-ball sized rocks that he fired at them, swinging the cloth round his head and releasing one end of it just as David must surely have done when he killed Goliath.

We unpacked our bags and put them into the tent, then we moved to join the others as we chatted about our rhino tagging project over a cold drink. The so-called White rhino, whose skin is actually grey, except when artificially daubed with whitewash, or more likely when it has been wallowing in mud of some other colour, has been given its inappropriate name because of a language switch between the Dutch of the earliest European settlers and modern English. The Dutch name was *witte renoster*, which soon became *witrenoster* in Afrikaans.

The *witte* meant "wide" and referred to the shape of the upper lip, which allows the animal to graze its favourite short grass effectively and move along like a lawn mower. English settlers who arrived later adopted the *witte* but based upon its sound turned it into "white." In a largely failed attempt to correct three hundred years of error, modern biologists, including the pre-eminent Jonathan Kingdon, have tried to persuade readers to call the animal the Grass rhinoceros, which nicely distinguishes it from the Black rhinoceros (which Kingdon aptly calls the Browse rhinoceros). The words *grass* and *browse* differentiate the two species on the basis of their feeding habits, as one might assume. The prehensile upper lip of the latter allows the grasping and plucking of shrubs and leaves from bushes.

The White rhino qualifies as one of the really impressive examples of conservation in action. The southern race, which once occupied an area in parts of what are now South Africa, Zimbabwe, Zambia, Angola and Botswana, had all but died out by the year 1900. A 1904 estimate had only ten animals left in the country, all of them in the Umfulozi area of Zululand. Mainly through the efforts of one man, big-game hunter Frederick Vaughan-Kirby, who was appointed in 1911 as the first game conservator in that part of the country, the species was brought back from the brink. In 1916 he reported twenty animals alive. From that nadir the numbers climbed slowly to something short of five hundred when in 1952, Ian Player, oldest brother of champion golfer Gary, got involved in the very earliest translocation efforts and movement of the animals to many parts of Africa, and indeed to zoos overseas. Between 1961 and 1972 White rhino had been moved to an impressive thirty-eight new locations in South Africa and eight other African countries, including Kenya, where they went to Meru National Park and became my patients when I lived in the area. Over and above these destinations, rhino also moved to seventeen different countries, including Canada, the UK and the USA.

In 1960 Player had enlisted the help of Dr. Toni Harthoorn, with whom I worked some years later on a cheetah that had broken both hind legs. Toni was a pioneer veterinary scientist working on wildlife immobilization and had worked out doses for rhino using forerunners of the types of morphine-like drugs that we were using on the Borakalalo animals and that I have used for thirty-five years in capturing wild animals. Toni was the inspiration for the title character in the Kenya-based television series *Daktari*, which is the Swahili word for "doctor."

Given that female White rhino deliver their first calves at about the age of five or six, are pregnant for sixteen months and deliver a calf only every two or three years, the increase in numbers was impressive and the level of protection from horn hunters must have been high.

Other races of the species, including the one known as the Northern White rhino, once ranged very widely. Rock art evidence shows that they existed in Morocco, Algeria, Tunisia, throughout the Sahara and into central and East Africa. When Douglas Adams of *Hitchhiker's Guide* fame visited Garamba National Park in what was then Zaire in the 1980s, there were twenty-two Northerns left. Today, there may be three left in what is now the Democratic Republic of Congo. There is a nucleus of seven pure-bred Northerns at the Dvůr Králové Zoo in the Czech Republic and three more, which are not breeding, at the San Diego Zoo. Idi Amin's reign of terror made sure that this race of rhino was exterminated in Uganda, and now the only members of the species that exist in that country are of the southern race, and they have only been introduced in the last five years.

Currently there are thought to be at least five thousand Southern White rhino worldwide, which is a testament to early conservationists like Vaughan-Kirby, Player and Harthoorn. Those early rhino captures, done when Player and Harthoorn were testing untried drugs and equally new ideas, took place before the concept of wildlife conservation had attained its present status and in a very different animal-welfare climate than today's. For instance, in 1936, when asked to set aside a special reserve for the last thirty remaining mountain zebras, General Jan Kemp, who was Minister of Lands in South Africa, is reported to have said, "No! They're just a lot of donkeys in football jerseys." What Kemp thought of rhino conservation does not seem to have been recorded.

The first part of the actual capture of most of the rhino at Borakalalo proved to be routine. Markus aimed the dart for the heavy muscles of the hind end; within a few minutes the animal's gait changed as its stride shortened; then it started to circle, crashing through heavy bush. After this, the next stage tended to vary considerably. Most animals

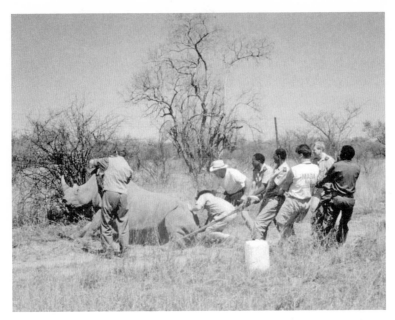
The team pulls on the hobble ropes to stop a drugged rhino.

simply blundered on, the gait becoming ever more collected, just like an old-fashioned Hackney Carriage or dressage horse, until the animal staggered a couple of times and fell onto its side or chest. At this point the ground crew moved in and began the monitoring and identification process.

In some cases, the steady decrease in gait length and apparent awareness did not materialize. If we were lucky, the animals would stop against a stout bush or tree. In some cases, no tree offered itself, and then my previous experience proved useful as we were able to get hobble ropes on the legs and trip up the patient.

Once or twice Markus had to top up the dose.

In all but a couple of cases, the rest of the procedure was pretty routine. While I checked the pulse and breathing, someone else notched the ears, and Rusty used a cordless drill to make a small hole near the base of the front horn. Into the hole went the tiny transponder, with its unique number that would identify that particular animal for a long time, at least while the horn grew from the base like a fingernail and was worn down at the tip, so the electronic gadget would, after a few years,

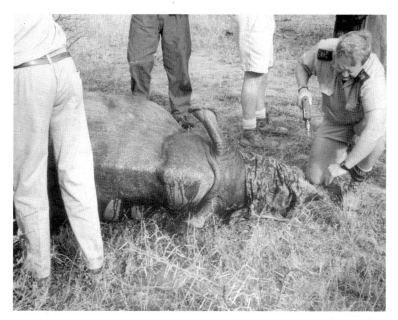

Rusty Hustler using cordless drill to make a small hole in the horn base. He will soon place the tracking microchip into the hole.

eventually rise to the top and fall out. Finally, the hole was plugged with five-minute epoxy glue.

Once all the long-term identification procedures had been carried out on the recumbent beasts, the final actions were to pour a good dollop of whitewash over each animal's back and to give it the drug antidote that would allow it to get up and trundle off, seemingly none the worse for wear. The whitewash was there simply to ensure that we did not catch the same animal again over the next few days, or at least until a rain shower washed it off.

We managed to catch three more animals on the afternoon of that first day, and by the time we had decided to call it quits, the camp beckoned. It was time to settle down, see how Jo was doing with her latest flower study and enjoy a cup of tea and chat about things of mutual interest. As tea-time moved to beer time, a pair of brown-hooded kingfishers flitted up and down the river, offering the chance for photography as the evening light once again proved to be ideal for capturing the scenery and wildlife around us.

Of course, as in any exercise of this nature, not everything went entirely smoothly. Indeed, if it always did, there would be little point in having an experienced crew working on the job.

The first two captures on the second day were pretty routine, but then a sub-adult gave us a few anxious moments. The first clue that something unusual was happening was evident when the young bull took a lot longer than usual to start his exaggerated gait or go into his circling routine. The ground-crew members were all nearby, but every time we approached to try to get a rope on him, he would break into a trot, indicating that he was somewhat aware of our presence, which is not normally the case once an animal has been darted. Eventually Markus was able to get a second dart, containing a top-up dose, into him, but even that did not do the trick. We caught up with the animal as he stopped against a small bush, the trunk no thicker than my wrist, which he would normally have brushed aside as a mere twig.

We moved in as a team and Markus said to me, "Keep me posted about this one. I'm a bit concerned about him."

I was already tuned to this need and had started to call out the heart rate every thirty seconds or so. The first reading was abnormally high, at over one hundred beats per minute, so I kept on counting, without any real pause.

Soon afterwards I called out, making sure that Markus could hear me above the other voices, "Up to 130 now, risen about thirty in under a minute."

Then it was, "180 and rising. I think we ought to quit."

"Ja. The rest of you get away, back to the vehicles. I'm going to give him the antidote."

A heart rate of 180 beats per minute is extraordinarily high for such a large animal, so the decision was an easy one. The first large dose went into the muscles of the hind end.

"What's he at now?" asked Markus.

"Still 180," I replied.

"Okay. Drop back, Jerry, and I'll get the rest of this into his ear vein."

Within thirty seconds the rhino was looking much more comfortable, his breathing noticeably slowing as we watched from behind a nearby tree. In less than two minutes he was on his way back into the bush. This sort of unexpected reaction occurs rarely, and no real reason for it springs to mind. It may even be an individual variation, but the capture crew has to be on the *qui vive* and be ready to deal with it promptly.

The other bit of excitement that day occurred with the very next animal, an adult cow. This incident was more a comedy of errors than any sort of crisis for the rhino. She had been darted quite near the park's perimeter fence, which relied more upon its high voltage wires than its sheer strength to keep wildlife in and cattle out. Of course, Murphy's Law at once came into operation. The heavily drugged rhino staggered into the fence and collapsed, exactly as one might have wished, had it not been for the little matter of the several thousand volts, not enough to kill either animal or human, but certainly enough to deter. The lowest "hot" line was below the recumbent rhino's level but not below any of the standing crew. The next few minutes involved Rusty and Ray and the junior wardens trying to roll the 1,800-kilogram immobile lump of sleeping flesh away from the wire without getting themselves zapped. They were not always successful, as Rusty's yelp and bound made plain. Once the cow was free of her entanglement, the rest of the procedure was routine.

After three days of steady work, Markus had to head back to meet some new animal arrivals at Madikwe, but we stayed on an extra day as the helicopter was still available, and it seemed to Ray to be a waste not to continue. Another vet took over the shooter's job and we carried on but not with quite the success that we had enjoyed when Markus was with us. Of course, the number of rhino that had not been tagged had now dwindled, so finding new ones was harder. On one occasion, as the chopper flew by, about two hundred metres away to the south an unmarked animal walked across fifty metres north of the truck in which Jo was sitting. The driver tried to call the pilot, but he discovered that the walkie-talkie was not working. He then tried to turn to find the other vehicle but found that his truck had a flat tire. The rhino remained untagged and undaubed.

Rhino conservation efforts that go back to those of Ian Player, and forward to those of Court Parfet, Anna Mertz, Ian Craig and many others, are direct links to species survival. That these efforts have had to be ongoing is because rhino horn has long been an expensive commodity in some market places.

Given that rhino horn is indeed closely analogous to fingernail in the way it grows, and even its composition, it is difficult to see how the media, especially the Western print media, which thrives on stories related to sex, can persist in writing that it works as an aphrodisiac. The truth is that it is much prized as an ornamental object, particularly for dagger handles in Yemen, for *objets d'art* in the Far East and as a component of traditional medicines in the Orient and parts of Africa. Historically, it was also used for the detection of poisons in food by Arabs, Europeans and Asians.

There are two small tribal groups who believe that rhino horn has aphrodisiac properties. In India's state of Gujurat, men use it by applying some ground powder to the penis just before intercourse, and in the Nakasongola region of Uganda, just south of Murchison National Park, it is believed by some that rhino horn ash helps stimulate sexual desire. Perhaps the shape of the horn, and the prolonged courtship and copulation engaged in by rhino (up to an hour has been recorded, with several mounts and ejaculations) are what leads to the misconception (to coin a pun). With typical throwaway humour, Douglas Adams of *Hitchhiker's Guide* fame, writing with Mark Cawardine in 1990 in the delightful yet sad book *Last Chance To See*, suggested that the aphrodisiac myth may be simply related to the fact that rhino horn is a "big sticky-up hard thing." I imagine that the only way it could actually work would be as a splint, but as most people realize, the brain is the most important sexual organ, and the power of suggestion is extraordinary.

In 1982 Esmond Bradley-Martin described in *Run Rhino Run* how expensive cups made from rhino horn were once used by European royalty for the purpose of detecting poison in food and drinks. Among those who are known to have engaged in this practice were England's Queen Elizabeth I, France's Louis XIV, and Rudolph II of Germany, who was the Holy Roman Emperor from 1552 to 1612. All of these people lived in an age when poisoning was a popular way of getting rid of unwanted rivals and enemies. It was thought that the horn could either neutralize the toxic substance or would effervesce in the presence of alkaloids, which are a common group of poisonous substances. According to a fourth-century Chinese pharmacist, "The horn is a safe guide to the presence of poison; when poisonous medicines of liquid form are stirred with the horn, a white foam will bubble up and no further test is necessary."

The Yemeni dagger handle market, which fifteen years ago may have taken up as much as half of all rhino horn being exported from Africa, has declined, but not vanished. Martin, who has studied and reported on the trade for the best part of twenty years and has written other authoritative texts on the subject, reported in 2003 that the number of rhino horn handles made for the traditional *jambiyas* (daggers) has declined sharply, mainly because of a shortage of rhino horn on the market.

However, the market has not entirely disappeared and Martin has traced the smuggling routes through Kenya, Tanzania and the Democratic Republic of Congo, whence the products go to Djibouti and thence to Yemen and its capital, Sanaa.

Another destination for poached rhino horn is the traditional medicine market in the Orient, which is considerable. Many plants and animal parts are used, and belief in the system is long-standing and widespread. The first written records of the use of animal parts in traditional Chinese medicine (TCM) date back over two thousand years, and oral records are evidently much older. Rhino horn plays a central role in several medications, primarily prescribed for the control of fever. It is not just in the Orient that rhino horn has been used for medical purposes, though. In Uganda, horn derivatives are believed to cure congestive heart failure and stroke.

Two detailed reports from the early 1990s that were prepared for the Trade Records Analysis of Flora and Fauna in Commerce (more easily known as TRAFFIC) show how rhino horn is both used and sold in Korea and Taiwan. In 1993 author Judy Mills found that 60 per cent of South Korea's doctors believe that horn is an effective medicine and 79 per cent believe it to be essential for a wide variety of ailments. In Taiwan, Kristin Nowell and her colleagues, both of whom were locals who could conduct interviews as "patients" or "consumers" and thus obtain information unbiased by the doctors' or dealers' concerns about detection of potentially illegal activities, reported in 1992 that the medical community recognizes differences between rhino horn from Asia and from Africa. The former is about ten times as expensive, averaging over US$60,000 per kilogram. They estimated that at least ten thousand kilograms of rhino horn were held in the thousands of licensed and unlicensed pharmacies during their study. Almost all of this was from African rhino, and the total retail value, in 1992 was in excess of US$70 million. The most expensive items, far in excess of unprocessed Asian horn, were the antique carvings, becoming ever more valuable as pressure is brought to bear against the use or ownership of rhino horn for any purpose at all.

Wu Yi-Luo, writing in *The New Compilation of Materia Medica* in 1757, stated that "rhino horn can cool down the heart, release waste from the liver, clean the stomach, reduce fever, remove the cold, clear the windpipe, keep away evil, detoxify poisons, cure typhoid and epidemic diseases, as well as cure symptoms such as jaundice, rashes, vomiting blood, excreting blood, delirium, abscesses, and lumps etc. It can also soothe the patient's nerves and improve his eyesight." That just about covers everything except vehicle accidents (there weren't many cars around in 1757) or knife and gunshot wounds.

It is easy to be pessimistic about the chances of success in efforts to derail the use of rhino horn and many other items of animal origin in TCM. Tiger bones are one such item, and there have been seriously worded articles in Asia espousing the farming of tigers for the express purpose of supplying medical needs. Indeed, in the *China Daily News* of September 8, 2005, there was an article recounting how the original tiger farm in China had grown to run five hundred animals in a tightly controlled system of records and production. There are a substantial number of farms in China where bears are kept in close confinement for the express purpose of extracting the fluids from their gall bladders for TCM use.

In a series of articles in the *Journal of Ethnopharmacology* and related publications, a group at the Chinese University of Hong Kong reported studies in which they used a rhino horn extract with or without mixed herbs in a TCM formula known as Qingying Decoction, to bring down fever in rats. They also reported that this stuff was effective without any horn, or with the substitution of water buffalo horn. Based upon the dose given to rats, a human would need over one kilogram of powdered rhino horn extract for a single treatment. As water buffalo are domesticated over vast areas of the India and the Orient and are common, it would be nice to think that if people must use horn, they might be willing to give the rhino a break.

A further TRAFFIC report by Simon Milledge in 2007 indicated that poaching and illegal rhino horn trading continues, with the main markets still in Yemen, and East and Southeast Asia. A total of 252 rhino were killed in Africa in the period 2000–2005. Of these, 151 were shot, but snares, spears and poisons were also used. During these years the weight of horn that entered the illegal trade was 102.4 kilograms, about fifteen kilograms per year, which is ten times less than the 165 kilogram annual rate during the last big period of rhino destruction from 1970–86. The worry is that since 2000 there has been a steady rise in the number of horns entering the illegal trade, which matches a new trend in commercial rhino poaching run by well-organized gangs instead of individuals.

This continued illegal trading is really no surprise, as both Judy Mills and Kristin Nowell concluded that the market is unlikely to vanish, with doctors in the Orient convinced that the product has no substitute for certain conditions.

IF THE POSSIBILITY OF POACHING IS THE MAJOR THREAT TO RHINOS, it is not the only one. Inbreeding is another obvious risk, perhaps made even more serious when one considers that the White rhino went through one serious bottleneck when Vaughan-Kirby reported on their status in 1911. To make sure that this does not happen again, even in the limited environment of a fully fenced park, it is possible to move bulls around from one location and breeding population to another, just as would happen in the beef industry. The ear notching technique can help identify individuals with their unique patterns, but nowadays DNA is a much more specific tool.

Over the four days at Borakalalo, we ended up catching and marking fifteen rhino, but there was one odd thing that I could not really understand. None of the tissue samples were saved. It would have been quite easy to place one small piece of ear tissue in a liquid nitrogen container and ship it to an appropriate lab for DNA analysis. In later correspondence with Markus I learned that this is now a routine practice for all animal captures, not just rhino.

After all, as the "wild" becomes increasingly small, and the human population grows by leaps and bounds, animals like rhino, as well as other megafauna, are going to end up in tightly restricted parks, or what amount to large zoos, and as such will need careful and detailed management. ✳

16

MADIKWE'S PAINTED DOGS

In which we learn about the successful rehabilitation of degraded ranch land; the integration of wildlife, livestock and local communities in South Africa; and witness a remarkable wildlife moment.

BEFORE HE HAD LEFT BORAKALALO, Markus had said, "If you like, when you get back we'll see if we can find the wild dogs. I'm worried about them, as we haven't seen the alpha male for about ten days. See you on Monday."

Of course the chance to see wild dogs was not one we were going to pass up, and our planned route was going to take us right past Madikwe anyway, on the way to Botswana and points north and west.

"Since we left Kenya," I said to Jo as Markus drove away, "wild dogs have taken a terrible hit through most of Africa, although they are now a top conservation priority in South Africa. They have been persecuted for years, but lately the situation has become even more dire.

They've suffered canine distemper outbreaks, almost certainly caught from unvaccinated dogs that roam free. Just like the distemper that killed so many lions in the Serengeti the early 1990s."

Three days later, driving rather more slowly than on the outward trip when we had followed Markus's dust cloud at breakneck speed, we headed west, stopping along the way to buy a supply of groceries in a supermarket. Here we made our first, somewhat astonished, acquaintance with a Braai pack, which is something like a barbeque pack in North America or a Barbie pack in Australia. As we would later see later in Namibia, the Braai pack is a popular and entirely meat-based combination of steak, chops and a coiled sausage, all done up in one package meant for one. It was certainly enough for both of us, with a generous amount left over. We left the supermarket and continued on our way.

Soon after we had passed through the Madikwe Park gate and turned left onto the gravel road, Jo spotted a bright red flash in a thorn bush to her left and we stopped to try to photograph a thrush-sized crimsonbreasted shrike about which our 1997 edition of *Sasol Birds of Southern Africa* states, "The striking combination of bright crimson underparts and black upperparts renders this species unmistakable." ("Shrike" was changed to "gonolek" in later editions of the Sasol guide.) Most of the time we could see little more than three to six metres into the thicket of 2.5 metre-high bushes that came right up to the drainage ditches. Delicate bright yellow flowers, a centimetre or so long, hung from the bushes like little light bulbs below a fuzzy pink collar. The curly seed pods, about three centimetres, were abundant and a close look showed us that the branches were well protected with masses of five-centimetre-long rapier-like thorns.

The view opened up as we crested a rise, and we stopped to watch a small herd of elephants meander across the road and disappear into the bush. Rounding a bend, we found Markus's Land Cruiser parked on the verge and saw him standing to one side talking to a group of men and women armed with pangas and rakes, just beside a freshly cut mass of the bushes we had seen so much of along the track.

"What's going on, and what is that plant?" I asked as he came over.

"I'm just checking with the crew about bush clearing. People from the local communities on the park boundaries come in every day and

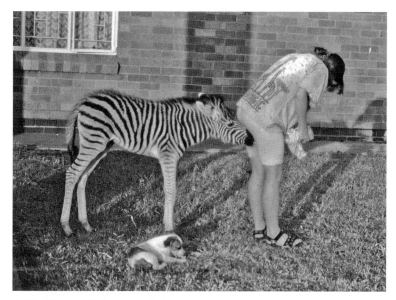

Michele Hofmeyr and the hungry zebra foal.

we try to clear as much as possible, at least fifty metres back from the road, so as to improve the grazing, and of course the visibility. And it may be pretty, but it's an utter pest. It's called sickle bush, and if it's not controlled it takes over completely if the land is overgrazed, as this was before the game park project started."

"Do any animals eat it?" I asked.

"Ja. It is quite a useful tree as the pods are eaten by game, but those wicked spines can easily pierce tires, so it's not a good idea to drive over it."

He switched topics. "Excuse me, I've got to go with Gavin," he said, gesturing to the stocky man standing beside the Toyota, "to film the release of the latest batch of hippo that have just arrived. I'll see you back at the house."

We soon arrived at Markus and Michele's home and got out to walk around to the verandah.

We were in for a surprise. As we came round the corner into the garden, the first thing we saw was Michele being butted up the rear end by a zebra foal. It was soon apparent that she was actually feeding the little thing and that she had a bottle facing backwards between her legs. As we laughed at and queried her about this bizarre sight she said, "I tried to hold the bottle in front of me, but he won't take it."

So, in this somewhat indecorous posture, she stood slightly bent over as he continued to suck. Of course, in any other position the foal would not have had the comfort of having its face in contact with something and its eyes and nose in the dark, which is how nursing hooved animals see the world.

With the feeding soon over we joined Michele for a cup of tea in the kitchen, where she washed out the foal's empty milk bottle at the sink and gave us more background about the bush clearing. "It's part of a poverty relief program run by Working for Water, an innovative program run by the Department of Water Affairs and Forestry. Here alone it has created 150 jobs for men and women. Team leaders have been trained as contractors and taught to run teams of fifteen people. Some of the team leaders have already talked about starting their own businesses to do outside bush clearing contract work when we don't need them."

"It sounds like a great program," said Jo. "How long has it been going on?"

Michele, the botanist in the family, gave us more. "This whole place, about 75,000 hectares, used to be a cattle ranch. It was overgrazed and the sickle bush—the taxonomic name is *Dichrostachys cinerea*—took over in lots of places, where it formed dense thickets. The only way to manage it is by cutting, applying a herbicide to the cut stump and layering the cut branches to protect the grass shoots. It has to be burned every three or four years, and with those two techniques combined the range can be maintained in good condition. Burning alone, though, won't do the trick, as its extensive seed banks can survive fire and may even be stimulated to grow as a result of smoke and heat. The trees are prolific seed producers and seeds persist for a long time in the soil. It also spreads by root suckers, so it is very invasive and extremely difficult to control."

"Sounds like quite a challenge."

"Ja, it's a serious bush encroacher on mismanaged land, and the place eventually became so inhospitable that even the cattle could no longer usefully graze in the area."

We went to get our stuff from the car and met a young trainee ranger, who was working on the wild dog project and living in the Hofmeyrs' guest cottage. She told us that she had been with Markus the previous day and that they had found the alpha male dog after picking up the signal from his radio collar.

Holding her nose and rolling her eyes at the memory, she said, "He was preddy stinky." She let go of her nose and her voice rose half an octave. "He was all the way down a big warthog burrow that the pack had been using as a denning site. He was stone dead, out of sight except for the tip of his tail, and I had to crawl in to pull him out. It was gross. Markus reckoned he'd been dead for a few days, but we don't know what he died of."

Markus turned up a while later and introduced Gavin, who had finished filming the unloading of the park's latest arrivals and wanted to use the rest of his limited time to get some footage for a fill-in program on wild dogs that was virtually finished and in the final editing stage.

"Would you like to come and see the wild dog puppies now?" asked Markus. We needed no second invitation and were soon inside the Toyota, Jo somewhat crammed in the middle seat, astride the gearshift, Gavin holding on in the rear bed of the truck, keeping his head down to avoid the worst of the dust.

As we drove through it, Markus told us about the park and some of the history of the wild dogs. "The land was purchased in 1991 by South Africa's North West Parks Board with the express purpose of developing a game reserve that would cater to an up-market tourist trade. Our official pamphlet, published by the board in 1997, makes the justifiable claim that 'the approach to conservation that has been adopted at Madikwe puts the needs of people before that of wildlife and conservation.'"

"It looks like it's been a success," Jo commented.

"I first heard about it in 1992, at that ranching symposium where we first met," I said. "How did you get the animals for re-stocking?"

"We did lots of translocations from all over the place. We've got another pamphlet, with the rather apt name *Operation Phoenix*, that describes the re-introductions. I'll let you have a copy when we get home. You'll see it's quite a story, but in short we brought in over eight thousand individuals of twenty-six species between 1992 and 1996."

"And the fence?" I asked. "It's pretty high powered, if you'll excuse the pun." I was referring to the large number of single strands of wire strung through off-set insulators at ground, belly and shoulder height, as well as up near the top of the 2.1-metre woven wire construction. "Must have cost a bomb."

"It carries about fourteen thousand volts in each line, on separate circuits, in case one shorts out. The guys from the same village as those bush clearers did the labour. In fact, the whole place was designed to give employment to the local people, which the board considers crucial."

"Top of the line specs," I said. "That makes it predator and elephant proof."

"And the dogs?" asked Jo, getting the business at hand back on track.

"We got the first ones from two different sources, three wild sibling males from a pack outside the western boundary of Kruger National Park and three sibling females from De Wildt Endangered Species Breeding Centre near Pretoria. It took only about a month for the two groups to integrate and form a pack as they were held in a quarantine boma. They were then released into the park proper, and after an initial few days of insecurity they began to hunt together and look healthy and alert."

"Did you vaccinate against anything?" I asked.

"Ja, we gave three doses of distemper vaccine and also rabies, but I'm not sure if any of them did any good, as they were domestic dog vaccines, and we don't know if they work in other canids. We also put radio collars on two of the males and one of the females, so it was easy enough to follow and study them. That's how we found the male, of course. He was too far gone to be of much use for post-mortem, but I sent some bits into the lab anyway."

"How did the pack get on?" I asked, eager to learn more about them.

"One interesting thing soon emerged. They quickly learned about fences, and used them, especially where there were corners. When hunting, they drive their prey, especially impala, which makes up about 50 per cent of their diet, into the barrier where they can easily be brought down."

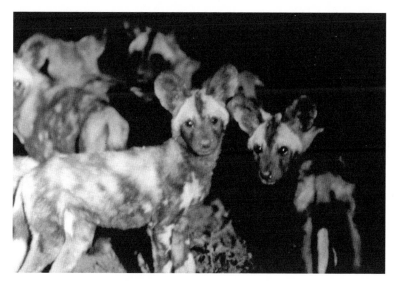

The wild dog pups hear the approaching adults.

"How did they get on with breeding?"

"The first year the pups either died young or the females miscarried, we don't know which. I've written it all up in a pamphlet that I can give you if you're interested. Hierarchy within the group changed a couple of times, and the first successful litter of pups is about a year old but not vaccinated, of course, as we decided not to put them through the stress of capture. Then we had another breeding success in July, and we're going to see the new litter, a dozen youngsters about ten weeks old. I think I'll be able to find them easily enough, although none of the litter has a collar."

I knew that at that age they were too young to go on hunting forays and were likely to have been left at a strategic spot by the adults. We hoped to see the entire pack as they came back from the hunt. It was obvious that Markus had spent many hours on this, his pet project, and it was therefore no real surprise that he knew, with remarkable accuracy, where the new litter of pups was going to be. We spent a fascinating hour, in the gathering dusk, watching them sitting under a tree, the creamy-brown, white and black of their coats like a box of delicious chocolates spilled in a pile among the greenery, the black ears moving like mini radio receivers. There was no roughhousing or

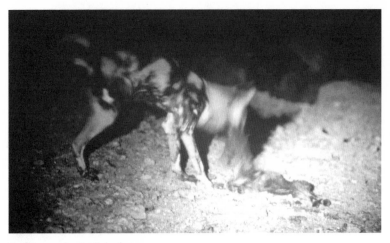

The Africa-map female kills her first pup.

play, but one or two of the more forward ones sat up and looked at us or stood and stared into the distance.

I slipped out of the front seat, in order to give Jo more room, and using the tire as a step I vaulted into the flat-bed at the rear and leaned against the top of the cab next to Gavin where I inserted a new film into my Nikon using the only remaining thing I had in my pack, some very fast 1000 ASA Agfa film. As the light dimmed, Markus turned on his powerful spotlight and the pups were ringed in a halo of bright light.

Suddenly their attitude changed as first one then two, and finally all of them, pricked up their ears. Then a couple of the boldest left the safety of the group and headed toward us, crossing right in front of the vehicle, no more than five metres away as Gavin set his camera rolling.

It was obvious that the adults had arrived and that the pups had heard them and were coming to greet them, no doubt in the hope of persuading them, with the well-known pattern of submissive begging, to regurgitate a bolus of food that they could feast upon. Right in front of the vehicle a pup approached an adult, ducked low and made a huge grin. But instead of receiving a meal, its next few seconds were its last. The adult, actually a yearling with a distinctive mark like an inverted map of Africa on her right hip, picked up the pup by its head and with one chomp bit down and killed it.

We stood behind the cab in the back of the Toyota flat-bed or sat more or less gob-struck as the larger dog proceeded to tear the pup apart and start to devour it, eventually leaving only a hind leg and part of the skull. The still photos are a bit blurred but no less dramatic for that.

Over the next hour and a half the Africa-map female—for that is what she was, Markus knowing every dog in the pack from his very frequent studies—and one helper proceeded to kill every one of the twelve pups, but they really ate only their first victim. Gavin had more unique footage than he could ever have imagined, for such an event has never been reported, before or since.

We eventually left, Markus remarking, "Ag, that was something, man."

As we headed back to the house, we tried to analyze what we had seen. The first thing was our emotional reactions. The principal ones were a mixture of horror, amazement and helplessness. Even if we had had a weapon in the vehicle, which we didn't, it would not have been right to shoot the killers. We had been witnessing a real-life wildlife event. It is even possible that such an event had occurred before, as we all knew that the wild dog had suffered a precipitous decline across the continent in the preceding two or three decades. There were thought to be several interconnected reasons for the decline, among them human persecution over many years, disease and a marked drop in the numbers of prey species.

Persecution of wild dogs, known by other colourful names like the Cape hunting dog and the painted dog, has occurred in several ways. European ranchers, carrying their cultural baggage, have stated that the way in which these predators kill their victims is cruel and that they should therefore be shot on sight. A quote from R. Maugham, written in 1914, sums up the attitude that prevailed at the time, and for many years afterwards:

Let us consider for a moment that abomination—that blot upon the many interesting wild things—the murderous Wild Dog. It will be an excellent day for African game and its preservation when means can be devised for its complete extermination.

Anyone who has seen film of a pack of dogs chasing an intended victim knows that they engage in a sort of tag-team chase that can go on for many minutes, over long distances up to several kilometres, which often ends in an exhausted antelope or zebra standing still while it is disembowelled. Jonathan Kingdon, renowned biologist and artist extraordinaire, has recorded dog speed bursts of up to sixty-six kilometres per hour, and sustained chases at forty-eight kilometres per hour. The method is efficient, although extensive research has shown that dogs may fail to catch their intended prey as often as 30 per cent of the time. Nonetheless, the anthropocentric view of the dogs' manner of hunting coloured people's attitudes for a long time, despite the fact that the dogs are killing to eat and exist.

There are also those who abhor and kill wild dogs because they are perceived as livestock killers. However, studies by long-time wild dog researcher Dr. Rosie Woodroffe, and others, have shown that only a minute proportion—around 2 per cent—of livestock killed by predators are actually taken by dogs, so their reputation may exceed their actual performance. In a study of wild dog predation in Kenya, Dr. Woodroffe and her colleagues showed that as long as wild prey exist, the cost of wild dog predation on livestock is very low at US$3.40 per dog, per year, but where wild prey were seriously depleted the cost rose to $389 per dog per year, with wild dogs repeatedly killing livestock. For instance, one Nanyuki-based farmer friend of ours lost 274 merino sheep in fourteen months to these predators, although there were plenty of buck on the property. My guess is that the sheep, being much less wary than their wild cousins after centuries of domestication, were simply a sort of "packed lunch" easy option for the dogs. For an extensive and thorough read about wild dogs I can recommend the 1997 International Union for the Conservation of Nature's Canid Specialist's publication *The African Wild Dog: Status Survey and Conservation Action Plan*, in which Dr. Woodroffe and others wrote chapters that cover anything and everything relevant to the subject.

Finally, dogs are killed for totemic and medicinal uses. In this case, the humans who take them are not using guns but more traditional methods, particularly snares. Harriet Davies and Johan du Toit, writing in the journal *Oryx* in 2004, revealed that over half of the people they surveyed in Zimbabwe reported knowledge of traditional use of wild dogs or their parts. Wild dog fat is reported to treat tetanus; wild dog brain is fed to domestic dogs so they become better hunters; and the end of a wild dog's tail, again fed to domestic dogs, was related to make them run faster and to magically make the tracked animal lose power.

Like many other animals, wild dogs have a symbolic role in African society, which is easy enough to understand given their hunting prowess, endurance and cooperative techniques. The cannibalism we had witnessed was obviously an aberration and anything but cooperation, and it was important for all of us who had seen it to find an explanation.

Markus and I began to try and reason it out.

"The adults had obviously not eaten. Their bellies would have be sagging if they had had a meal. I don't think they've had a successful hunt for some days," he said.

"But I doubt that the one animal killed from hunger. More likely some sort of disease, maybe rabies or distemper," I replied.

"Ja, I agree. We'll have to try and dart one or two tomorrow and put them in the boma so that we can work them up and watch them. We'll come back and pick up the pups as well."

Soon after breakfast the next morning, and after calling Norman Matabula, the dapper chief park warden, Markus outlined the plans. We set off, this time armed with a rifle, a dart gun, immobilizing drugs and a post-mortem kit.

The first task was to collect some bait. One unsuspecting impala, taken from the area of the park where hunting, as opposed to photography and tours, was the main activity, soon met its end. Back at the dog-kill site, we fixed the impala to the tow bar on the truck, using a stout rope tied short. In moments, the dogs appeared, and in the daylight it was evident that they had still not had a meal, as their bellies were tucked right up. They began to tear at the carcass, pulling and trying to drag it into the bushes. We soon identified our Africa-map killer and had a dart in her hind leg. The alpha female, easily identified by her radio collar, was acting rather strangely, hanging back from the pack, and so she, too, began to feel the effects of the drugs as Markus showed his skill with another well-placed shot.

We loaded the dogs into the back of the Toyota and went on a search for the pups. All lay within twenty metres of the spot where the first victim had been killed. Most had been dispatched with a single bite to the head and then left, but one had been partly dismembered. The picture of their bodies lined up near the truck, now not at all cute, tells its own tale.

The next step was to head back to the quarantine site where the dogs had been held when they first came to the park. It was here that they had been vaccinated against a range of diseases that were known to be risk factors, including distemper, which had been diagnosed in wild dogs in several areas of Africa, no doubt jumping from unvaccinated domestic dogs owned by herders living near or in the parks. Another of the vaccines given to the dogs had been against rabies, an ever-present risk to all mammals in Africa.

We then examined the adults and put them into the boma, watching carefully to make sure that they recovered uneventfully from their drugs. I was surprised at how rough their coats felt, even through my protective gloves.

Next came the post-mortems on the pups, which did not tell us much beyond the fact that the pups had obviously not eaten for a while. Markus later sent send samples off to a government lab, but they would take time, and Jo and I had to go on to Namibia, where I was supposed to be working in a few days.

We stayed with Michele and Markus for a couple more days, naturally visiting the quarantine boma each day to see how the dogs were faring but not seeing anything significant in the way of abnormal behaviour. They readily ate the meat that was dropped into the pen.

We also travelled with Markus as he made his rounds of the park and kept in touch with the staff. In his Toyota, we climbed a steep hill that had a water tank at its top, and Markus set up his radio antenna to check on several recently released animals. He and I, with Jo well back, climbed a tree, where I readied my camera, and he tried to call out a Black rhino that he wanted to check.

Anna Mertz, who founded the rhino sanctuary at Lewa, has described the various sounds that Black rhino make as they communicate, and it was the "squeak," a most unlikely noise for such a large animal to

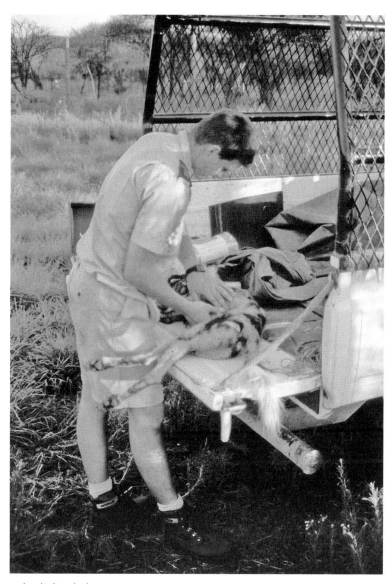

Markus checking the dogs.

make, that Markus used. After four years of almost daily contact with Samia, the calf Anna raised from the age of two days, she has been able to pinpoint about twelve variations of squeak in the rhino's lexicon. In her fascinating 1991 account *Rhino at the Brink of Extinction*, the sound is represented by Anna as "eeeak," and she found that to get rhino to come to her call she had to hold the last syllable steady. To my ears the noise is not unlike a lower pitched mew of a domestic cat. To accompany the mew, Markus broke off the occasional twig, trying to suggest to the animal that he was in fact either a rival or a potential mate who was feeding nearby. It may have been that Markus did not make quite the right one of the twelve variations on "eeeak," or perhaps a swirl of wind came by as we perched three metres off the ground, and the rhino decided that our smell did not match our sounds. The rhino did not appear that day.

After this, Jo and I had to move on, still not knowing why the wild dogs had done as they did. We had an appointment in Namibia's Caprivi Strip to join Mike Briggs and members of the Namibian Wildlife Department do some work on lions.

It was two months almost to the day, and we were back in South Africa, before we heard more details on the dogs. As we had expected, but had not dared to voice too firmly, the dogs had contracted rabies. Strain identification had proved that it was the jackal form of the virus, and it is reasonable to speculate that the alpha male, the first to die, had had contact with this main carrier of the disease in Africa in some sort of fight near, or maybe even through, the park's fence. By the time we got back to Madikwe five months later, all but three of the original pack of twelve were dead.

There can be little doubt that the virus that causes rabies had set up shop in a part of the Africa-map dog's brain that controls behaviour, particularly the well-known behaviour that sets the pattern for group caring for young in a pack animal. Instead of greeting the approaching pup and regurgitating food for it—had she had any in her belly—she perceived the pup as either a nuisance to be swiftly dealt with, or a food item, and she was doubtless hungry. Either way, it was all over for the pup and its littermates. As rabies had taken hold in the pack, it is likely that the pups would have contracted the disease, as well, and would have died soon anyway.

Not surprisingly, I soon got myself to a medical clinic and asked for a booster vaccination against rabies. Although I was, and am, thoroughly vaccinated against this most deadly and incurable of virus infections, a top-up was going to do no harm and would supply some peace of mind.

It did not take Markus long to track down some more wild dogs in need of some space to roam. A pair of males from Kruger National Park joined four hand-raised pups from Botswana and the survivors of the outbreak we witnessed to make up a new pack, while another was established when five animals from De Wildt Cheetah and Wildlife Trust were moved to Madikwe. Markus wanted to cover his bets. If one pack should fall afoul of the same problem, there would at least be some insurance. All were vaccinated, of course, but the ever-present threat of rabies, especially in any new pups that may be born and cannot be vaccinated, remains a worry.

I later found time to read Markus's pamphlets, which gave some more insights into his fascination with and dedication to the wild dog project. His was the first successful translocation of the species; at least it was until disease took over as the main restriction, much as he had predicted.

Most people think that in pack animals, such as the wild dog and the wolf, an alpha male and female do all the breeding, while the reproductive urges of the others are suppressed. Markus had, with his daily observations, witnessed something quite remarkable and completely different. The subordinate males had enjoyed, if that is the right verb, brief periods of ascendancy while the females were in heat. As Markus wrote:

> The hierarchy changed almost daily with a new alpha male establishing himself after winning a fight...During this period of tremendous change, all three males mated with the alpha female during her heat period. Interestingly, though, although the male hierarchy changed frequently, only the alpha male of the day would mate with the alpha female.

Another fascinating observation of this changing interaction was that the lowest-ranked male, which was normally timid, lost his shyness, but only when he was top dog. As soon as he fell from grace, he reverted to his standoffish behaviour.

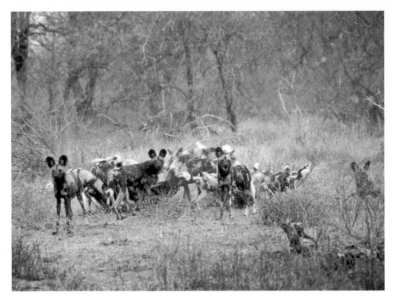

Wild dogs—one of the most beautiful sights in Africa. (Photo by Cobus Raath)

MICHELE AND MARKUS HAVE LEFT MADIKWE and are both now working in Kruger National Park, Michele in charge of public relations for the scientific services department, so she no longer has to feed young zebras from either in front or behind. Markus is chief veterinary officer for the park, which involves him in many things including Tb research and translocations. But he has not lost his interest in the wild dogs of Madikwe, which still thrive and continue to breed, although they did suffer another rabies outbreak in 2000. None of the vaccinated adults died, and three of the eleven unvaccinated pups also survived. More dogs have been introduced, in order to ensure the genetic health of the packs, and Markus concludes, in his most recent report, that it is "accepted that wild dog introductions in small numbers will need constant monitoring and even frequent introductions to sustain the populations." He also states that regular vaccinations will have to be a part of the program.

Markus's Madikwe model has become the accepted norm for wild dog introductions throughout Africa. In 1997, as reported in the IUCN document mentioned above, there were only from three to fifty-five thousand wild dogs, in perhaps six hundred to one thousand packs, remaining in Africa. The time may come when Markus's method, or a further modification of it, will become a key tool in conservation of the species.

The attitude to wild dogs has changed a great deal since 1914. Although many small holders and farmers still dislike them, a lyrical sentence written by David MacDonald in the preface of that IUCN report sums up the alternative attitude:

> To nominate one sight as the most beautiful I have seen might, in a world filled with natural marvels, be considered disingenuous. Yet, of images jostling for supremacy in my memory, it is hard to better the bounding forms of African wild dogs, skiffing like golden pebbles across a sea of sunburnt grass at dusk. ✳

17

THE
PREGNANT
LION

*Jo and I find ourselves camping
in Namibia's Caprivi Strip as I join
a team working on lions and hyaenas.*

ONE TROUBLE WITH LIONS is that while you are conducting a pregnancy test, you need always be aware of what you can learn from the lion's front end. It is there that the first signs of awakening from anaesthesia will occur.

The pregnancy check was fairly routine, as the swollen belly of the lioness made her condition pretty obvious, but it was reassuring to feel the hard masses of at least two cubs inside her. As I gently pressed down with my right hand against the slight upward pressure of my left hand underneath her, I felt one of the cubs move.

I fervently hoped that none of her relatives were lurking in the grass and watching me. As for her head, all was quiet.

My examination of the lioness that night followed a practised procedure conducted by the men I was with. I certainly wouldn't have been able to be as up-close-and-personal with her if I was without the aid of some bait, some drug-filled darts and the support of a team.

Here I was, in October 1997, working with a team led by veterinarian Mike Briggs of Chicago's Brookfield Zoo, who for most of his career has had a special interest in wild carnivores. Another team member was Kallie Venske, the heavily built, grizzle-headed chief warden from Etosha National Park. The three of us, sitting in a four-wheel drive vehicle started out our evening waiting for a call over the two-way radio from Lue Scheppers.

Just before dusk Lue, a tall blonde rough-hewn Namibian game warden, had gone ahead of our group, shot a warthog for bait, and tied it to a nearby tree with a length of two-centimetre diameter cable. The cable would prevent any lions that showed up from pulling the carcass away and out of the limited range of Lue's dart gun. We then all joined up, and Lue unloaded loud speakers from the back of his vehicle and tested the system as we stood, watched and listened. Once it was all set up, the rest of us moved off about a kilometre, in order to minimize potential disturbance to any incoming lions, and left Lue in his vehicle.

By 2:00 A.M., we'd been listening on and off to tape recordings of lions fighting over a kill for six and a half hours. A series of grunts and snarls had come over the air, just as if a pride of lions were scrapping over a carcass. Played over loud speakers fit for a small rock concert, the sounds were supposed to attract any lion within miles.

"You're just using the lion tapes," I had said, "not those of lions and hyaenas fighting over a kill that the South Africans favour."

"Ja, we have had good success with this version, so we stick to it," said Lue. "What I usually do is to sit quietly until I am fairly sure that the lions are on the bait, feeding well, and then I turn on the red spotlight, which doesn't seem to bother them, so that I can fire the darts."

Lue's technique is not new. Hundreds of lions have probably been darted in this way since detailed studies of lion biology that required them to be immobilized, including radio collaring, were first carried out over twenty years ago. When the hoped-for pride arrives, they are darted from the vehicle and do not appear to take much notice of the red spotlight that is used by the humans to work by. Darts strikes are probably perceived as mere pricks, or maybe taps from a rival wanting to get at a choice part of the carcass.

The technique is also not without its risks, most of which are for the people involved. It's important to make sure that all the animals in a pride have been darted before anyone gets out of the vehicle. There's also the danger that animals from other prides might come in after hearing all the growling. One member of the study team must be alert and make sure that no animal is more awake than is safe, although in our case that night, with just two lions to watch, this was not a problem. I imagine that with a dozen immobilized animals lying over a larger area the situation would require careful monitoring. The risks of the actual drugging are minimal, since drug technology has advanced to a sophisticated level. Once the animals are down, routine health checks can be carried out. Once those are done, the team should remain with the animals until they wake up so that no potential rivals attack them.

When the lions arrived, Lue darted both animals from the safety of his Land Cruiser. Soon, the lions were lying on their sides, bathed in a pool of light coming from the vehicle parked no more than ten metres away. Ten metres farther on the light faded rapidly and beyond that lay who-knows-what in the pitch dark of the African night, a sliver of the old moon just appearing over the horizon, not enough to make any difference.

My burly bearded colleague, Mike Briggs, approached the animals with commendable caution, prodded them with a pole he kept in the vehicle and pinched the upper ear of each in turn. Their lack of reaction was reassuring and meant that we could all get out and start work. I followed Kallie from my somewhat uncomfortable seat astride the gear shift, stethoscope in hand, and checked the vital signs of the lioness. Heart rate, sixty beats a minute, six breaths in thirty seconds. All was well.

I heard Lue say, "That's one dart, I'll get the other one. Then I'll get my rifle and keep an eye on things, but I don't think there are any more out there."

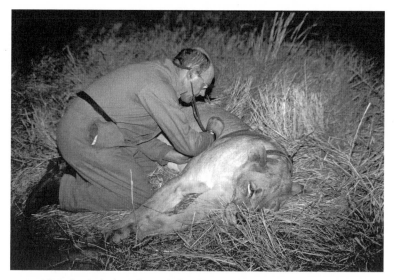

2:00 A.M.: the author checks the vital signs of a darted lion in the Caprivi Strip.

He pulled the six-centimetre dart from the lioness' shoulder and walked over to the male lying not more than two metres away. Another aluminum-bodied dart was glinting in the glare of the truck headlights as it stuck up from his hip, the orange tailpiece clearly visible. Lue leaned over and, with a scalpel in his hand, made a nick in the lion's skin, just beside the dart, and pulled it out.

Next came the pregnancy check. As she lay on her side I put my left hand under her abdomen, pressed up gently and simultaneously pushed down with my right hand.

"That's a pretty easy call," I said to Mike, who was standing beside me. "You could even feel some movement in there." I let go and pointed to her abdomen.

"Not exactly rocket science," he said as he knelt down beside her back leg, needle holder and blood tubes in hand.

"Can you hold off the vein for me Jerry?" Mike asked as he removed the cap from the needle and leaned forward. I turned sideways, put one hand under her hock and pressed down with the other on the vein as it coursed across the bone just above the joint. Mike slipped the needle into the vein with practised ease and we watched as the succession of tubes filled up with dark red blood.

"I suppose you do a full panel," I said. "Do you run any hormones as well?"

"Yeah," he replied. "We pull the blood, extract the serum, freeze it in the liquid nitrogen and get it back home for a full range of things."

"Any particular diseases you're interested in?" I continued, thinking mainly of the canine form of distemper. The disease had first been recognized in lions only three years previously, some two thousand kilometres northeast of us in Tanzania's famous Serengeti National Park. There were also several other cat viruses whose antibodies have been detected in the species that Mike would be checking for.

"Yes, we want to do a full panel, but we very much want to find out if this population of lions can be safely used as semen donors for other areas, or for captive lions in zoos, so the disease thing is pretty important."

We were in a remote corner of Namibia's Caprivi Strip, which we had reached after travelling from South Africa via Botswana and meeting up with Lue, a who was our local contact in Katima Mulilo, which lies on the banks of the Zambezi River, not far from Namibia's easternmost border with Botswana.

"After you get your shopping done," Lue had said, "just come back on to the main road and then go straight until the first left, about 150 kilometres from town. Follow that track until you see the sign to Lianshulu Lodge and check about the track to Buffalo Camp with them. Mike and I will be there in a couple of days."

We headed out on the newly tarred road, which stretched as far as the eye could see in an absolutely straight line, rather like some of the grid roads in my home province of Saskatchewan. One difference between the two was that here the road was lined on both sides with heavy bush, instead of vast fields of crops, making the view very limited. Another difference was that there was not a single turn-off of any sort until we reached that 150-kilometre mark.

We were headed to a campsite that had once been popular with hunting guides to await the arrival of Lue, Mike and Kallie, who were studying lions in the area and would join us in a week's time.

While on a visit to the Brookfield Zoo in 1996 I had met up with Mike, a long-time friend from numerous zoo and wildlife veterinary conferences. It soon transpired that I might be able to join him on one of his projects, as he was conducting carnivore research in Namibia and would be there just about the same time as we were scheduled to be in southern Africa at the start of my sabbatical leave from the university. We were now in the second month of that leave.

A quick look at the map of southern Africa will show that Namibia has an odd shape. The odd bit is the Caprivi Strip, which drives due east, like an old-fashioned bloodletting lancet, at the extreme northern corner of the country, toward the heart of the region. The reason for this narrow extension to the boundary has nothing to do with tribal affiliations and everything to do with Victorian-era politics. At the 1890 Berlin Conference, the Germans, who had colonized Namibia—which was then called South-West Africa—gave up their claim to sovereignty of the east coast island of Zanzibar in exchange for access to the Zambezi River and Africa's interior. The strip, about four hundred kilometres long, was added to South-West Africa and named for the German chancellor who rejoiced in the name of General Count Georg Leo von Caprivi di Caprara di Montecuccoli.

At its narrowest, the strip is no more than about forty kilometres wide, but near the eastern tip it widens out as its western and southern borders become the river that is variously named (according to which country it flows in) the Kwando, the Linyati and finally the Chobe. This river divides the strip from Botswana before it joins the Zambezi just above Victoria Falls. It was into the tip of the strip, the blade of the lancet, that we were headed to work in one-thousand-square-kilometre Mudumu National Park, one of the three national parks in the region.

Over 430 species of bird have been recorded in the park, and the mammals that may be seen there, according to guide books and web pages, include small populations of the swamp-dwelling sitatunga (which we had never seen), as well as red lechwe, elephant, buffalo, roan, sable, kudu, impala, oribi, zebra and wild dog, with spot-necked otter, hippo and crocodile in the waterways.

When we met him Lue had said, "Buffalo Camp is no longer used by either tourists or hunters, but we like it because it is right on the riverbank, only about a twenty-minute drive from the lodge, has lots of shade and is peaceful."

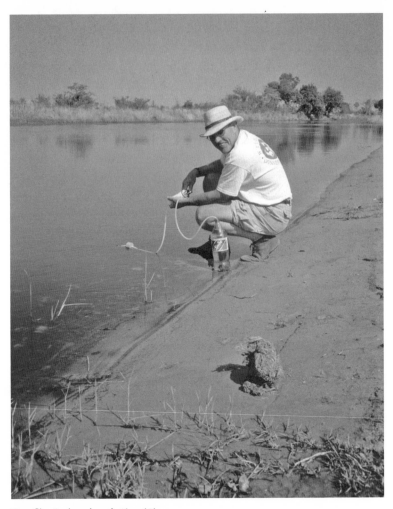

Water filtration hazards on the Linyati River.

Worried about the fact that we were driving a small sedan rather than something more substantial with four-wheel drive, the lodge manager accompanied us to the old site, which was a real boon, as we could easily have missed it. Africa had claimed its own, and there were no obvious signs of previous occupation at the camp. However, the site had been well chosen. It lay about five metres above the river and was shaded by three large and leafy fig trees whose roots could be seen in the bank where the water had eroded the soil. The slight

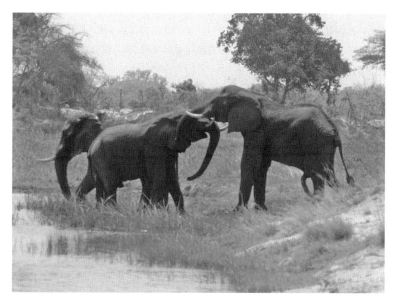

Elephant in musth at the Linyati River.

elevation gave us a steady breeze, and at any time of day one would be in shade.

Not twenty metres away, the river was easily accessible along a sandy beach, and here we had access to fetch water, although we soon learned to choose our moments for doing so.

On our second day in camp a herd of about one hundred elephants came down for a midday drink and splash, just upstream. We sat in our easy chairs and watched through the leaves for over three hours as the young submerged themselves and charged in, out and around, between and under adults, while the older ones rolled and splashed.

About half-way through the proceedings I noticed a big bull heading for the river with a determined walk, and whispered to Jo, "Check out that guy: he's got an impressive erection. See its s-shaped curve?"

I suggested we check though our binoculars for the telltale waxy secretions from the temporal glands on the side of the bull's head, behind and level with the eye. I reckoned he was probably in musth, and the secretions might help confirm my guess, although in African elephants secretions from those glands are seen at other times as well, and even in females.

We lifted our binoculars, more or less in unison. The secretion showed up clearly, and through the lenses the penis became truly impressive.

"Is that the same as musth in Indian elephants?" asked Jo.

"Just about. It was Joyce Poole, whom we met at Pilansberg, who worked it all out in Amboseli. He's too far away to see if there is any green stuff dripping from his penis, which Joyce saw before she had fully worked out the musth thing. She even called it Green Penis Syndrome. Their testosterone goes off the scale, and they get dangerously aggressive. They chase off younger bulls and gain access to females in heat. If there's another bull in musth down there, we could see a hell of a fight."

As it turned out, all the other bulls backed off, and the latecomer began to pay close attention to one particular female.

For several hours after this show we could not get water that was even slightly clear from the river. The soil stirred up by all the bathing and the enormous volume of vegetable matter left behind by the animals combined to make it impossible. Passing the suspended organic particles through our filter proved too much for it, and it clogged within moments.

The other thing that disturbed the water, but for a much shorter time, was the passage of a fan-driven air boat carrying heavily armed members of the Botswana border patrol. We sneaked a picture of them as they headed upstream. It would not have been wise to let them know what we were doing.

For our baths, we simply went down to the beach, checked for crocs, filled a large plastic bowl, and sluiced each other off in total open-air privacy amidst the sounds and smells of Africa.

Eventually, Lue and Mike arrived. The final member of the research team was Kallie Venske, who arrived a couple of days later. We soon found out that they all had a prodigious capacity for two things: beer and meat, in various forms. The chosen beer was Castle, the South African brew in its pale golden can, and the meat was a Braai pack, just like the ones we encountered recently in South Africa, one of which each of them consumed, in its entirety, every evening. Vegetables probably made up no more than 5 per cent of their camp diet, and the offer to share our greens was not quite mocked but certainly turned down. They did show us how to make camp bread in the three-legged cast iron pot that is called a *potjie*, using as a yeast source what else but beer?

Mike, heavily built to begin with, and showing some belly evidence of his liking for beer, showed me his impressive array of equipment.

"We've got liquid nitrogen for storing blood and tissues, particularly for DNA banking, as well a good microscope, semen-freezing equipment and of course drugs and other medical inventory," he said.

"How many lions do you think we'll get?" I had asked.

"It would be nice to get ten or so. There are one or two around here that I've done before, so I hope we catch up with them, and then there should be others."

For three days nothing happened. And it wasn't as if we were simply swanning about trying to find lions. That would have been quite fruitless and completely unproductive.

For two nights after the team had assembled, Lue spent the dark hours sitting in his truck, about one kilometre from camp, fruitlessly waiting as the odour of the kudu that he had shot became stronger and stronger in the African heat and his tape player, which we could clearly hear, did its thing. We simply stayed in our tents and got our eight hours of sleep. Finally, on the third dawn, we heard the growl of his diesel engine and he arrived in a cloud of dust to announce that we had our first capture.

Naturally, we all piled into the vehicles—all except Jo, who slept on after a brief wake-up—and drove back to find just one immature male lion, with a radio collar attached, who had finally either heard the noises or smelled the bait. We collected all the usual samples, but Mike already had enough data from two previous years of study to know that there was no point in trying to collect semen, the testicles of this youngster not yet being well enough developed. Even the animal's DNA was known, but we thought the serum samples might yield something new, if the patient had contracted some disease agent since he was last handled.

After breakfast it took no time at all for the team to decide to look elsewhere, and so we packed up and moved on. Jo and I were told that there was absolutely no chance of our little sedan being able to get across the semi-desert sandy terrain through which we were headed. We would have to ride in the open back of Mike's Land Cruiser. The dust billowed up over the tailgate and enshrouded us for the entire trip. We could see the sun only as a bright haze. Within moments I don't think either of us had been quite so filthy in our lives.

The new camp was located in a beautiful grove of twenty-metre-tall trees that had grown up entirely because a queen termite, at some distant time in the past, had landed and started her new colony in the sand, thereby stabilizing the light soil and allowing seeds to take root. The entire area had similar groves, each about half a hectare in size, scattered at intervals of about two hundred metres for many kilometres in every direction.

Bathing was a bit more of a problem at this camp. Although close, the river here was fairly steeply banked, and the only access to it was down the narrow paths that had been created by hippos as they entered and left the water. Our technique for bathing here was to stand at the top, slightly to one side of a run. One of us would quickly go down to the water's edge and fill the plastic bowl with a small bucket. Then, as we both kept a lookout for crocs, we would sluice each other as before.

In order to search for lions, we took longer trips away from camp and sat for long hours just waiting. When we arrived at Lue's chosen location, this time with the aforementioned warthog carcass, we chatted for a while as the electronic equipment was unloaded from the back of the Land Cruiser.

Lue asked, "What is your wife doing while we are out here?"

"Sleeping soundly I imagine," I replied.

"She isn't scared?"

"I don't think so. We do lots of camping in bear country at home, and we've been in Africa many times."

He seemed impressed, but we had already determined in our own minds that he was somewhat of a male chauvinist. Perhaps he was finally coming to terms with having a woman in camp, something with which he had been patently uncomfortable at the beginning of the trip.

We suffered two long and sleepless nights, with not a lion in sight. Jo had also missed some sleep, as lions roaring quite close to our base had disturbed her, although they were across the river from us.

"Hoping that it might work for lions as it does for bears at home, I grabbed the tea billy, a torch, a spoon to rattle in the tin and Jerry's filleting knife," she said when we returned. At least it made her feel comfortable. Now Lue was definitely impressed.

It was on the third night that we got the two lions. Lue was in charge of watching out for other lions, or maybe even hyaenas that might be on the prowl and could have heard the tapes. There are records of as many as a dozen animals of one pride being darted and studied at one time, but this never happened for us. We had no trouble collecting and freezing the male's semen. We tried to lure lions for two more nights, but without success.

The reasons for the scarcity of lions in that part of the Caprivi Strip were not long in emerging. A senior government bureaucrat had signed an order allowing cattle herders to shoot lions that were killing their cattle, even inside the park. The fact that the cattle were grazing illegally inside a park did not seem to warrant any consideration, and we had no idea how many lions had been killed under these circumstances. To add to our problems, the lions were somewhat shy of humans, as just across the river from our camp on the old termite mound, we could see the palm-thatched roof of an up-market safari hunting camp run by Botswanans.

On the sixth night, we drove a much longer distance, around some lakes, because Kallie had received radioed news that there was a dead elephant being scavenged by lions and hyaenas and we might be able to achieve something there. Lue and Kallie disappeared for about two hours as Mike, Jo, who had decided to join us as a change from sleeping, and I waited in the second vehicle. Suddenly we saw the headlights, and before we were out of the cab, Lue and Kallie were pulling spotted hyaena bodies out of the back of the Toyota. Four animals were lined up side by side and we began to work on them.

At this point it is relevant to remind the reader that a hyaena, or maybe more than one at a time, can very easily get right inside the carcass of an elephant. It is also necessary to note that the particular

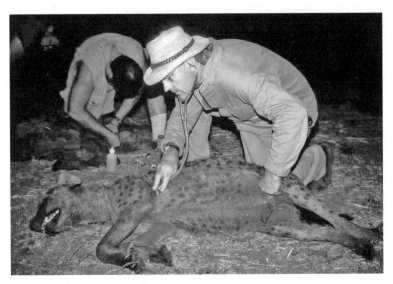

The author checks the heart sounds of an adult hyaena.

elephant these hyaenas had been feasting on had been dead for at least four days, "cooking" in daytime highs above 30°C, and that the pack had been feasting on it from day two. Then there is the little matter of temperature and decomposition. To add a little spice, one of them had vomited in the back of the vehicle, and the product of this action (rotten elephant meat) was generously smeared over the coats of the other three. In case anyone has not yet got the message, these hyaenas stank. Phenomenally.

Putting aside the little matter of olfactory sensitivity, as, after all, a vet is occasionally subjected to powerful smells, there was one thing I particularly wanted to see close up, which is the unusual arrangement of the female sex organs.

There has long been a myth that spotted hyaenas are hermaphroditic, misinformation that is likely due to the unusual arrangement of the external genitalia. Only recently have Laurence Frank and his colleagues at the University of California at Berkeley shown, in a series of sophisticated experiments, how it is that the female genitals develop so differently than those of other mammals, and how, therefore, the myth may have developed and persisted. However, not all ancients held the belief. Among those who debunked it was Aristotle, who

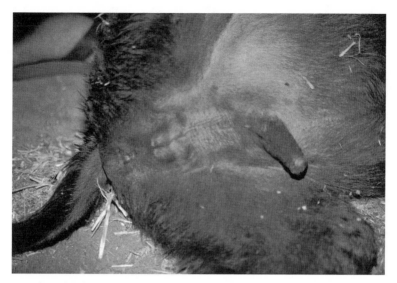
External genitalia of a juvenile spotted hyaena.

lived from 384 to 322 BCE and who is considered by most to have been one of the great natural historians of all time. A. L. Peck's 1970 translation of Aristotle's *Historia Animalium* has the following sentence: "The statement has been made that the hyaena has both male and female sexual organs; but this is untrue." Even if Aristotle's actual descriptions are a bit convoluted, he does write: "In fact, the sex-organ of the male is like that of the wolf and the dog"; and ends up with a clear statement. "The female hyaena has a uterus as the other female animals have which are of that sort."

I knew, from diagrams and photos, why the hermaphrodite myth had persisted, but here was an opportunity to see it first hand. I was in luck. We had an adult male, an adult female and two juveniles in the group. The adult male was easy to identify, penis in its sheath and testicles tucked up close to the body but freely moving in the scrotum, not unlike a dog's. The adult female's organs showed clearly why the hermaphrodite myth developed. First, she had no genital organs like those of the bitch or mare below her tail. No vulva, in fact. Second, there was a pair of hard fibrous round masses under the skin where testicles would have been had she been a male. Third, she had a sheath, very like that of the male, but of course no penis inside it, merely with an opening at the tip. The sheath is, in fact, the clitoris. Finally, and the dead giveaway that she was a female, there were two large nipples, obviously used, on either side of the sheath. The youngsters showed why a cursory examination could easily fool the less than careful observer. The sheath was plain to see, as were the two hard lumps behind it, but in neither of these juvenile females were there testicles, but just those fibrous immovable masses. As these animals had never borne litters, there was no mammary development, so the nipples gave no clues.

For the acts of mating and parturition, the elongated clitoris can create problems. While hyaenas have no doubt worked out how to breed, giving birth through the narrow channel has its risks. Stillbirth is not uncommon, the skin often tears, and as many as 18 per cent of first-time hyaena mothers die giving birth.

The work of Frank and his colleagues has shown that the unusual arrangement of the reproductive organs, and all that follows, goes back to hormonal events that occur very early in the life of the fetus. Of course these events still do not, and probably cannot, answer the question as to which came first, female dominance in hyaena society or hormonal changes in early pregnancy. Another example of the chicken and egg question.

It is extraordinary, knowing what we know about hyaenas and their organs, that I was able to find an article on the web that had been published in *Travel Africa* magazine online in 1998. The author was one Angus Begg. In it he stated that on a nighttime game drive, a young Kruger National Park ranger called Willempie "explained that the hermaphrodite hyaena has both male and female sexual organs and that the female is bigger than the male in order to protect the cubs from the father, who has a tendency to eat them." I just hope that it is Begg who misunderstood or misquoted the information, or that the editors made a typo, as I know that South African game guides and rangers go through rigorous training before qualification, and I cannot imagine that the hermaphrodite story persists as "fact." Perhaps Willempie presented the story as a myth, and the author wrote it down thinking it was fact.

After the interesting, if stinky, experience with the hyaena, we continued failing to find lions, and it soon became obvious that attempts at lion capture in the area were going to be unproductive. Jo and I said farewell to the rest of the team and headed for the fabled Okavango Delta in Botswana for a bit of a break from the grind and filth of three weeks of camping rough. Kallie headed back to Etosha to see how much damage had been done to the lodge kitchen that had caught fire while he was away, and Mike stayed on with Lue for a couple more nights of effort, just in case the luck turned.

I FOUND HOW THE REST OF THE TRIP HAD GONE when I next saw Mike a year later at the 1998 zoo and wildlife veterinarians convention in Omaha.

"Yes, we did see another lion, but not quite as we had hoped," he told me over a beer in the hotel lounge. "We were only about four miles from where you left us and had decided to just sleep in the open, not putting up the tent. Suddenly, about midnight, there was the most god-awful racket, a mixture of snarls, howls and grunts, and then a big male lion chased a terrified hyaena right through the camp, between the fire and our bags. We didn't get a lot of sleep after that."

Mike also told me that upon Kallie's return to Etosha, where we heard that the whole canteen had burned down, he was subjected to a nasty shock. He had been summarily dismissed and accused of setting the fire to the canteen (a bit difficult to do when you are three hundred kilometres away). Mike said that that a political appointee with almost no experience of park management had superseded Kallie. Welcome to the world of politics. ❋

18

TIME OUT IN BOTSWANA AND NAMIBIA

Jo and I take some time out to relax and do some touring, as well as try to set up some future research work. A San man shows us how ostriches are important in his culture, but he has trouble believing my account of ostrich medicine.

IT WAS TIME TO TAKE A BREAK FROM CAMPING, especially the rough camping that we had been doing as we sat and waited for those lions in the Caprivi Strip. We had not seen the bottom of a glass of water for over three weeks, as anything we filtered still retained the colour of fairly strong tea (actually a mixture of mud and hippo dung), and the very thought of a cold lemonade or possibly the potential hedonism of a dish of ice cream determined our next move.

Only an hour or so west of our encounter with the hyaenas, we turned south and headed into Botswana again, exchanging South African Rand for Pulas. On our first border crossing we had fallen for the

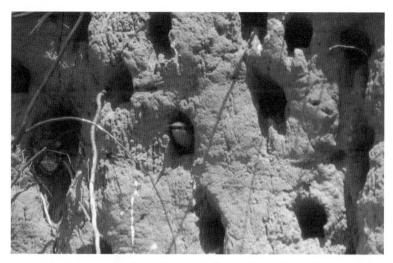

A carmine bee-eater emerges from its nest hole, unaware that a monitor lizard has paid a visit to its neighbour.

old "We have no change, so I'm afraid we can only give you 190," when we had given them 250 Rand.

"What is the real rate?" I had asked.

"One hundred and ninety-five."

This time we were prepared for the lack of change, which may have been real, or maybe a convenient way to make a few cents or more on a daily basis if repeated often enough. We handed over the exact amount needed for a round sum in the local currency.

Drotsky's Cabins, on the west bank at the head of the Okavango Delta, was the first place that we came to, and we could not have made a better stop if we had had hundreds to choose from. Jan and Eileen had a cabin for us, and we definitely spent an unreasonable amount of time in the shower washing our filthy clothes and ourselves.

There were several magic moments in the next few days. The first morning, cruising slowly downstream in the lodge boat, we came upon a nesting colony of the aptly named carmine bee-eaters. This must surely be one of Africa's great sights. There were hundreds of these glorious birds flitting in and out of their nesting holes in the sandy bank and briefly resting on an overhanging tree. Of the numerous photos I took

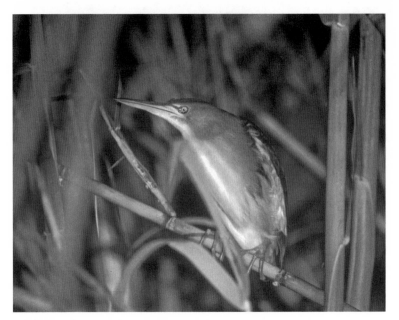
Little bittern in the papyrus, Okavango River.

of this place, where we spent the best part of an hour, one shows, upon careful viewing, the principal non-human predator of the birds. While we were watching and photographing and marvelling at the subtle changes in blues and pinks, a monitor lizard lay motionless at the mouth of a nest hole where he had presumably been feasting on eggs or young chicks. No more than one metre to his left a mature bird sat at the mouth of its hole seemingly unaware of the danger.

We sat that evening and sipped a cold one in the bar, with the sun setting blood red behind us. A steady stream of great white egrets settled in ones and twos on the papyrus as delicately as a *corps de ballet* as they came in to roost. I enthused about the bee-eaters to Jan. He responded with some information that brought us back down to earth.

"There a sad side to this," he said. "Poachers come at night with weighted nets. They drop them over the face of the bank and in the morning the birds emerge, just like you saw them. They can catch hundreds at one go. Whole colonies have been wiped out."

"What do they do with them? asked Jo.

"Eat them."

We saw many other birds near the water and naturally took a pile of photos of African fish eagles, in the process learning how it is that so many really good pictures of these glorious birds, which are seen by many as the icon of Africa, are taken as they swoop on a fish. The boatmen on the delta were adept at placing a shortish piece of papyrus under the skin of fish that they have purchased in the local market. The papyrus floats, and the eagles act as though trained, like winged Pavlovian dogs. As the boat approaches a roosting bird, the helmsman starts to make an eagle-like cry and waves the fish over his head. Meanwhile the photographer has specified where the bait is to be thrown, with due regard to lighting conditions, lens length, background and so forth.

The fish is thrown, lands in the water and floats; the bird swoops and grabs; and the photo is taken. With motor drives, auto-focusing lenses and fast film, the memory is sealed.

One boat trip was not going to be enough, and the next day we travelled this way on another boat trip to photograph the eagles with new acquaintances Ian and Pepe Shaw, who were near the beginning of what would be a year-long honeymoon that had started in South Africa's port of East London, whence they had shipped a long-wheelbase Land Rover that they had had kitted out in England for an extensive African safari. Ian owned a restaurant in London's Covent Garden and kept in touch with the staff by e-mail through his Apple laptop and the satellite above the South Indian Ocean, which he could dial into with the dish that was part of his safari kit. He and Pepe would travel widely, camping most of the time, except when, like us, they needed a break and a laundry stop. As a passport to village campsites, they had packed a couple of dozen soccer balls, which they inflated and then invited the villagers, especially the children, to join them.

As Ian put it, "Half the time the children and young men want to play soccer, the other half volleyball, with one exception. In one village in western Zambia all they had wanted to do was play 'kick the ball into the river and chase it.'"

After four days at the cabins, we moved on to another lodge owned by the Drotsky family, from which we embarked on a poled dugout canoe (called a *mukoro*) deeper into the delta. We saw masses of birds,

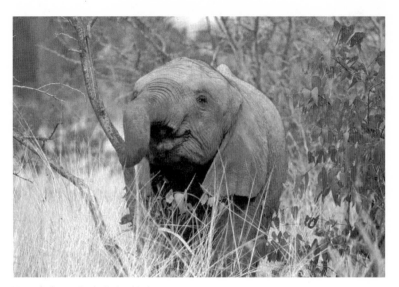

Young elephant at Etosha National Park.

each species identified for us by the boatman. We camped on an island under a tree from which we hung our mosquito net, the sky huge, dark and star-filled above us, the Southern Cross clearly visible and the Milky Way a hazy streak right across the dome above. Not an artificial light anywhere to pollute or dilute the effect.

Thence it was back to Namibia and the next leg in the sabbatical tour, where I was to set up a liaison with the veterinary staff at the headquarters of the Etosha park in the community of Okaukuejo, where Kallie Venske had just been given his nasty surprises: the fire and then the firing.

Etosha has been described as one of the great, and sparsely enjoyed, wildlife experiences remaining in Africa. It is the jewel in the crown of the Namibian park system, with restaurants, super rondavels (circular cabins, usually thatch roofed), shady campsites and all the facilities that one could want, including places to wash clothes, a shop and a post office. One of the features of the park is that at each camp and lodge site there is a large floodlit water hole, with a safety barrier around it and several powerful spotlights.

The park once contained an enormous lake fed by the Kunene River. Its name, Etosha meaning "the place of dry water," is a memo-

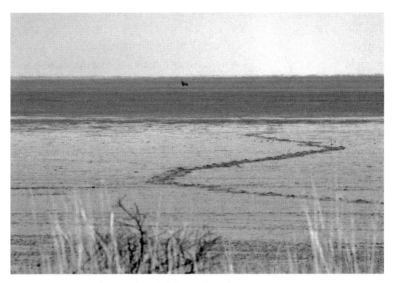
Only the zigzag tacks confirm that this gemsbok in Etosha Park is not a mirage.

rial to the fact that the pan dried up thousands of years ago when the river cut a new course. In the dry season, when we arrived, the vast bone-dry salt pan covers five thousand square kilometres. The heat shimmering off the surface created a hazy effect and, had it not been for the footprints zigzagging out onto the salt behind the animal that we could see a couple of hundred metres away, we would not have been certain that the grey body, with its black-and-white face and long straight horns, was a mirage or a real gemsbok.

The plan was to spend two or three days getting to know the park staff at this time, in late October, and make arrangements to return in February 1998 for a month during the wet season, when many animals throughout the park are found dead (usually from anthrax) and a good deal of veterinary input would be needed. However, the political events in Namibia made us change our minds, and we found plenty of other things to do.

On our first night, after dinner, we sat and watched the water hole near our tent for over an hour and saw a show that rivalled anything you could see on the stage, with a fine mixture of comedy and drama, almost Shakespearean in breadth. The spotlights trained on the area for the express purpose of facilitating viewing made things quite clear.

The show started rather slowly, as three elephants appeared out of the gathering dusk and began to drink and spray themselves. A couple of giraffes were standing nearby, unsure if the elephants were going to let them in. The giraffes were definitely apprehensive, and it soon became apparent why, as there was a good deal of noise from lions roaring quite close by. One of the giraffes then plucked up the courage and came in for a drink, bending in the ungainly manner of his kind. However he was soon interrupted by a herd of about forty elephants, which appeared like grey ghosts, completely silent, and took over the waterhole for a while.

They did not get things entirely their own way, though, because four Black rhino turned up and got sort of mixed up with the elephants. The rhino group appeared to consist of a mother, her large offspring and another youngster of perhaps six months of age, as well as an unrelated sub-adult. The first farcical moment in this drama happened when the youngster mock charged a very large old bull elephant, who was about fifteen metres away from him, quietly minding his own business. The mock charge consisted of the rhino bobbing up and down like a four-legged basketball, making sure that mother was close, and shaking his head at the elephant. Luckily for junior the old granddad decided that this nonsense was not worth bothering with.

Quite soon after this, a single black-maned lion turned up and tried to get a drink. He had no luck. He was chased off by the solitary sub-adult rhino and did not reappear while we watched.

The giraffes and rhino then had a drink together, as the elephants gathered to one side were a bit tentative, but then the elephants decided to get serious. Many of them got into the water and had a high old time rolling about and trumpeting. There were several small babies, including one of only a few months of age that did not really know what to do with his trunk.

A group of three female lions and some cubs turned up during the water show at which point the next item of farce occurred. Many of the elephants had left by this time, and the lions came to the water hole on the opposite side from the remaining elephants and tried to get an undisturbed drink. It was not to be. A teenaged male elephant decided to strut his stuff, like a young Prince Hal, and came right around the water hole to threaten the lions, most of which got the message. One cub, more daring than the rest, hung on but was finally routed when the elephant got within about eight metres. Having made his point, the teenager wandered back to his group. However, as soon as he had gone a safe distance the lions returned to finish their drinks. Of course the young elephant saw them, and not content with having shown off once, he had to charge around the edge of the water and go through the whole bravado thing again.

We watched all this from the relative safety of a wall about fifty metres from the near edge of the pool. Every few metres along the path on top of the wall, signs admonished people not to camp here but to return to the official site. We later heard that one unconvinced tourist once decided that the top of the wall was a great place to spend the night. It was not a good decision as, tragically, he became a lion victim. The warnings were for real.

After three nights of camping we headed south from Etosha and visited several well-known tourist spots, including the amazing petroglyphs at Twyfelfontein, where our guide, Patrick, professed to a working knowledge of seven languages, including Japanese, German and French, as well as a burning desire to get a place in a tour-guide school in Johannesburg.

Along the way south to the Namib Desert, we called in at a park-cum-lodge called Intu Afrika. The whole place was a massive series of sand dunes, with a fine tourist lodge in their midst. Drinking chilled white wine at dusk amidst red dunes and scattered thorn trees was a great start to the visit. The highlight for us, though, was the visit to a San (formerly Bushman—part of the Khosian group of people) camp that is occupied more or less permanently by family groups of this ancient culture. Members come and go as they please, and lodge visitors are invited to visit if they wish. The managers of the lodge, Michael and Bets Daiber, both anthropologists, were making every effort to give these diminutive people a meaningful life, as their culture has been devastated by modern technology and government indifference, or sometimes downright hostility, as seems to be the case in Botswana.

Michael speaks the clicking language of the San people, and with him acting as interpreter, we met the group and introduced ourselves, the San giving us their biblical names—Anton, Joseph, David, Anna, Francine and Marie—which they then challenged us to repeat.

Anton, his milk-chocolate skin wrinkled like aluminum foil that has been crushed and opened up again, was the oldest male and became the spokesperson. He talked of ostriches.

"We use the shells for water storage in the desert," he said. He then mimed a digging effort. "We dig a hole in the sand, put in the shells full of water and cover everything. The water stays fresh for a long time. The wind soon hides our work, but we know the place."

As he pointed to the delicate necklaces of Anna and Marie he said, "We use the broken pieces of shell as jewellery."

He went on to described how well-adapted ostriches are to the desert.

"They even provide milk for their young. When the chicks are new they follow the mother and peck at the milk she passes." He mimed again, his left hand, fingers and thumb joined in a point pecking at the ground.

Rather than contradicting him, since birds do not produce milk, I held my tongue as he continued and went into what was obviously his main party piece.

"To catch ostrich we build a trap."

In no time he had built a small corral, no more than about twenty centimetres across, with sticks about thirty centimetres long sticking straight up out of the sand.

"Then we take some string, either from the bark of a tree or from an animal sinew, loop it around the top of the trap, stick in a piece of wood with a small branch to hold the string in place and pull it tight to a branch like this one." His stage had obviously been used before and was handily placed next to an acacia bush. He bent down a stout branch and tied the other end of the string to it with a quick knot.

"We put in some bits of ostrich shell"—he picked up a few chips from the pile where the necklace makers had been working and scattered them into the mini-corral—"and the trap is ready. When the ostrich comes along it cannot resist and reaches in to get them."

His mime changed as his whole body became an ostrich. He hung both arms down a few centimetres from his sides, palms backwards,

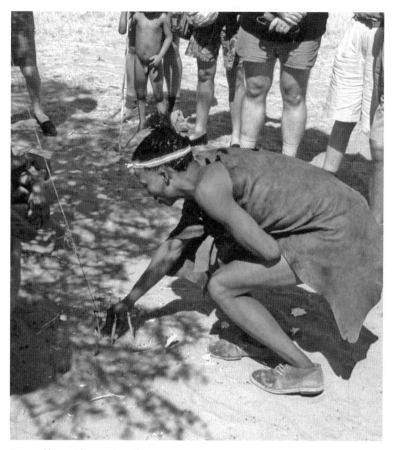
Anton and his ostrich trap at Intu Africa.

elbows loose. We were at once convinced about his "wings." Then he bent over and began to waddle, just like an ostrich inspecting the ground, and approached the trap again. He turned slightly and his right arm became a neck, the hand now a bird's head, with pointed fingers extended and thumb joining them in a point like a beak, exactly in the position that I used to use when casting shadows of a dog's head onto the walls of my children's bedrooms.

The head and neck went into the trap, grabbed a piece of shell that was tied to the key piece of wood and pulled up. The locked sliver of wood released, the branch above sprang up, the string tightened around his wrist and he was caught in the noose.

"The bird is now finished," he said. "It fights and struggles"—he obviously enjoyed this bit of the mime as his scrawny body, arm attached like a long neck, went dancing around like a dervish; indeed, just like a chicken with its head chopped off—"and as the string tightens his head soon comes off. He then runs around aimlessly until he crashes into a tree and we can then find him dead and get some delicious meat."

"What happens if he has chicks?" asked one of our party.

"Oh they stay with him and we can kill them easily."

Ostrich farmers, and at least two unfortunate veterinarians of my acquaintance, are well aware that alarmed ostriches are inclined to panic. If bird IQ could be measured, the ostrich would rank well below the turkey. Almost certainly in single figures. If they get their necks down between a couple of fence posts, and are then startled, they will pull straight back, which, if the fence posts are as wide apart as their necks, but considerably narrower than their heads, is detrimental to their well-being.

When his act was over and he invited comment, I tried to explain how ostriches are attracted to white objects, of almost any sort, and how I had even had a sick bird peck at the white toecaps of my rubber boots. I explained that the white of the "milk" was really a sort of bird urine (there was no point in getting too technical). The droppings of "milk" would indeed teach the chicks to peck at the ground, and they would thereby get nourishment from the other components in what the parent bird had passed and then learn to eat other things that might be on the ground nearby. Ostrich farmers are well aware of this fact and often use eggshell chippings mixed in with starter pellets to get new chicks to start feeding.

The old man was already looking pretty skeptical before I then explained, through Michael, how I had medicated sick ostriches in hospital by putting antibiotics inside marshmallows, which ostriches promptly eat. His look of skepticism turned to amazement as he asked, "Why would anyone want to give medicine to a sick ostrich?"

I covered this by talking briefly of the large-scale farming of these birds, not just in Namibia but also in many other African countries, and indeed in other parts of the world. At the time the prices being paid for breeding pairs were huge, tens of thousands of dollars, which would have probably been meaningless, so I just said that they were worth a lot of money.

"You have seen that other birds produce white stuff from the back, and they do not feed the young with that," I then said.

Anton then spoke briefly and Michael turned to me and said, "He says that you, too, must be a bushman. That's quite a compliment; I've never heard him say anything like that before."

"Not as good as you," I replied, looking straight at the old man.

Next morning we headed out for a walk with another member of the San community who was wearing no more than a jock strap made of duiker hide. However, I did see him take off his shorts before he left his compound; it seemed that his traditional and hyper-simple garb had now become a costume for the benefit of tourists. At one point on our guided walk, he had just shown us a few tracks in the sand, and we had identified the animals either through our field book, or by the size of the tracks, when he suddenly seemed to abandon us, sprinting off some twenty metres to a bush. Here, he extracted the bush's root with his digging stick, replaced most of it, and the plant above it, and rubbed his stomach while rolling his eyes, miming that it was for use as medicine for a sore gut.

From Intu Afrika it was onward for a few days near Swakopmund on the Atlantic coast and then a visit to the sand dunes and water hole at Sussusvlei.

At the coast we had one of the most unpleasant camping experiences of our lives. We set up our tent at a place we now recall with wry smiles as Mile 72. We were the only people there in an area that had over one hundred numbered camping spots. As we tried to cook a meal, the wind off the Atlantic seemed a bit strong, so we put our stove in the lee of the car. That was not enough, so we piled all our luggage between the car and the heat source. We even stood our camp beds on edge within half a metre of the cooking pot to reduce the affect of the wind on the stove. None of this was good enough, though, as the wind got stronger and the tent tried to take off. Only by placing the Gaz cooker about thirty centimetres upwind of the metal stand for our pans could we get anything even remotely warm. As if this performance were not enough, we "enjoyed" the doubtful privilege of ingesting about fifty grains of sand with each mouthful of what passed for supper. We had planned, and even paid for, a two-night stay, but to hell with the fee. We headed off early next morning to Swakopmund and the really comfortable Strand Hotel. Thank goodness they had a room for us.

The first thing that caught our eyes north of town was the Rössmund Golf Course. It was, at the time, almost all sand, but by 2007 it has become one of only five fully grassed desert courses in the world. At each tee box there was a patch of planted grass. The caddy—every golfer has one—carried a one-metre square of green carpet. Before the development of the full-grass fairways, the ball would be hit and when it reached the spot where the likes of Tiger Woods and Mike Weir would expect another hundred yards of roll, it simply plugged into what was really the world's biggest bunker. Of course, the carpet now came into play. The ball would be set on it, and the next shot taken. Depending upon the power and skill of the golfer, this process would be repeated a few times until the ball finally landed on the grass that had been planted, and no doubt extravagantly nursed, within some twenty metres of the green and its flag. Once on the grass, the usual rules of golf would come into play.

In Swakopmund we went to get the jammed tent zipper—no doubt affected by the Mile 72 winds and sand—fixed. The store owner, Peter, answered us in an almost pure Brooklyn accent, and we fell to chatting.

"I was a crop sprayer in the USA, a taxi driver in New York and worked in the garment trade in Montreal. You ever been there? Interesting city," he said. "When I retired I came home to Namibia. Within two months I became an instant paraplegic when my car was hit from the side. The only thing to do was to start again. I wasn't going to sit and mope, so I started this business. We employ half a dozen people, all handicapped in some way."

A fine man and a good example of not indulging in self-pity over unalterable circumstances.

After Swakopmund we continued our tour of Namibia with a must-do visit to see the amazing 1,500-year-old, two-leafed plant known to us only as *Welwitchia mirabilis*. This extraordinary plant gets its only mois-

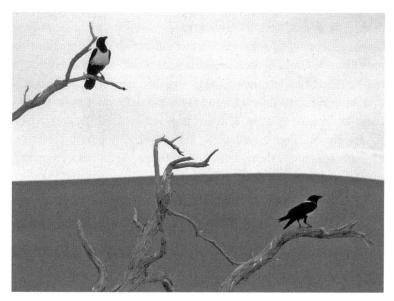

The yin and the yang. Pied crows at Sussusvlei, Namibia.

ture from the early morning mist that falls on it or the surrounding sand, so its root system spreads in a very wide circle around the base. One particular plant, about three metres from side to side, and just over a metre at its tallest, is thought to be the granddaddy of them all. It is fenced off so that visitors like us could not walk around it and possibly damage the delicate root system that lies just millimetres below the surface. The leaves grow and split, which gives the plant an appearance of having multiple greenery, but in fact the split ends of the two leaves all twist, coil and intertwine, making it look like a particularly bad hair day.

Following our homage to the *Welwitchia*, we continued on our trip and took another early morning walk into the oasis water hole of Sussusvlei, set amidst the dunes of the Namib Desert. Signs of animal life were restricted to desert-hardy gemsbok and a pair of pied crows perched on the dead trees beside the pan. The gemsbok can survive under the harsh conditions of desert areas because of adaptations that include their ability to dig down at least twenty centimetres and find roots and tubers, as well as their ability to raise their body temperatures by as much as five degrees Celcius on hot days or when short of water, which reduces fluid loss through sweating. The elevated temperature, to as much as 45°C causes the blood to heat up, and this would be dangerous for their brains if there were not also a special mechanism in their skulls to cool the blood before it reaches that sensitive tissue.

We tried the spiky melon fruits (that the gemsbok use for moisture) growing on the bushes along the path but found them too bitter. Later we learned that the Khosian people also used them as a vital source of water, but baked them first, to make the fluid palatable. They are apparently the precursor to the large juicy watermelons that we see in our supermarkets today.

After the trip south through Namibia, we turned east again into South Africa and spent a couple of nights with Hendrik and Gio van Eck, whom we had met six years previously when I was on a fact-finding tour about the world game-ranching industry. Hendrik had been a member of the United Party that opposed apartheid in the South African parliament in the dark days of that policy's ascendancy. Hendrik and Gio run a mixed farming/ranching operation near Campbell an hour or so west of Kimberley, in the Northern Cape province.

The ranch is mixed in a way that is familiar to many South Africans, where the term does not mean a mixture of dairy or beef cattle and crop growing, as it likely would in the northern hemisphere, but rather a mix of traditional livestock and game management. Altogether, the wild and domestic livestock are managed on almost 7,500 hectares. The land is harsh and dry and receives precious little rainfall. On it, the van Ecks run Dorper sheep and a large-scale hunting operation, which involves thirteen indigenous hoof-stock species such as wildebeest, impala, kudu and gemsbok that are not farmed so much as ranched, in that they are enclosed behind a game-proof fence, are offered mineral licks but are otherwise left to fend for themselves. As far as the owners are concerned, the hunting operation serves both as income and as a management tool to keep a balance between animal numbers and available feed, in the absence of predators.

Each client pays a license fee to the government, as well as a fee to the van Ecks. They are guided by ranch staff and all hunting is done on foot. Hendrik has introduced an extra element in the business in that the families of the guides become involved when meat packing and processing takes place. Hunts can be for trophies, at top prices, or for population control, when for instance a young person, accompanied by an adult, can be given the chance to go on a first hunt for the pot for a very reasonable fee.

GAME FARMING, OR HUNTING, is an integral part of land use in Africa. There are about six thousand licensed game ranches in South Africa, roughly one third of them members of the South African Game Organization, and regulations apply as to which species can be placed on the land. Many of the regulations are also concerned with the type of fencing that is used.

At Madikwe, where we observed the wild dogs, for example, there is a complex mix of high-tensile netting and many strands of electric fence, which means that they can keep any species, up to and including lions and elephants, on the property. The van Ecks have a much less expensive perimeter fence, which does not permit the keeping of predators or pachyderms.

Across South Africa there is an integrated and sophisticated industry that comprises all the sectors of any ranching operation of traditional livestock. Stocking densities, disease control, round-ups, auctions, translocations, hunting, venison sales and so on take place on a regular basis. Some ranchers breed endangered species, while others specifically aim to breed disease-free stock. There is a veterinary group allied to the industry through the country's professional veterinary association. Detailed, thoroughly researched and annotated texts have been produced, such as *The African Elephant* [or *Rhino* or *Sable*] *as a Game Ranch Animal*.

As in many parts of Africa, wildlife no longer roams free in South Africa as it did in former times. Whether they are kept in national, provincial, municipal or private game parks, much of South Africa's wildlife now has to be closely managed. In many parts of the continent, especially where human populations have expanded (or is that exploded?), with the land taken over by pastoralists or crops, there really is no longer room for wildlife to exist. In most parts of the continent an extra complication to the existence of wildlife has occurred with the invention of cheap and readily available automatic weapons.

As one Texas oil millionaire and philanthropist put it to us, when we visited his ranch and asked about the potential of returning some of his herd of scimitar-horned oryx to their native range in Niger, "There's no point, they've already been shot out once, and when everyone and his brother owns an AK-47 they wouldn't last a month." ❋

19

A TRIP TO ZANZIBAR

*Jo and I take a trip to the East African island of
Zanzibar, which is still caught in something of a
time warp. A surprise family connection, a Swahili
puzzle and a fishing trip with a difference.*

AT 11:30 A.M. ON TUESDAY AUGUST 25, 1896, the Sultan of Zanzibar,
H. H. Seyyid Hamed-bin-Thwain, died. Within half an hour his cousin,
Seyyid Khalid-bin-Barghash, proclaimed himself Sultan and seized the
palace. At the time, Her Majesty Queen Victoria's government ruled
the roost in the Indian Ocean through the power of their navy. Disap-
proving of Khalid, the English suggested that he "retire quietly." This
he refused to do and mustered his supporters, some seven hundred in
all, in the palace courtyard, where he had the ancient cannons primed
and shotted. The warship, the HHS *Glasgow* (built in Dunbarton, just
downstream from that Scottish city to which my father and I both
have connections), which he had "inherited" from his predecessor was

equipped with nine-pounder guns (muzzle loaders) and was ready for action in the harbour. She was up against five of Her Majesty's ships, the *Philomel*, the *Racoon*, the *Thrush*, the *Sparrow* and the *St. George* under Rear Admiral H. H. Rawson.

Edward Rodwell, Kenya historian and long-time newspaperman, tells the story of several ladies who were eyewitnesses to the events that followed. The ladies, including Mrs. Cave, the acting consul's wife, and a Mrs. Corning, were invited out to breakfast by Admiral Rawson's wife. The sultan had been warned that failure to capitulate would lead to a bombardment that would start at 9:00 A.M. on the Thursday morning. It did, with one minute's grace. The cease-fire was ordered at 9:45 after the palace flag was shot down. The *Glasgow* had returned some fire with her nine-pounder guns, but they were quickly silenced. By 10:45 she had sunk, her three masts and some rigging being the only visible remnants of her existence. Not surprisingly, Khalid became persuaded that he had made a false move, and he fled to the German consulate, whence he was removed to German East Africa (later Tanganyika). On August 27, Hamed-bin-Mahommed, a brother of the late sultan, was installed as sultan by Consul General A. Hardinge.

Shortly after the *Glasgow* sunk, a twenty-three-year-old naval lieutenant, newly commissioned to HMS *Cossack*, was standing on deck as the ship sailed into Zanzibar harbour. Using the dry plate camera that he had been given to him by his professional photographer father as a going-away present, he took some pictures of the vessel and the ruined palace and harem, even writing in his elegant hand that the men walking in front of the remains of the harem were chained slaves. The photographs lay hidden for over a hundred years.

Our own trip to Zanzibar, 101 years after the short military exercise at Zanzibar, was by no means as grand as that of the young naval lieutenant, although we did have a camera with us.

Jo and I had travelled overland as two of sixteen passengers on a smart truck-turned-bus with a tour company through Zimbabwe, Zambia and Malawi into Tanzania, where I could once more use my Swahili to converse.

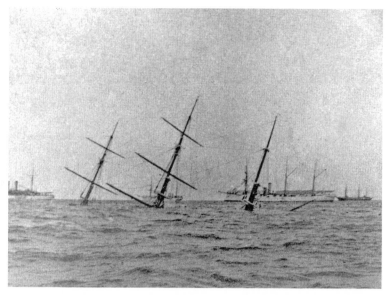

The SS *Glasgow*, the flagship of the Sultan of Zanzibar, sunk by the British Navy in 1896, lies in Zanzibar Harbour the day after the bombardment.

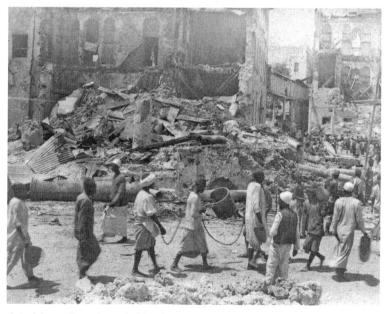

Chained slaves walk past the wreck of the sultan's harem's quarters after the shortest war in history.

We had left the bus in Dar es Salaam, which I had last seen during a rugby tour with the East African Scorpions in 1973, and after a night's sleep we boarded a morning ferry that was packed to the gills with all sorts of people, including many tourists, as the cacophony of languages attested. One tall slim Maasai, at least a couple of hundred kilometres from his ancestral home and cattle-herding culture, was working on deck, still clad in his traditional red *shuka*. The majority of the passengers were local coastal people. The Muslim men wore their brimless cloth hats, and most of the women were shrouded in black *buibuis* that rendered them virtually invisible, as their creed dictates, although the occasional flash of a bright cotton print skirt could be seen below the hem of the outer, more sombre, skirt. How and why black became the standard for this garment, given the heat, has always been a mystery to me.

The first surprise we had when we landed was that we had to have our passports stamped in the immigration shed at the port. Tanganyika and the island state of Zanzibar were united on April 23, 1964, and both adopted the name by which the country is now known—Tanzania—in October of that year. Despite this, the island's governors have obviously decided to cling to one last bit of their history, hence the extra passport check.

After an excellent biryani chicken lunch, we roamed the old town, now called Stone Town, with its narrow streets and fascinating history, ending up in the Anglican cathedral, which was built in 1873 on the site of the old slave market. The story goes that the altar was built right on the block where the infamous sales took place, and there is little other evidence of those ghastly events, except for one small low-ceilinged cell, where slaves awaiting their fates were crowded like packing cases in a warehouse.

For the next five nights we stayed in a simple hotel on the very northern tip of the island. The food was good, the beach was gorgeous, the beer and fresh lemon juice were cold and we could do as little, or as much, as we wished.

We snorkelled over the coral heads after sailing sedately on a dhow. We walked along the shore and chatted with the boat-builders, who were using tools, such as a bow drill, which must have been used in their craft for centuries.

Walking on the beach around us were tourists of other nation-
alities who seemed to have taken no notice of the requests by tour
guides, and indeed on notices posted at intervals in several languages,
asking us, particularly women, to respect the local culture and at least
wear a skirt and blouse. Most objectionable, to me, were the women
whose spandex bathing suits left absolutely nothing to the imagination, either below or above the waist.

One early morning, when the fishing boats came in, I walked up
to the local auction site at the top of the beach, where a small crowd
had gathered and two or three somewhat battered small lorries were
jammed together under the shade of a group of casuarina trees. A gov-
ernment-appointed auctioneer sonorously and sedately sold off the
night's catch. There were none of the frenetic run-together words of the
North American members of this ancient form of selling. As swordfish,
barracuda and others that I could not recognize came on the block, each
word was clearly audible, the current price was plainly stated, and the
fish sold just as readily as by any other method I had ever witnessed.

After the sale I chatted with the auctioneer and asked him about
his trade, the general state of the market and other related subjects.
Of course his version of Kiswahili was much more refined than my
own, which had never been *safi* (pure, classy) but had always been of
the up-country variety and was no doubt somewhat eroded by time.
A couple of times during our chat we came up empty. When he asked
me about my work, I explained that I was a vet (using the term *daktari
wa ngombe*, which literally means doctor of cattle). I had to then refine
this by saying *lakini si wa ngombe wenyewe, lakini wa wanyama wapori*,
which means "but not of cattle themselves, but of wild animals." Had
I known the true Swahili term for a vet I would have said *mwenye
elimu wa marathi za nyama*, which translates as "owner of knowledge
of disease of animals."

He then asked me a question that I failed to understand. "*Mambo
vipi?*" *Mambo* meant "things, affairs or conditions," according to context
and was easy, but *vipi* had me stumped. Only later, when I asked our
Tanzanian guide what it meant, did I learn that it is a very local term,
used widely in Zanzibar, and to some extent along the Tanzania coast,
which can be loosely translated to mean "what sort." All he had really

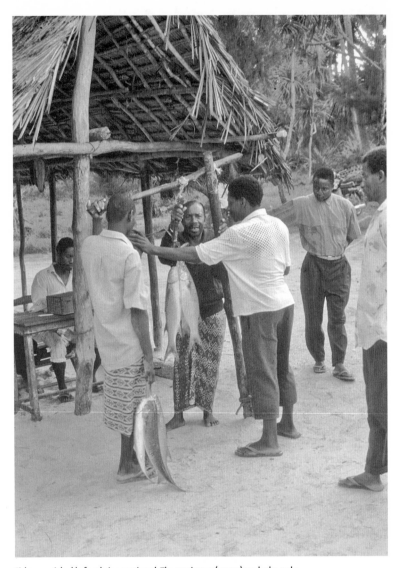

Fish are weighed before being auctioned. The auctioneer (centre) reads the scale.

been asking was what my work consisted of. Of course, we had circum-vented the language block, as one usually can in Swahili, and once he understood that I had worked with lions, elephants, rhino and the like, he asked another question, which was simply, "Why?" My best tactic seemed to be to use the example of something he would certainly know about, which was the death through disease of a large number of lions (almost one thousand of them) in Tanzania's world-famous Serengeti National Park. When I explained that the disease had been studied and diagnosed by people like me, he seemed satisfied.

"I am going to the Serengeti right after we leave Zanzibar. Maybe I will see a sick lion there," I told him.

"Yes, I remember something about that a few years ago, but I have not heard anything for about two years," he replied.

By now a small crowd had gathered to listen and join in. I guess not many tourists speak Swahili, or maybe it was the crude "up-country" Swahili that caught their ears, although none were impolite enough the say so. Because I knew that it would excite some interest I told him and the men nearby about darting, or as I clumsily put it "giving injections with a gun," to capture large creatures like elephant and rhino.

"What kind of medicine do you use to make them sleep?" asked a tall skinny guy to my right.

"The same sort that the doctor uses if you have to go to hospital for an operation, but much stronger." The men nodded, seemingly satisfied with the explanation.

Each evening, as the tide came in, we watched groups of ten or a dozen women wade out into the shallows, still fully covered in their buibuis, and form a circle before dropping a net into the water. Highlighted against the setting sun it was no doubt a scene that had been enacted for hundreds of years.

As I watched the women fishing I saw a couple of men pull up their dug-out canoe on the shore and realized I was missing out on an opportunity. I have been accused of having 10 per cent heron blood in my make-up. At least I never travel without fishing rods, so I approached the men about the chance of spending half a day with them. We set off early next morning, and after they had put up a small lateen sail, we moved sedately out to sea, beyond the reef, until they decided that they had reached a good spot. Down went the homemade anchor, joined with various lengths of rope of differing diameters, and we set up our hand-lines, with heavy lead weights at the ends. None of the lines were of less than twenty kilograms breaking strain, and each of the half-dozen hooks attached to little outrigger lines was baited with a small lump of some sort of fish. In the next five hours we pulled up about fifteen fish, none bigger than about three kilograms (6.6 lb). The most striking, and largest, was a gloriously red specimen with yellow fin tips and bright golden-yellow spots scattered over its body. Within about fifteen minutes of its being landed the colours had faded.

It was a spectacular day. We were well outside the reef, and to our east lay miles and miles of Indian Ocean, next stop possibly the Seychelles, or, if one missed them, many more miles to Indonesia. To our west, low on the horizon, Zanzibar and the Tanzanian coast. There was a gentle swell running, and as the day wore on the swell picked up.

I am not the world's best sailor, at least not when engines, especially diesel engines, are involved. The last time I had gone deep-sea fishing had been with Chris Nicholas, owner, sometime barman and occasional chief bar customer of the Ocean Sports hotel at Watamu on Kenya's glorious sandy coast just south of Malindi. We had been ferrying a moderate-sized fishing craft back to Kilifi. At first I did well, but then the fumes got the better of me and within a very short time I had lost my breakfast overboard. Within seconds a barracuda was hooked. Soon afterwards we got into a school of tuna. I was between vomiting bouts, sitting on the fishing chair, when my rod bent sharply. Even the adrenaline surge of the fish was not enough to quell my stomach, and I had to give up the rod to Chris. For a while after that, as Chris trolled back and forth through the school, passing close to the gulls feeding on some unseen fry as the tuna took them from below, it seemed as if we caught a fish every second time I puked. I suppose that I was chumming the water. At any rate we caught five before it was over. Give me a quiet trout stream or a canoe any time.

I can go all day in a good blow in a yacht, as long as I am working the sails. Sitting in a narrow hollowed log, with about ten inches of freeboard, anchored with a lump of unidentifiable machine part a long way below, is, in my book, something between the diesel engine and the yacht. I began to feel a little queasy, and, knowing that the fishermen would find my weakness completely incomprehensible, I wondered what to do. Then I remembered a simple lesson that I had learned from Jo. In one of her early acupuncture classes she had been shown the pressure point for motion sickness and had passed the tip on to me, so

I dug out my Swiss Army knife and opened the Phillips screwdriver blade. This I applied to the spot, three fingers width above the crease in my wrist and between the easily palpable tendons. After holding on for about five minutes the queasiness disappeared, and I was able to concentrate once again on my fishing. Once again the Swiss Army knife had come to the rescue, but this time the lack of drama would probably not have worked for a *MacGyver* incident. I continued chatting with the fishermen, father and son, who were very happy to accept us$15 for the day, particularly as I took none of the catch away when we returned to shore.

The next day, I was a landlubber once more when Jo and I joined our group in a standard tourist visit to a small farm. Not for nothing was the island of Zanzibar favoured by traders for many years. The Sultan of Oman shifted his capital to the island when he realized that the slave trade was developing into a major cash cow. Apart from the slave trade, there were also spices. In the nineteenth century, some 90 per cent of the world's supply of cloves came from the islands of Zanzibar and nearby Pemba, and Zanzibar town was the centre of the spice trade in East Africa.

"Who dares to try these little green peppers? They are the hottest on earth," said Ali, our local guide, a smartly dressed young man of Indian and Arab extraction.

I have heard this claim made in other parts of the world, but a test would require tasting, and this was not a competition in which I cared to partake. I had my own brush with hot peppers as a very small boy in the garden of a house in Moshi, on the slopes of Kilimanjaro where my father had been posted in 1943. There, at the age of two, I had discovered the joy of tomatoes direct from the vine and had been strictly told not to pick them. Of course the ban had not worked, as most two-year-olds are quite serious about stretching the rubber band of parental discipline to see how far it will go. This time no parental comment was needed about my infraction, as I made the mistake of picking a small luscious red fruit and popping it into my mouth. One bite, so I no doubt thought, would release the tasty juice, and I could go on to the next plant. There was indeed a release, but it was mostly the release of loud screams as the red hot pepper fired up my taste buds. This account is taken from one of those pseudo-memories that become part of family lore, repeated at intervals for many years (including of course to the first girl I took home to "meet the folks"), especially by my mother, who had had to try and help my ayah quell the screaming and keep me from waking my baby sister Brigid.

While the rest of our group went into town to do some more touristy stuff and curio shopping, Jo and I hired a taxi and visited the Jozani Forest Reserve, a small patch of just over twenty-five square kilometres that lies more or less undisturbed in the centre of the island. On the edges of the forest, there is a mahogany plantation, but this soon gives way to a pristine mix of large trees, vines and a wide variety of bromeliads and orchids, in what is known as a "ground water forest"—one of the last of its kind on the coast. Our guide was Charles (who never gave us his surname), a tall very dark Swahili man.

Right away we saw a black bird, about the size of the red-wing blackbird of the swamps and marshes of home, but with no red-wing flash. This one was all black, and had a tail about as long as its body, with a fork at the end. Charles said, "A Drongo," to which I added "Fork-tailed." He was now on his mettle and commented, "You know your birds." Which was not really true, as the identification was hardly difficult. Then we all spotted a little yellow and green jewel, no more than about four inches long, the underparts bright yellow, the head and upper breast iridescent when a ray of sun cut through the canopy and the feathers glinted. A collared sunbird.

"Look there," he said with excitement, "it is a Fischer's turaco. See the white stripes above the eye and the red peaked crest with its white edge." We checked our copy of Stevenson and Fanshawe's *Field Guide to the Birds of East Africa* and found out why Charles had been so animated. The text is marked with a black dot as being one of the species "often the quarry of keen birders" (for which we do not qualify in the obsessed "twitcher" sense of the word).

Back in the more open section of the park, where logging had been carried out and some cattle grazed, we came upon a troupe of the island's race of red colobus monkeys, just hanging out in an almost leafless tree. Charles said, "They are called *kima punga* in Swahili. This means 'poison monkey' and is used because they strip the leaves of the tree they are in."

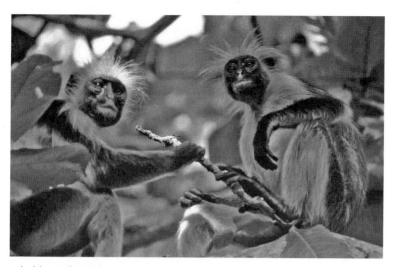

Red colobus monkeys in the Jozani Forest Reserve, Zanzibar.

David Elsworth, writing in *Swara*, the magazine of the East Africa Wildlife Society, gives a further explanation of the monkey's Swahili common name and a different spelling of the adjective, which he wrote as *punju*, quoting a traditional Zanzibari belief that dogs that eat these monkeys will lose all their hair. I tried to get to the bottom of the language puzzle, as the only Swahili word for "poison" in my dictionary, or my vocabulary, is *sumu*. *Kima* is Swahili for monkey—although technically for a different genus (the *Cercopithecus mitis* group), which Charles may not have known.

Since hearing Charles call the monkeys *kima punga*, I have tried to verify the meaning of *punga* and *punju*, and even a hybrid *punja*, but despite reference to several Swahili-English dictionaries, including three that I found on the internet, I was unable to find a direct link to poison, although there is a translation of *punju* meaning "snake-bite." The puzzle was finally solved when freelance biologist Tom Struhsaker told me, via e-mail, that in his 1959 edition of the Oxford Swahili-English Dictionary the word is sometimes "spelled as *punyu* and it is a medicine prepared by wizards composed of a plant and animal bits which when mixed with food causes constant coughing and a fatal illness." As some Swahili terms are unique to Zanzibar, and do not appear in general dictionaries, it may be that the word has a very local meaning relating to the monkeys and the trees, which Charles, of course, knew.

Finally, no visit to Zanzibar would be complete without a walk along the seafront at Stone Town, where food vendors have set up their tiny stalls—which are no more than about a metre long, with a cooking unit and a shelf—where one can get a range of delicious island foods. We watched locals playing the ancient game of *Bao*, as it is known locally. The object is to move two parallel rows of stones (seeds, marbles or anything similar will also do) along the side nearest one in such a way that they can capture those opposite. Some boards have six, seven, eight or ten fist-sized hollows in two rows, others in four rows. It sounds simple, and played at slow speed it seems so. Experts play at great speed and know many moves ahead which pile of stones to pick up. The clicking sounds just like that of the ancient Chinese game of Mah Jong. Woe betide the tourist who believes that he or she can take on a local for money.

The game we occasionally play on our own board is known as *Kiothi*, the Kimeru name of the game by which we first knew it when our friend, Andrew Botta, introduced it to us. Our board came with marble-sized seeds of the caesalpinia tree *(njothi* in Kimeru). *Caesalpinia* is a genus of prickly scrambling shrubs with bi-pinnate leaves and vicious recurved spines. According to a note in Michael Blundell's *Wild Flowers of East Africa*, the seeds, which develop in long bristly ovoid pods, float well on the sea and can remain viable after spending two, or more, years afloat.

Our board has ten hollows on each side, with one larger indent, known as bomas, into which captured stones are placed at each end. The object is simple, to capture more stones (representing cattle) than one's opponent. But it's not that simple. To win by just one stone is the most difficult and thus is akin to ten wins by other margins.

There are traditional permanent Bao or Kiothi sites in many parts of Africa. Among them, in the area where we used to work and live, is one near the top of the flat-topped mountain known as Ol Olokwe, which is a landmark north of Isiolo and on clear days is visible from the slopes of Mount Kenya. There are several of the game sites in Meru District, where Jo and I met and married. Two are in the Lewa Wildlife

Conservancy, one near the town of Kianjai north of Meru town and one that we visited in 2005. We drove east of Meru, over very dusty roads, toward the southern end of the Nyambeni Hills, where hundreds of hectares of new patches of tea bushes had replaced the native forests that we knew in the 1960s. We climbed up a steep path, with our guide Johnson Mugambi, an urbane and successful business man, whose paternal home was in Meru but who had moved to Nairobi and become one of the many highly successful upper-middle class of the new Kenya. Also with us as we climbed a steep path between the tea was the land owner, Peter Kaberia, and his brother, as well as about fifty of the local children. Finally we came upon a large rock—it must have weighed at least fifty tonnes—on the flattish top of which were a series of hollowed out depressions, two rows of ten and a larger one at each end. None of the children had ever heard of the place, but they crowded round as Peter and his brother Anastasio played a mock game with seeds that Anastasio had appropriately brought along. As I set up my camera, I wondered to myself if a scene such as this had been played out before, when the site might have been used for tournaments, and an audience had gathered, not to watch two white-skinned *mzungu* (more interesting for the kids then the game), but perhaps to witness the outcome of a contest of some sort.

In the age of the internet there are now websites devoted to this ancient game. I doubt that the exponents whom I watched in 1968 playing in the sand, as they waited for a cattle auction to begin near the desert oasis of Laisamis in Kenya's Northern Frontier District, would need the rules laid out for them. They simply ground out the right number of depressions in the sand with their fists and started to play, their hands moving too fast for me to follow, as they picked up and dropped the pebbles that they used instead of the njothi seeds. Canadian Len Lemoine, who transcribed the Kiothi rules into English for Andrew Botta when he was teaching in Meru, mentioned to me that he had even seen the game being played with pebbles on the beach in the Caribbean.

In Zanzibar, local young men touted the boards for sale and offered lessons at the café as we sat and sipped our fresh lime juice. After our harbourside supper we boarded a night ferry and headed back to Dar es Salaam and the next phase of our journey, a trip to the world-famous Ngorongoro Crater and its equally famous neighbour, the Serengeti, where part of the extraordinary annual wildebeest migration takes place. I was anxious to see if there were any rhino left in the crater, maybe to see some lions in the park and get some sort of feel for the effects of the massive distemper outbreak that had done so much damage to their population three years previously. Our ultimate goal was reuniting with Kenya, where I had begun the veterinary career that had led to my work in the field of wildlife medicine.

OH—THE NAVY LIEUTENANT who had preceded my Zanzibar visit by 101 years was Francis Evans Percy Haigh, my grandfather, who later became an engineer captain and had a great deal to do with the development of torpedoes leading up to and through the First World War. Trying to guess what sort of camera he used to capture the sunken *Glasgow* and its surroundings is quite a challenge, but it will certainly not have been the same as my Nikon. After looking at the old picture, Saskatoon professional photographer John Waddington told me that it was almost certainly a Schoviell Dry Plate Outfit. These cameras were developed in the late 1880s in Europe and revolutionized photography for the keen amateur (just like digital has replaced film). The dry plate technology made it possible to transport the film, store it for long periods, and avoid all the problems of the wet plate systems that preceded it.

Percy's father was Edward Mackeson Haigh, who was one half of the professional photography partnership Moira and Haigh of London's Portman Square. His business card carries a portrait of a Catholic bishop on one side and the inscription *Photographers & Miniature Painters to the Principal Sovereigns of Europe* on the other. It is fun to speculate that Edward Mackeson may have given his son a camera as a going-away present when he was commissioned into the Royal Navy in 1894.

Edward Mackeson also had maritime experience. For their honeymoon in 1860, he and his new wife Emma, my great grandmother, headed off on a six-month sailing ship trip to Australia and back. She was the only woman among nineteen men. She must have been a tough and determined soul.

As for the surfacing of the photographs of the sunken ship one hundred years after their taking, one of my cousins, Sue Langford, found them among a collection of memorabilia that our grandmother had stored in her husband Percy's naval trunk. In a spirit of enquiry Sue sent them to the Royal Naval Museum at Portsmouth, on England's south coast. The curators were more or less ecstatic about them, as they had no visual records of those events, although there are a few in other collections. The written history is well documented, but Percy Haigh's pictures, the originals of which are now in the museum, round out this little slice of Victorian colonial history. *

20

SICK
LIONS

Jo and I journey to a somewhat soggy Ngorongoro Crater, where we reminisce about a cold night to remember at the crater and an unusual way to promote wine. Fighting lions in Samburu National Reserve, lion diseases and disease control efforts from Scotland to East Africa.

OUR TRIP TO NGORONGORO CRATER AND THE SERENGETI IN 1997 was memorable for one principal reason, which had nothing to do with wild animals and everything to do with rain. The year 1997 was the year of the BIG El Niño. The rains had arrived early, and with a vengeance. It poured every day, and the roads quickly became a rust-red quagmire. Huge queues of heavy trucks lined the mud roads like a scene from a stretched-out wrecker's yard or a war. Some were merely mired. Others had gone one worse and were on their sides. The best part about the soggy situation was that as paying passengers we did not have to worry or do a thing about it. Wherever there were villages, mobs of young men gathered to push, grunting and heaving as

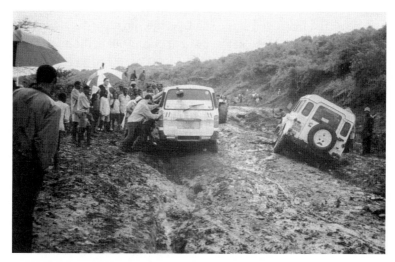

On the road to the Ngorongoro Crater. El Nino rains made a mockery of road conditions.

the mud-caked vehicles slid sideways and every-which-way out of trouble.

We arrived much later than scheduled at the crater rim and spent a very damp half-hour in the dark putting up our tents on a grassy patch of ground that had only a few trees scattered around the clearing. The major challenge was to avoid the copious number of not-quite-fresh buffalo manure patties that lay around like soggy unexploded land mines.

During the night Jo woke me with a loudly whispered, "What's that noise?" Within what was surely no more than thirty to fifty centimetres from the tent wall, I could hear something chomping on the grass and the occasional rumble of a stomach.

"Sounds like a buffalo," I replied.

The morning light proved me to have been right, except that the "a" had been an underestimate. Judging from the number of really fresh patties, a large herd of these massive black animals must have decided that the grass in the clearing was to be the main course for their nighttime feed.

At least we had been warm. Our first trip to the crater had been over Christmas twenty-seven years earlier. At an elevation of 2,500 metres on the rim, with the incredible panorama of the world's largest crater spread out below us, the far lip seemingly kilometres away, we had stood and marvelled at the sight. As the sun dipped and the heat went out of the day, we soon had the tent up and put in the mattresses and sheet that had served us so well on the dry plains of the Maasai Mara. The heat continued to vanish, and for much of the night we lay, dressed in every stitch of clothing we had, and shivered. There was only one thing for it. After our early morning drive into the crater, we paid a visit to the lodge and begged for help, which was readily given. For the next two nights we wrapped ourselves in warm blankets that had been loaned us.

Naturally, we tried to repay the kindness in some way, but the charming manager would have none of it. We decided that the least we could do was to have dinner at the lodge, and so we headed straight there after our game drive. The most memorable moment of the drive had been the rhino encounter. Our guide had already primed us.

"This rhino does not like vehicles. If he charges you must stop at once. If you try to drive away he will hit you."

I urge the reader to remain calm if a tonne of angry rhino were ever to come at you from twenty metres, going from stationary to full throttle in three strides. For a fraction of a second I thought about putting my foot down, but the guide repeated his order, this time with greatly increased volume, and I stopped side-on to the massive beast. He got to within what seemed like three centimetres of the door, and I could swear that I would have been able to count the hairs in his nose, had I had a mind to do so. Having made his point, the rhino snorted, stood for a moment longer, spun round and trotted off, tail held high, about fifty metres before turning sideways and taking another look at us, the intruders.

At dinner that night I had browsed through the menu as we waited for our food to appear. One item on the wine list caught my eye. "Try our Dodoma red. Made by the monks at the monastery it has the subtlety of a charging rhino." We passed on that one.

Now, after our second visit to Ngorongoro, we went on to the Serengeti and found that it was no drier than the crater, and several roads were impassable. We saw no rhino, and our only encounter with lions was a lucky one for the occupants of a stranded Land Rover. We had seen the stationary vehicle about a kilometre away and assumed that there might be something worthwhile to see. Of course we were right.

Three big lions, one with a black mane, were lying half asleep about ten metres away from the Land Rover. We drove up alongside, and at once the driver, an American with a slow southern drawl, called over.

"Can you pull up close to the hood and give us a jump start? My battery died when I stopped to see the lions, and we can't get going. I daresn't get out to check it."

"How long have you been here?" asked our driver.

"About three hours. We wondered if anyone was ever going to show up."

He had made the right decision. Lions are not only powerful but over short distances they are quick.

While we did not see sick lions in the Serengeti we had a close-up view of a lion fight, and its consequences, a few months later in Kenya's beautiful Samburu National Reserve, one of our favourite haunts from courting days many years earlier. A fight between two domestic tabbies is an impressive thing to watch. Scaled up a hundredfold and morphed into a gang fight among females fighting over a male, the fight becomes epic. The battle we saw was almost certainly the result of the continued destruction of lions, especially males, by people.

We were about half a kilometre south of the Uaso Nyiro River, driving along sandy tracks as we emerged from the groves of fever trees that line the riverbanks. With us in the Land Rover driven by Moses, our Kenyan guide, were our long-time friends Paul Sayer and Olwen Owles. Suddenly, Olwen spotted a group of lionesses heading our way over a slight rise. They were alternately trotting, walking and occasionally stopping briefly.

"They are on a mission—they look so alert—I wonder what they are staring at?" she said.

The answer was not long in coming. Moses said, "Look over there, just near those bushes straight in line with Ol Olokwe. There's another lioness."

We turned our heads to the north and had no trouble locating the animal as the mountain is such a well-known landmark, once seen, never forgotten. No matter how far away from Africa one goes, its flat top, rising three hundred metres above the surrounding plain, at once appears in the mind's eye when the name comes up.

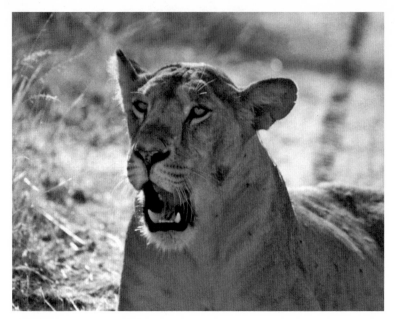

An alert lioness checks out the invaders.

Suddenly there were four, not just one, lionesses to the north, and they set off toward us, advancing in what military strategists would call line abreast.

The two groups met about one hundred metres away from the Land Rover in a confusion of snarls, biting and striking with incredible ferocity. One animal was at once in trouble as she was bitten somewhere low down on her left front leg. In less than a minute a large black-maned male appeared from the bushes nearby and trotted over to the scene of the fracas. He must have said something like, "Now, now, girls, that's enough, cut it out."

Whatever it was, it instantly worked. The females stopped their fight. One group—"the home team"—sat down and the other, the "invaders" and presumably those we had first seen, headed back south.

"That one's in trouble," I said, as the victim of the bite took two very pain-filled steps and sank down out of sight. We drove round on a narrower track to see if we could spot the injured animal, but the bushes were too numerous and we never knew what became of her.

"Have you seen that sort of thing before?" I asked our guide.

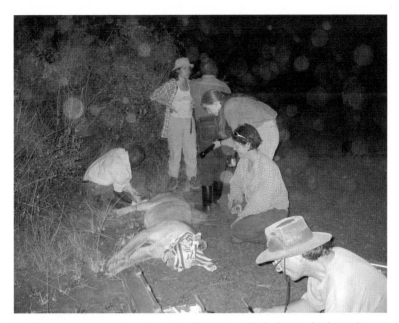

Canadian and Ugandan students examine an injured lion in Queen Elizabeth National Park. Dr. Ludwig Siefert prepares an injection for treatment.

"No, but I heard from other drivers that it is occurring, and we think we know why."

"Is it anything to do with the settlements?" asked Paul. He was referring to the dozens of corrugated-iron-roofed huts that dotted the surrounding hills, all something new since the 1970s, when we had last visited the area.

"I think so. The men spear the males. They want males particularly because of the manes, and so the females do not have enough men to meet their needs."

He gestured with his chin toward the departing animals.

"The other group probably came looking for a mate, and ran into more trouble than they expected."

The number of lions that are injured in giant cat fights can only be guessed at, and the number that recover is also mere guesswork. When two different group of students, in different years, who were studying with me in Uganda's Queen Elizabeth National Park were able to treat a lioness that had been severely injured in a fight, it was undoubtedly a

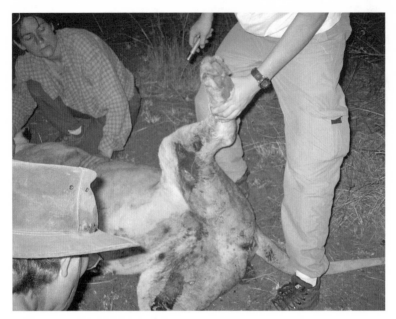

The same lion showing extensive bite wounds on the inside of the legs.

memorable event (for the students; the lion was immobilized and probably knew nothing of the event except for the initial prick of the dart and the drug-induced hangover afterwards). The first one, a lioness with extensive tears and deep bite marks in both rear legs, was treated with much wound cleaning and heavy doses of antibiotic. The students christened her Canada, in honour of the Canadian flag bandana that they used to cover her eyes while she was under the influence.

The second lion, a young male just beginning to show his adult mane, had a deep cut in one pad and was profoundly lame; lame enough to have had little chance of hunting successfully. He, too, was treated with antibiotics and wound cleaning. Whether the lions would have survived without the antibiotics and treatment we administered is a moot point.

Large- and small-animal veterinarians may be called upon to treat or diagnose disease in individual animals or whole herds or groups. It is only lately that wildlife veterinarians have begun to study diseases of lions and other big cats and a good deal of information has been accumulated. Much of the early information on big cat diseases came from

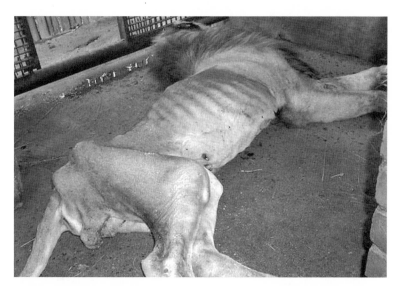

An emaciated lion that has died of tuberculosis lies on the post-mortem room floor at the Kruger National Park headquarters. (Photo by Dr. Markus Hofmeyr)

lions that had died in zoos, often in countries outside Africa. It is no real surprise that lions do indeed suffer from diseases, although they cannot be reported until someone actually goes to the trouble to look for them. As the great Canadian physician William Osler wrote, "Every outbreak begins with a case." The odd case of some disease in a large lion population will have little effect upon overall numbers, especially in a species that used to be as abundant and prolific as this one.

Infectious diseases that are known to impact lions include several virus conditions known in domestic cats, as well as anthrax, the nasty bacterial disease that sometimes occurs in wildlife populations during rainy seasons and is an indiscriminate killer of many species, not to mention the little matter of its being of major interest to governments concerned with the possibility of bio-terrorism. Lions, of course, get it when they scavenge the carcasses of prey species that have succumbed. There are probably not many cases, but in South Africa's Kruger National Park, cases of lions dying of anthrax have been seen. In Uganda's Queen Elizabeth Park, four habituated leopards that we had frequently seen in previous years all died of anthrax in the outbreak of 2005.

One virus that does not appear to have any lethal effect upon lions is the feline form of the immunodeficiency virus FIV, closely related to the human HIV that is so devastating the African continent with its AIDS pandemic. Lions are infected with FIV in many regions, but no associated disease has been documented.

Not surprisingly, human society has had negative effects upon lions, in terms of disease, some of these indirect. The most dramatic occurrences of infectious diseases that have impacted lions in Africa in the last twenty years have direct links to human activity and common diseases of domestic animals. Two such diseases, one bacterial, the other viral, have had significant effects.

In the Kruger about twenty years ago, tuberculosis spread from infected cattle and moved into the park from the south. The first species to fall victim were the buffalo. Their habit of congregating in large herds, sometimes as many as one thousand head, and then dispersing, as well as running and creating mini dust storms, has proved to be just about the ideal way of spreading this disease, which is easily disseminated when an infected animal coughs. Of course lions and other large predators prey on the buffalo, and if a buffalo weakens because its body is riddled with Tb, there is no one there to tell the lion to stay away because of the health risks. Inevitably Tb has spilled over to the lions, and Markus Hofmeyr has told me that some twenty or twenty-five cases are seen each year in the park. The situation is getting worse as the disease gradually spreads northward.

It is obviously impossible to treat wild buffalo, or lions, for Tb, so the only hope here is to try to develop some measure of control through test and slaughter. Such a program has been instituted, but it is a massive and probably impossible undertaking.

The other disease of lions that has arrived indirectly has come from human inaction, rather than action: a failure to vaccinate dogs against a common and often lethal virus condition known as canine distemper.

Pastoralists the world over have dogs as companions and often as working assistants. Contacts with wildlife are common with these groups. The most famous of the tribes whose lands surround the Serengeti and Maasai Mara parks are the purely pastoral Maasai, but they pose less of a risk to wildlife than the Wakurya and the WaSukuma who are both pastoralists and planters. The Wakurya and WaSukuma and their dogs live at much higher densities, and the dogs are not traditionally vaccinated. This might not have mattered, and indeed probably didn't for a long time, until the virus itself underwent a small change and in 1994 was seen to have had a profound effect on a new host—lions. It was this situation that I had discussed with the auctioneer in Zanzibar. By the time I talked to him in 1997 it had become apparent from blood sample surveys that at least 85 per cent of the lions in the Serengeti had been exposed to the virus.

It is estimated that by the end of this particular epidemic, as many as a third of the lions, perhaps one thousand of them, had died in the Serengeti and Mara areas. The virus had jumped from the domestic dogs and had first been seen in jackals and wild dogs at the start of the outbreak. It is thought to have wiped out the latter in the region, and it also affected hyaenas. In 1994 lions started to die, and it was not long before the cause was confirmed.

The first report came from an observant tourist who was a paying passenger in one of the many tour company balloons drifting almost silently over the Serengeti and saw dead lions below him. Very soon afterwards, American veterinarian Dr. Melody Roelke, who was working in the park, was able to get some fresh carcasses and carry out necropsies. She was able to get some samples to wildlife pathologist Dr. Linda Munson, who has a worldwide reputation for her work with big cats. It was Linda who confirmed the unexpected finding that the canine virus had found a new host. There is a dramatic, but grim, movie clip shown on the Glasgow Veterinary College website, taken by modeller Professor Ray Holborn, of a lion in the Serengeti in the throes of a grand mal seizure, which is one of the classic signs of distemper.

There is now an active vaccination program for the domestic dogs all around the Serengeti, and as long as this continues some measure of control will exist on the spread of the disease into wild populations. Dr. Sarah Cleaveland, of Edinburgh's Royal Dick Veterinary College, has dedicated her career to understanding and controlling diseases that involve wildlife, people and domestic animals. One of her biggest projects has been to spearhead a program among the herders around the park in which domestic dogs are also vaccinated against distemper and another lethal disease—rabies. She hopes to find out if her successes with the dogs will translate into control of distemper in the lions, as the number of cases in domestic dogs should diminish markedly as the vaccination program is established, thus reducing the chance of transmission to lions and other vulnerable species.

When we visited the Mara in February 2005, we met a herder as we sat under a thorn tree and had a picnic lunch. I asked him, "*Mbwa walipigwa sindano?*" (Have the dogs been given their needles?)

He replied, "*ndiyo, wote.*" (Yes, all of them.)

Large-scale vaccination of lions and hyaenas against distemper is pretty impractical, although some animals could be dart-inoculated. Still, the vaccine was originally developed for dogs, and it was therefore imperative to see if it would work in lions. The vaccine was tested by wildlife veterinarian Richard Kock and his colleagues and found to fulfill two basic criteria. First, it did no harm; second, it caused some apparent measure of protection as judged by the antibody responses of the patients. The gold standard test would have been to take two groups of lions, one vaccinated, the other unprotected, and expose both to a strain of the virus known to be virulent in lions. This was not done, for obvious welfare and common-sense reasons.

The distemper that made such an impact in Tanzania also caused problems in other parks. At about the same time as it was running amok in the Serengeti, distemper was detected by a soft-spoken Ugandan veterinarian named Dr. Margaret Driciru some six hundred kilometres to the northwest, including two hundred kilometres across the open water of Lake Victoria, in Uganda's Queen Elizabeth National Park (QEP). Seventy-nine per cent of the lions she surveyed had antibodies to the virus. Deaths, nervous signs and another classic clinical manifestation of distemper, the so-called "hard-pad" of the feet, that is seen in dogs, were all reported.

Ten years later, Margaret started post-graduate work on a population of lions not much farther north, about four hundred kilometres from QEP in Murchison Falls National Park. She found clear evidence of several other diseases that affect domestic cats. Almost half of the lions she immobilized had ulcers, gum disorders or tooth abnormalities; over a third of them had cauliflower-like masses on their tongues;

over 90 per cent had antibodies to a condition called Feline Respiratory Disease Complex, which can be caused by one of two viruses, a herpes or a calici virus. Indeed the incidence of this condition is on the rise throughout East Africa, some 70 per cent of big cats now being recorded as having been exposed. Perhaps most interesting, none of the lions in this study of Margaret's showed any evidence of ever being exposed to distemper.

These various findings are a worry. The lion population in Murchison is small and they are genetically isolated from any others, separated by not only distance but also by dense human settlement. The animals are under constant pressure from poachers, who not only seek to protect their stock but are also in the market for lion parts for medicinal purposes, and the total population is not increasing. There are signs of inbreeding, with a skewed sex ratio of cubs (3:1 in favour of males), and Margaret speculates that inbreeding in what is essentially an island population could be causing a greater susceptibility to disease agents. Margaret goes on to make some predictions based on one or two different models. The worst scenario could be the arrival of distemper, which could take out almost four hundred animals, 85 per cent of the population, as they are probably fully susceptible.

THE INCREASE OF KNOWLEDGE about lion diseases is, in part, because people have become more aware of disease issues and have ever more sophisticated tools with which to look for, diagnose or treat them. It can also be ascribed to other factors, such as human activity or inactivity. Of course lions have also caused trouble for humans through the ages, and it this subject to which I turn next. ❋

21

LIONS AS TROUBLE

Lions and other Big Cats as predators of humans.
I relate personal encounters.

THERE IS NO DOUBT that lions have been predators of humans and their stock for as long as the three have been in contact. An early and graphic example comes from an ivory panel at Nimrud, the ancient Assyrian city located in modern-day Iraq. It dates from the eighth century BCE and shows a man being grabbed by the throat by a lion. His chances of survival would have been virtually nil. Other accounts of lion predation or interactions go back to the beginnings of recorded history, mentioning warriors and kings such as Xerxes and Tutankhamen and their problems or hunting prowess.

In 1899 missionary teacher Albert B. Lloyd wrote about his travels in Uganda in a book whose title must qualify to be, in twenty-first-century terms, as politically incorrect as one can imagine. It is called *In Dwarf Land and Cannibal Country*. He frequently refers to the problem of predator attacks upon villagers. It is obvious, from reading his accounts, that both lions and leopards were a constant threat to life. The latter could and did gain access to people during the night and were able to remove single victims without people sleeping nearby even being aware of what was happening. Lions would often attack in daylight. They would simply lie concealed in the tall grass and seize people going to fetch water or walking on narrow trails. The natives lacked firearms and probably did not have the lion-hunting traditions of the Maasai and their kin, which must have created hazards that we can hardly imagine. In today's terms it would be like crossing a busy highway wearing earplugs while blindfolded, never knowing when a car was going to try and deliberately run you over.

Lloyd tells of an event in the kingdom of Toro, in what is now western Uganda, which he probably recounted in detail because of its unexpected outcome. Two lions had killed many people, and Lloyd himself had tried, unsuccessfully, to kill them with his advantage of a gun. A party of villagers had been out hunting antelope for the pot, and as they returned home, he continues:

> *Walking in single file through the long grass, the man at the end of the line was suddenly seized by the lioness and instantly killed and carried off. The rest of the party made off with all haste, excepting one little boy, the son of the man killed, and he, amazingly plucky little fellow that he is, actually turned back, and, armed with nothing but a small spear, followed the blood-stained track through the thicket. After a little while he came upon the lioness in the act of devouring his father. Without a moment's hesitation this brave little chap rushed at the huge beast, and the lioness, becoming aware of his approach, left the prey and sprang upon the boy. By a merciful Providence the spear the boy carried entered its breast, and by the animal's own weight was forced right into its body, piercing the heart, and the great creature rolled over stone dead. The boy was utterly unharmed. Rapidly withdrawing his little weapon he went and knelt by the mangled remains of his father, and while bending over him in his sorrow the male lion came roaring through the ticket. The grief-stricken*

lad sprang up and with almost superhuman courage rushed towards the second lion, waving aloft his blood-stained spear and shouting, "Come on, come on, I'll kill you also!" But the lion was so discomfited by the unexpected approach of the lad that he turned tail and fled, leaving his partner dead by the side of her mangled prey. The boy then went home to his village and called his friends to come and bring the dead lioness to the king, and this was done. The brave little fellow was suitably rewarded by Kasagama [the Toro king] for his wonderful pluck, and he made him his own page.

An incident in 1904 that helped South Africa's Kruger National Park gain international attention also involved a lion attack on a human. A ranger named Harry Wolhuter was dragged almost one hundred metres by an old male lion after it had attacked his horse and he had fallen. With great presence of mind and fortitude he killed it with his knife. The incident is celebrated to this day in the history of the park, and the knife and the lion's skin are on display at the park headquarters at Skukuza.

A more modern and better-known account of lion predation on humans is related in J.H. Paterson's story *The Maneaters of Tsavo*. He describes the harrowing experience of the railway crew who were working on the Uganda railway during a nine-month period in 1898 and 1899. The two lions involved have been mythologized and reported to have killed something close to 140 men during this period. The true number of victims was probably closer to twenty-eight, still horrible enough, and they were certainly not the most voracious or efficient of their kind. Other man-eaters were described by David Western, in his lyrical *In the Dust of Kilimanjaro* in 1997. Western records how George Rushby, ivory hunter turned game warden, claimed to have destroyed the man-eating lions of Njombe, in Tanzania, that had killed more than 1,500 people.

In his 1973 book *The Gardeners of Eden*, Alistair Graham quotes from a Uganda Game Department report: "Even entire districts were affected '...where lions had established complete mastery over the inhabitants, where most of the population had either been killed or fled.'"

Kenya's history would have been very different had Lord Delamere not survived a mauling before he became the iconic figure and *de facto* leader of the settlers who were at constant loggerheads with the administration in the early 1900s. A contemporary diary from that era records how there were seven graves of lion victims in the Nairobi cemetery in 1903 and how the postmaster emerged from his house to meet a young lion asleep on his front steps. At a time when the numbers of immigrants probably numbered in the few hundreds and there were seven mzungu lion victims buried in the cemetery, how many more had there been among the native population throughout the country?

The carnage continues today, an ongoing example being in Kruger National Park. Mozambiquan refugees, desperate to flee the poverty, disease and hopelessness of a country still trying to deal with the aftermath of civil war, have tried to trek through the unguarded border between their country and the hoped-for greener pastures of South Africa. Their path leads them through the barrier of the sixty-kilometre-wide park full of wild animals. The lions in the park have taken advantage of this situation, and no one knows how many would-be immigrants have failed to run the gauntlet and ended up as prey.

In the late 1990s a lion turned up unexpectedly in Lake Nakuru National Park in Kenya, which no doubt increased the drawing power of this wonderful place, already famous for its huge numbers of birds, especially flamingoes. An unsuspecting female ranger walking near the main gate was soon killed. The lion was shot to prevent further killing of people, especially as the park borders right onto settlement land, the main gate is only a couple of kilometres from the town of Nakuru, and the park fence is not predator-proof.

I may have come close to being prey myself on a few occasions, but only once did I know for sure that I had had a brush with an attack. It was in 1968, when I was out walking in the long yellowing grass near the frontier town of Isiolo in Kenya, shotgun in hand, that my adrenal glands suddenly received an unwanted stimulus. I was with friends Frank Douglas and George and Irralie Murray, and we had taken a day off work to visit the Isiolo Quarantine Area to see if we could bag some guinea fowl and yellow-necked spurfowl for the pot.

After a tasty picnic lunch of egg sandwiches, cold sausages and to-matoes, washed down with tea, we had resumed our walk. Irralie had stayed back in the Land Cruiser and we three men were weaving our way north and east, our backs to the view of Mount Kenya's peaks that we had been admiring during our rest. The weaving was unavoidable, as the myriad thorn bushes made straight lines impossible. Most earnestly avoided were the wait-a-bit bushes. As anyone who has ever been caught in one of these will attest, you do indeed wait a bit if your clothes or skin get snared. The deadly little thorns, each curved like a scimitar, face in different directions, so as soon as you think you are free of one, its neighbour slams into you. It is impossible to emerge from the thicket without bleeding.

Frank and I had just gone round each side of a wait-a-bit when a covey of yellow-neck flushed. We got off three quick shots between us and were walking forward to pick up the birds when I saw the rear ends of three lions bounding away, no more than sixty metres in front of me. Burly mustachioed Frank commented quietly, as we stopped to settle our racing hearts, "I wonder if they were waiting for us?"

There was no need to reply. We both knew that the shots had scared them off. Had they had one of us in mind as a potential feast? I'll never know, and I'm not complaining either.

The predatory nature of lions does not change when they are held in captivity. My guess is that it is hard-wired. Visitors to zoos may have noticed that even caged lions change their demeanour when they see a small child, something I witnessed most clearly at George Adamson's camp in Meru National Park when I took some friends to meet him in the late 1960s. George was the former game warden and Kenya character who had been involved in the *Born Free* stories told in book and film. He and his estranged wife, Joy, had two separate camps in the park. George had sited his camp below the imposing rocky outcrop known as Muguango, on top of which has now been built the stunning tourist lodge, Elsa's Kopje, named for the lioness star of the stories. My friends had their three-year-old daughter with them, and we sat and enjoyed a cup of tea as George sipped the White Horse whisky we had brought (it was always best to go prepared when visiting George). Girl, the lioness and film star, wandered into camp and came over to the wire mesh enclosure to greet us, and then suddenly she noticed the child. Her hackles came up, her eyes half-closed and seemed to shoot beams, and her whole body language changed to "alert." The youngster probably looked just like a tasty morsel.

Of course the lion's predatory behaviour around humans and humans' aversion to the depredations of predators is nothing new, is not limited to Africa and will no doubt continue for the foreseeable future. The specific tale within the story depends only on which continent the predators are predating and therefore the species involved.

Lions have also been an issue in India. As Jim Corbett told in his wonderful stories, tigers and leopards were a huge problem for the people of the Himalayan foothills. When the lions of the Gir forest in the sate of Gujurat changed their eating habits and took to killing cattle, the villagers naturally objected and were soon poisoning them.

Mountain lions (panthers or cougars) have been extirpated from eastern North America, with the exception of a remnant and fragile population in Florida, whose main predator is the automobile. In western regions of North America, cougars, and even bears, occasionally prey upon people, often solitary joggers.

Wolves, which have been recorded as people-killers in Eurasia, have long since been eliminated from most of Western Europe. In North America their reintroduction to several states in the northern part of the USA from Canada in the 1990s created a considerable controversy. The strong words voiced by a Wyoming rancher, captured on film during a town hall meeting about the translocation of some wolves into that state, may be a bit over the top but are understandable. She said, during an open-floor session, "Wolves are the Saddam Hussein of the animal kingdom." She was worried about the impending arrival of the wolves because of their likely effect upon her family's livestock, not on humans. I have used that clip in teaching exercises on several occasions to illustrate to veterinary students that wildlife issues are far from simple.

If lions have been predators of humans throughout the ages, they have also competed with us for resources, mainly, of course, for our cattle. ✻

22

LIONS
IN
TROUBLE

*Lions and other predators of livestock. Maasai
ceremonies, snares, poisons, witchcraft,
traditional medicine, population declines and the
roller coaster of conservation. Where does the
future for lions and other large predators lie?*

IN MY GENERAL PRACTICE DAYS OF THE EARLY 1970s, there were
several occasions on which I heard about the outcome of visits by
hungry lions to cattle and sheep ranches. I saw the consequences of
one such visit during a trip out of Nanyuki, which took me north and
east round the slopes of Mount Kenya toward Timau, on a farm visit
to one of my major cattle clients.

The morning had been bright and clear when I rolled out of bed and
took the almost reflexive peek through our bedroom window at the
five-thousand-metre peaks of Mount Kenya, which stood out as dark
silhouettes back-lit by the dawn light. In Canada a common opening
gambit of any conversation concerns the weather. In Nanyuki, and

especially on the Laikipia Plains, where just about every house was built with a view of the mountain, the gambit might just as easily be the state of the peaks: clouded, clear or "there must have been quite a storm up there, lots of new snow."

A couple of wispy clouds gathered around the mountain's shoulders while Mutua and I planned our day. Mutua had just returned from a week's leave at home and had picked up his new, and first, pair of glasses, making things much easier for him, but he had not had a chance to check the appointments diary, so I had filled him in.

"We have about three hundred head to 'preg check' at Kisima and then after lunch we have two dogs to spay, so I hope we get done in decent time," I said.

Pregnancy checking of cattle was the bread and butter part of my practice, and as long as there was no serious drought, I could be sure to check at least two thousand head a month around the district. I had to be sure of my accuracy, as any animal that was not pregnant was likely to be sent for slaughter the next day, but after several years of pulling on an arm-length plastic glove and feeling through the rectal wall for the relevant bits inside the cow, I had become reasonably adept. It was almost as if my hand, rather than my brain, knew its way around and could feel uterus and ovaries, or if the calf was well grown, even its individual parts, most often the head.

We had pulled into the handling yards just after 8:00 A.M. to be greeted by a decidedly jaded Tony Dyer and at least a dozen of his farm labourers, all of whom were of the Meru tribe. After greeting Tony, I said hello to the men in their own language.

My Kimeru "*Mugane,*" ("Hi, everyone") was followed by "*Muga sana*" (the emphatic singular form of greeting) from those standing nearby.

Tony quickly explained his tiredness. "Morning, Jerry. I'm afraid I've been up all night after those lions. We finally got them though."

"How many?"

"Five of the brutes. I've been after them for three nights. They're the ones I told you about at the polo club on Saturday. They've killed sixty sheep, but last night we finally caught up with them."

It was now time to get on with the job and determine how many of the black Galloway cattle were going to deliver calves. It was also possible to predict with considerable accuracy the date the births would occur. The handling system was cleverly designed. The animals were brought into a circular corral that fed into a single raceway that led some thirty metres slightly uphill to a swing gate that could draft each animal into one of four holding chutes. As soon as the cow had entered the chute, a bar was slipped behind its legs, and it was caught. Once the swing gate had been closed, I could step behind the row of cattle and get on with my part of the proceedings. As I felt the reproductive tract of each animal through my protective gloves I called out my findings. It was just a case of calling the numbers out to Tony. The herdsmen called out the cow's ear tag number, I called out the weeks "eight to ten," "sixteen to twenty," and so on. Moving along the line I could check each animal in under thirty seconds. By the time I got to the end of the line, more animals had been brought into the first couple of chutes.

There was only one problem. If Tony had not written down the call by the time I was on to the next animal in line, I had forgotten what my fingers had told me. On this particular morning we had to go a bit slowly at first, with a few repeats, because Tony was exhausted after his all-night shenanigans, but Mutua soon picked up the slack, and now that he could see properly, he began to write down my calls and relay them if needed.

After an hour, I needed a break, a change of glove and a rest for my arm, so I clambered up the rails to sit next to Tony and paused to admire the panorama below our almost 2,800-metre viewpoint. The cattle yards were located just above the sloping airstrip of the farm. Such was the slope that all planes landed uphill and took off down, whatever the wind direction. Just beyond the strip lay fields of yellowing wheat and the odd line of trees along fencerows. Then the land dipped and dropped out of sight until the hills surrounding Isiolo came into view, slightly hazy as the heat of the day began to affect the view. Isiolo, almost 1,500 metres lower down, was only about thirty-two crow-fly kilometres away. The unmistakable flat top of Ol Olokwe, over eighty kilometres due north, stood out clearly three hundred metres above the plain.

I picked up the thread of our earlier lion discussion.

"Five's a lot. How did you manage that?"

"Oh, with a driver and a spotlight. The only reason it wasn't six was that the last one took off before I could get a shot in. The blighters are a serious nuisance; they're always killing cattle and horses. One gang of three killed all of our children's ponies just in front of our house a few years ago."

This simple statement belied the fact that to shoot five lions quickly, before any of them could panic and run off, required very considerable skill.

Tony was, at the time, the chairman of the East African Professional Hunters Association and would remain so until the group disbanded in 1977. He acknowledges having shot twenty-eight stock-killing lions over a period of about fifty years. When we chatted in 2005, he said, "Lions have this strange urge, particularly after the first heavy rain after a long dry spell. They've got to go off and kill some cattle." He added with a wry chuckle, "It's the rites of lionhood."

Above my desk I still have a framed cable sent in 1972 that in my mind simultaneously sums up the problem and wins a prize for brevity. It said, STALLION KILLED BY LION STOP OPERATION OBVIATED STOP EVANS.

The sender was Jasper Evans, who ranched near Rumuruti, some one hundred kilometres north of Nanyuki, and the cable arrived just in time to prevent my long and dusty ride over murram roads to treat his stallion.

Jasper's problems did not stop there. When I had lunch with him thirty-three years later, he recounted how a lion killed three of his camel heifers on consecutive days before he shot it.

"I think we disturbed it each morning before it could get a proper feed and it would not come back in the daytime, or return to its kill."

It is not just lions that cause such trouble. One of my clients and rugby teammates was short stocky David Dewar, manager at the Italian-owned Suguroi estate that lay below the Aberdare Mountains. As we walked beside the Ngobit River on our way to check out some trout pools one day, he said, "We lost fifty-four sheep to a leopard last week, over three nights. As far as I'm concerned the bloody things should be re-named 'the greater spotted sheep-eater.'"

"Did you get the bastard?"

"Yeah," said David, "finally got him in a trap last night. The game warden came and took him away, but unless they move him a helluva long way I'm sure he'll be back. If he is, there'll be no second chance. I won't be calling the game department."

Over lunch on another of my client's farms I learned more about the dimensions of the predator problem.

"You probably heard about Tony's five lions in one night last week," I said as we started on our mushroom soup.

"You know," said my host, "when cheetahs turn up they can give you just as much trouble as lions."

"How so?"

"Well, last week we lost twenty-eight sheep in a single night, and this was the last straw. We had lost ten over the preceding few days. I was out checking to see if the wheat was ready to harvest when the combine driver, who was with me, saw a cheetah running through it. I got out my rifle and took a pot at it, but missed. I fired twice more and finally got it, so we went up to pick it up. We found three cheetahs, all dead, strung out in a line."

"That's some shooting," I said.

"Just luck," he replied.

"Well, David calls leopards the 'greater-spotted sheep-eater.' I suppose cheetahs would be the lesser-spotted."

"I'd agree. Good name," he said.

He is not one who boasts and made no further reference to this remarkable display of marksmanship, but I knew his reputation as a fearless exterminator of marauding buffalo, and that is not a species that gives any second chances.

When I reminded him about this conversation over thirty years later, the farmer asked me not to name him because in the intervening years the cheetah has become an iconic figure and is listed as vulnerable in the IUCN's red data book.

It is not just large-scale farmers and ranchers who have trouble with big cats.

Charles Chevenix Trench, who served as a district commissioner in northern Kenya in the years before independence in 1963, tells, in his entertaining 1964 book *The Desert's Dusty Face* of a meeting at which Chief Leparachao of the Samburu summed up the attitude of many of Africa's pastoralists to their cattle.

"We love to collect cattle as white men love to collect money," said the chief. "Why don't you get rid of all your surplus money? You like to keep it in a bank: our cattle is our bank." In response to a question from a government administrator present at the meeting, who asked whether one hundred good cattle would not be worth more than two hundred living skeletons, the response was, "I'd rather have a thousand, starving until God gives us grass. If a man has a lot of cattle and some die, he still has plenty left. But if a man has few cattle and some die, how will he and his family live?"

Small wonder, then, that among cattle herders the lion is merely seen as a pest. It is surely no leap of faith to accept that the famous lion hunts of the Maasai evolved because someone had to do something about the depredations of these powerful carnivores on the things more highly prized than wives or any material goods among the men of the tribe: their cattle.

Confirmation of the status afforded to cattle by the Maasai lies in the possibly apocryphal story that they once believed that all the world's cattle belonged to them by divine right. When the Kenya government issued postage stamps showing Maasai herders and their beasts, the Maasai considered it to be an official confirmation of their long-held beliefs. If lions were seen as a menace to their only means of livelihood—more than livelihood, as cattle meant status, as well as the ability to purchase wives—then they would naturally need to be dealt with. Who better to hunt them down and eliminate them than the young men of the warrior class, the *moran* or *murran?*

In her 2006 thesis based upon studies in Kenya's Maasailand, Leelah Hazzah distinguished two basic reasons why Maasai hunt lions. The best known is their ritualized *Olimayio* ceremony, when young men pass into manhood. The other is for revenge and is called *Olkiyioi*.

The no-doubt somewhat romanticized version of Olimayio involves the encirclement and spearing of a male lion. A group of warriors surrounds the animal as it stands at bay and will provoke it to charge. The man it charges falls down beneath his shield but is sometimes clawed to death. The rewards for being involved in this exercise include the privilege of wearing a lion-mane headdress on ceremonial occasions, and the man who gets the headdress is the one who drops both spear and shield to catch the lion by the tail while the others spear it to death above their comrade. The true technique is almost certainly somewhat less glorious, as the lion is likely to break out of attempted encirclement and is speared with one or more of the 2.4-metre-long spears until the final act, which may indeed involve tail-grabbing. There is no arguing that whatever happens, the whole thing is certainly very dangerous.

Leelah established that Olimayio is a manhood ritual for the moran, which takes place in the wet season when the young men have returned from their wide-ranging search for cattle grazing. The ritual and its outcomes provide enormous prestige. Only spearing is used, and the trophies (ears, paws, tail, mane and nose) are always removed. Olkiyioi, on the other hand, can involve anyone and any method (spearing, poison, guns). Trophies are rarely removed and season is not a factor.

For those who lack guns, or choose not to risk life and limb using a spear as a weapon, there are other and sadly easier ways of dealing with lions. Snares are indiscriminate, but effective, as Myles Turner relates in his 1987 book *My Serengeti Years: The Memoirs of an African Game Warden* about the sixteen years he spent there as deputy chief game warden. The book could easily have had a sub-title like "Poaching Wars," as the author makes constant reference to snares, which are one of the tools used by poachers. The situation has not changed. In fact it may have escalated.

In 2005, within a couple of months of his graduation from the Western College of Veterinary Medicine, Patrick Garcia, who had been with me in Uganda earlier that same year and had experience with wildlife in both Mauritius and Madagascar, was given the chance to work on a film in the Serengeti–Mara area. He witnessed the dying moments of a lion caught in a snare that had tightened about its belly. This was just one snare victim of several species that the crew saw, all deep inside the park. The pressure of poaching is constant and unrelenting.

Another effective, and completely indiscriminate, way to kill lions, as well as other carnivorous species, is to poison them. There are two types of poison that have worked over the years, and both are extremely easy to obtain. One group, the organochlorines, were, until banned in

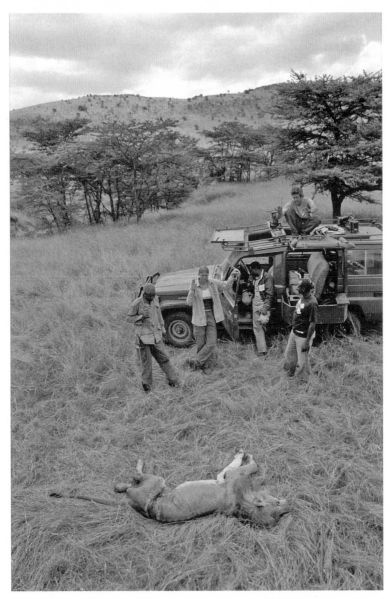

The end of the lion, Serengeti National Park. A film crew comes upon a sorry sight. (Photo by Dr. Patrick Garcia)

2001, a vital part of cattle management wherever ticks and tick-borne diseases created problems for livestock owners. Farmers up until this time would kill ticks by actually poisoning them. When used as intended the poisons were diluted from the potent parent compounds sold in any agricultural store and were either put into a plunge dip into which the cattle were driven or sprayed onto the cattle with a pump. The other type is carbofuran, which is sold to control insects in field crops. A quarter teaspoon is enough to kill an adult human.

All one has to do to kill lions, or any other predator, is to inject small quantities of the undiluted poison into a carcass and leave it out for the intended victim. If the poison kills off a hyaena or two, or maybe a bunch of vultures that have come to feast, that will not be of much concern to the poisoner: indeed it may be seen as a bonus. Worse yet, the chemicals seem to taste good, at least to dogs. Many a vet in East Africa has had to treat a dog that has licked some drops of the diluted cattle dip from a farmer's boots.

The organochlorines are just as poisonous for humans as carbofuran, and one small boy may owe his life to the fact that I had had to treat a few dogs during my practice days in Meru in the late 1960s. During our courting days, Jo had been confronted with a three-year-old whose father had brought him, late at night, to the hospital where she was on duty. With considerable presence of mind, he had also brought the little yellow tin from which the boy had sipped. The tin showed a picture of a cow and had the word KUPATOX, printed on the side. *Kupe* is the Swahili word for tick, so the name was entirely appropriate. Through the nurse he had explained that the lad had drunk some of the chocolate-coloured sweet stuff, no doubt tempted by the bright container. Jo's scribbled message, carried by a staff member to my house at 3:30 in the morning, had rousted me out of bed and got me to the hospital in record time after I had picked up my *Veterinary Toxicology*, which gave a clear description of the protocol for treatment in animals. Jo's innate skills with intravenous injection into a patient whose uncontrollably violent fits, every couple of minutes, would rip out the intravenous lines, saved the little boy's life.

In the 1950s the lions in Uganda's Lake Mburo National Park, which is surrounded by the traditional lands of the pastoral Ankole people, were poisoned out, only to reappear, it is thought as refugees from Rwanda, in the early 1990s. Again a poisoning program by herders began, and the last lion in the park was seen in 1997. This killing bout was a reaction to the lions' predation of cattle, which were grazing, presumably illegally, inside the park. This was exactly the same sort of revenge killing that my students saw in Uganda's Queen Elizabeth National Park in 2005. Luke Hunter, a carnivore specialist with the Wildlife Conservation Society, recorded another poisoning in QEP in 2006. In that case the victims were five spotted hyaena, two genets (a small slim long-bodied spotted carnivore, weighing under three kilograms) and even a buffalo calf that he assumed had been grazing near the poisoned carcass.

Accidental deaths also occur, as reported in an *Associated Press* article of October 23, 2007: "last week, five rare Asiatic lions were found electrocuted on the edge of western India's Gir National Park. Authorities said the lions were killed by an electrified fence that a villager had put up illegally to protect crops near the sanctuary." This item appeared under a headline about a terrifying mental image in a report about elephants that had been electrocuted after they went berserk following the drinking of copious quantities of rice beer and uprooting an electric pole.

If the Olimayio spearings were for ceremonial purposes and others for revenge or prevention of livestock predation, they were not the only motives for the killing of large predators. The killing of lions has played a large part in other cultural activities in Africa. Along with many other components, from a variety of plant and other animals, their parts have been used by witch doctors for generations, as Joy Adamson's illustrations in her *Peoples of Kenya* show clearly. There is hardly a picture of a warrior or witch doctor that lacks animal parts.

Dr. Margaret Driciru, in her 2006 thesis, documented many elements of the use of lion and leopard by the people around Murchison Falls National Park in Uganda. She reported that lion or leopard skins were reserved for royalty, either as costumes or as seat covers, and when chiefs died they were buried in leopard skins. If a member of either the Alur or Banyoro tribes of Uganda killed a leopard and gave the skin to a king, they were rewarded not only with his blessing but also with two bulls and a goat. On the other hand, members of the Labour tribe, whose totems include both lions and leopards, are not allowed to use any part of either species.

Lion and leopard tissues also have an important role in other witchcraft and traditional medical practices. Claws and teeth are extensively used. Margaret writes that skin, teeth and claws are "used as herbs for protection against people who may be their invisible enemies." A lion-tooth necklace is deemed to have "magic powers of protection." Lion fat is probably the most popular medicinal component, so much so that its sale has spawned substitute fat products from other animals. It has been promoted for use in back ache, burn wounds, rheumatism, tuberculosis, cosmetic bleaching and for use when dislocations are being massaged. A lion's heart is a prized item, giving its consumer what else but bravery? The heart is also used for treating heart disease in people and the bones are consumed for treatment of pneumonia and fractures. As for the leopard, Margaret learned that the skin may be used secretly by witch doctors for strong medicine because of its association with magic powers, and other people believe that the skin may be useful for the treatment of measles, while the bone is useful for whooping cough and arthritis of the knee.

While studies of diseases and witchcraft continue, several scientists have been studying other elements of the lion story. Kenya has among the most active predator research programs anywhere in Africa. The Laikipia Predator Project and the Kilimanjaro Lion Conservation Project are both directed by Laurence Frank of the University of California, Berkley, who has been engaged in this field for thirty years. The Laikipia Project (LPP) is based at Mpala Ranch, only a forty-five-minute drive from my old home in Nanyuki. The Kilimanjaro Lion Conservation Project (KLCP) is based on Mbirikani Group Ranch between Amboseli and Chyulu National Parks.

In a 2003 article titled "Once There Were Lions," in *Swara*, the magazine published by the East African Wild Life Society, Frank shows how the pace of predator extermination has changed with time and technology. He writes:

> *Historically, herders lacked the technology to rid themselves of predators: it took the Europeans millennia to get rid of lions, wolves, and bears. With better technology this took two centuries in eastern North America, and just a few decades in the American West. Twenty years ago, large carni-*

vores were still abundant in Kenya and much of eastern Africa, but with
cheap and effective poisons and the ubiquitous AK-47, Africa's predators
may largely disappear in our lifetimes.

At that time an AK-47 could be had in some parts of Kenya for the
price of three goats, about US$100.

In that same *Swara* article, Frank also shows how widespread the
attack on lions and other predators has become. He writes:

> *Even the lions of Masailand are disappearing. While the Masai might once*
> *have been natural conservationists, young men with spears have reduced*
> *to a handful the lions of Nairobi National Park. Poisoning and spearing*
> *have decimated that population. The same is happening in Tanzania's*
> *Ngorongoro Conservation Area. And there have been poisoning incidents*
> *in the Mara.*

In 2005 a different story about a seemingly brighter light in a grim scene
appeared in *Swara*. It described The Predator Compensation Fund,
which was developed in mid-2003 by consensus among the Maasai
members of the Mbirikani Group Ranch (MGR), Richard Bonham, a
native-born Kenyan and self-described committed conservationist and
local tourist-lodge owner, and Thomas Hill, an American entrepreneur
and philanthropist. It was the last two named who wrote the *Swara*
article.

The fund deals specifically with the MGR, which lies between Kenya's famous Amboseli, Tsavo and Chyulu Hill National Parks. The
ranch, 1,200 square kilometres in area, is home to ten thousand Maasai
pastoralists and to tens of thousands of their livestock. The authors
work closely with Laurence Frank and his team and told how they have
been instrumental in bringing about a major shift in thinking among
the MGR members.

Initially, when they first met with the herders to discuss the lion
killing and see if a way could be found to change things, Hill and Bonham were given short shrift. As they relate it, one elder said, "I think
we should kill off all the lions, once and for all. Our people would be
far better off." The pair was often told, "I cannot afford to lose even

one cow to a lion, not one. My cattle are worth far too much money."
These views show an interesting change of attitude. The cattle were
now a means to an end, the end being the acquisition of material
goods, or payment of things like school fees, or for the wealthy, the
"cattle barons," more expensive items like Western-style houses or
cars.

The compensation fund, which no doubt took an enormous amount
of time to hash out in meetings too numerous to count, boiled down
to three essential elements. It meant that no lions were to be killed,
rangers were to patrol and compensation was to be paid to any MGR
member who lost livestock to carnivore predation. The rangers even
included some women—a real sea-change for this tribe.

By 2006 this dream-like compensation fund, at least in the greater
Tsavo–Amboseli area, and particularly Amboseli National Park, had
become a nightmare, or perhaps it was an illusion all along. The lights
were obviously a swirling mirage, a migraine.

It seems as if not all the elders in that 2003 meeting were as sin-
cere as would have been hoped because, in a May 2006 report about
lion-killing in the region, Laurence Frank and his team have a telling
paragraph that relates the inadequate attempts at policing and pun-
ishment that have occurred outside the MGR. It is worth quoting in
full:

> In recent years the Amboseli-Tsavo Game Association has arrested nearly
> all the young men involved in spearing lions. However, in no case have
> they suffered serious legal consequences. They have usually been let out
> on minimum bail, and then either evidence is "lost," prosecutions fail to
> materialize, or judges have been bribed to drop charges or impose trivial
> fines. In several cases, the game scouts who arrested offenders were se-
> verely published by the community: the elders took their wives away from
> them. In summary game scouts have paid a much higher price for their
> enforcement activities than have morans for their offences.

The story was picked up by *National Geographic* and thus received
worldwide attention, which filtered back to Kenya and created quite
a stir.

Almost all of the lion killings described by Frank occurred on the Olgulului Group Ranch, which virtually surrounds Amboseli National Park. In particular, nine lions were killed inside the park boundary. As the lion population in the area heads inexorably to zero, the numbers killed seems to accelerate.

As Laurence Frank put it to me in an e-mail, "The wives were returned right away, once the game scouts learned the penalty for actually doing their jobs!"

Seamus MacLennan, who is one member of the Chyulu-based KLCP team, has developed a detailed set of figures that show the decline, both generally throughout Africa and specifically in the Amboseli–Tsavo study area.

In 1950 the number of lions in Africa was reputedly around the half million mark, although no one can vouch for this estimate. In 1975, the year that I moved to Canada, there were an estimated 200,000 lions on the continent. By 1990 the numbers had halved. In 2002 the figure was 39,000, and at the end of 2006 there were only 28,000 left. In fact, all of the figures are estimates, but there is no doubt about the trend.

The reduction in lion numbers in the Amboseli–Tsavo area is startling and MacLennan's figures for last six years provide some focus. At least 116 lions, and probably many more, were killed between 2001 and December 2006.

There are several key points about these numbers. First, the deaths are certainly nothing more than part of the story because the moran will boast of their exploits when they kill with spears, so the information is readily available, while more lions will have perished, unnoticed, in one of the all-too-numerous snares that abound, or through poisoning.

Second, of the kills up to May 2006, the sex was reported in fifty of 108. Almost twice as many females as males were speared. If any of those females had small cubs, they will have died, too, and the effect upon the overall population will have been much more pronounced than if the victims had been males. More lions were killed in 2006 (twenty-five of them) than in any of the preceding five years, even in the face of a rapidly declining lion population.

Third, as Dr. Frank put it in a January 2007 e-mail to me, "lions are in very deep trouble in Kenya. Unless the government gets serious,

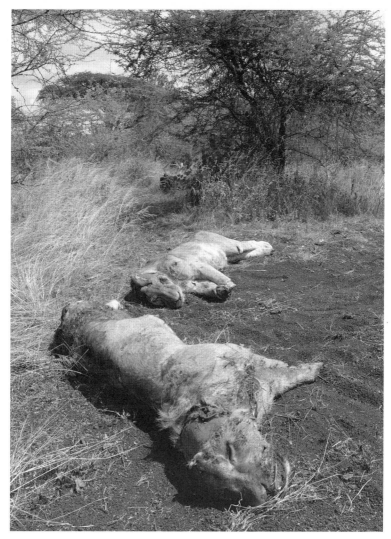

Two dead lions in Maasailand. The manes were cut off by the killers. (Courtesy Amy Howard)

lions will be extinct in Masailand outside the Masai Mara, in a very few years."

However, on a positive note, in the eight months following that May 2006 publication, and two months after the pessimistic e-mail, a massive change of heart occurred among the MGR people. In March 2007 Frank wrote a report for the Wildlife Conservation Society very shortly after being present at a remarkable event where he and his team witnessed hundreds of young warriors meet to celebrate the end of lion-killing as a manhood ritual.

In the report Frank states that in much of the region (Kenyan Maasailand) the picture is even worse than before. But the story is quite different in the MGR. He writes, "There have been what can only be described as sensationally positive developments." The lion population of the MGR has increased by 67 per cent. Only one of the 2006 lion spearings in the Amboseli-Tsavo area took place inside the MGR and the elders severely punished the youths involved. (The other killing was due to a snare).

Two important ideas led to the change in attitude. The first has been the production by members of Frank's team of an educational video in which the narration is in the Maa language. The film has been widely shown using donated equipment. As Frank puts it, "The great majority of pastoralists have never seen a TV, let alone a film, so this is a very powerful way to reach people with a conservation message."

The second idea has been the start-up of the Lion Guardians program (known locally as *Simba morans*). This program involves the conversion of young men "the great majority of whom are uneducated and unemployable, from lion killers into paid conservationists and community educators."

There have been two encouraging spin-offs from these initiatives. The morans themselves have formed the Mbirikani Moran Conservation Society, which is led by their chief. Then in June of 2007 a delegation of MGR members spent six weeks at the San Diego Zoo when the new Wild Animal Park was opened. This most certainly raised the profile of the conservation efforts in their homeland. The most recent news from the program remains upbeat. Long may it do so.

Meanwhile the KLCP is expanding its range and activities. Seamus MacLennan is branching out to study lions on neighbouring group ranches, which are beginning to get involved in schemes like the Mbirikani Predator Compensation Fund. Seamus is also expanding hyaena research.

Ogeto Mwebi, one of the graduate students in the KLCP, has been studying the difference between herding practices in the Tsavo–Amboseli region and those of the Maasai pastoralists in Laikipia. In the latter, the cattle are counted before being moved into bomas at night. In the Kilimanjaro area, the cattle are often not counted and are frequently left out at night, which inevitably leaves them open to predation. Mwebi found that during a trial period when experienced herders looked after the cattle of people who had experienced high losses, no livestock were killed. Hopefully the message about secure night bomas will get through to others.

Finally there has been a strong interest in taking the messages to other countries in Africa because, in the words of Luke Hunter, and as all members of the African Lion Working Group, a like-minded group of scientists who work on lions, well know, "conflict with people is now the gravest threat to the lion."

Attempts to curtail the destruction of lions can best succeed if the people affected by them can see an economic benefit to their efforts. Communal ranches like the one at Mbirikani have embraced so-called eco-tourism, because for them to succeed they need wildlife, especially lions, which are a major (perhaps the major) tourist draw.

In South Africa there are a large number of predator-proof fenced parks, just like the one at Madikwe, and lions can thrive in these, although their populations have to be controlled. If their numbers aren't controlled, and if the lions remain disease-free, their populations can increase very rapidly, perhaps by as much as 20 per cent a year. With nowhere to go outside the parks, the lions would soon overwhelm the prey resources.

A revenue-earning way of controlling lions in fenced parks has been through the sale of hunting licenses, and hunters may pay a good deal to have the chance at lion. When we met at Mpala in 2007, Laurence Frank, in shorts and sandals and shielded from the sun by his well-worn leather hat, told me that a lion hunt in Botswana might cost US$140,000. This would probably include a healthy tip and all licenses for other species in a typical eighteen-day safari, as well as trophy fees for each individual animal, which, for the lion alone might be as much as US$15,000.

Some people find the notion of hunting to be thoroughly distasteful, but both Frank and Luke Hunter, who have dedicated their careers to conservation, recognize that sheer practicality may sometimes have to supersede emotion, a position with which I strongly agree. However, it is not always that simple. David MacDonald of Oxford University's Wildlife Conservation Research Unit has been involved in long-term lion research in Zimbabwe and Botswana. He and his team have recounted how excessive hunting of lions, especially around the borders of the word-famous Hwange National Park, have impacted the overall structure of their populations. Over half of their radio-collared animals were shot, the large majority (82 per cent) within one kilometre of the boundary. A third of the males were sub-adults, providing inferior trophies, and the overall effect has been to change the sex ratio of the populations, increase infanticide by males that take over prides, and disrupt pride structures and social dynamics. Another effect of the over-hunting of lions has been to create a vacuum effect that draws lions from the centre of the park to the much less safe perimeter, taking the place of lions that once had their territory there, where they, in turn may be subject to hunting if they wander that short distance across the invisible line. Right now there is a moratorium on hunting of lions in western Zimbabwe, but it has resumed in Botswana after a four-year ban.

While hunting on a ranch would be no more than the sustainable use of a privately owned animal, not much different than shipping a load of cattle off to the abattoir, there is an ugly side to it that has been controversial for many years. A small number of "ranchers" breed lions for what are called "canned hunts." The animals are held in small enclosures—I have seen them in pens that were no more than twenty metres a side—and then shot by paying guests. I avoid the used of the word "hunted" here. There is a difference between hunting and shooting. This practice is condemned unanimously by all except the South African Predator Breeders Association whose chairman was "very disappointed and shocked by the announcement" that canned hunts had been banned through an act of the South African parliament.

In Kenya no hunting is permitted, and other solutions have been tried. In the *Swara* piece Laurence Frank describes how radio-collared lions have been studied in the region. He estimates that to tolerate lions it costs commercial ranchers about us$350 annually in livestock per lion. The communal ranches in Kenya are less forgiving and lions do not last long in those areas. In both types of operation habitual livestock killers are sooner or later killed. The reason is not far to seek. While an average cost may only be us$350, a lion invasion on an individual farm can lead to some real problems. One Laikipia rancher friend of ours lost several head of cattle, with a combined worth well in excess of us$350, to a lone male lion. He shot it and returned the collar to the Mpala Research Centre anonymously. This was a classic case of an old principle that states, "the statistics may not be significant, but when it's you it's 100 per cent."

So, ONE WONDERS, where does all this leave us and where does it leave the future of the lions and other big cats in Africa?

One possibility is that they will become a ghost species, a mere memory in the mind of man. I saw a good example of this on a road sign at a junction not far from Pretoria, South Africa's capital city. If you turn to the right you can go to Leeuwfontein; go straight on and you will get to Kameelfontein. The former translates from the Afrikaans as "lion spring," but there is absolutely no chance of seeing a lion in the area, which is now a stretch of farmland and small communities. The Kameelfontein (camel spring) part of the sign tells an interesting, but slightly different, story. It has precious little to do with camels and everything to do with giraffes. The taxonomic name of the giraffe is *Giraffa cameleopardalis,* and the story goes that the early European settlers in South Africa, devout churchmen to a man, who took the Creation story absolutely literally, could find no reference to these tall and graceful animals in the Good Book. The closest they could come to it was another hoofed animal, and they assumed it to be a camel, which they had never seen either. Of course there are now no giraffes—or camels—at Kameelfontein, although presumably there were plenty there in the not too distant past.

One hopes that Tony Dyer's pessimistic prediction is incorrect. In *The Big Five* he wrote: "In the end the large national parks will be the

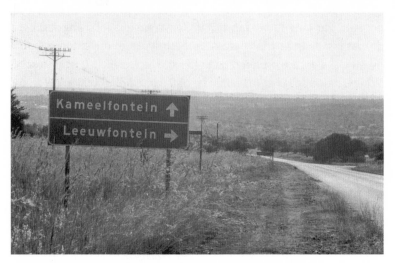

A road sign near Pretoria. Signs of things past.

only home for a lion." Maybe Tony was being overly optimistic, what with lion killings inside Amboseli, Nairobi and Queen Elizabeth National Parks, or maybe, with programs like the one at Mbirikani, there will continue to be a place for them as a symbol of so much, and a sight to stir the heart and set the hairs on the back of our necks a-tingling. ✻

2002–2007

ON THE
GROUND
IN UGANDA

The Pope has swept through Africa,
where 5 million people are already
infected with the AIDS virus, and
which expects by the end of the
century to have 10 million orphans
whose parents have died of AIDS—
and told them not to use condoms.

—BRENDA MADDOX

He who has tasted honey will
return to the honeypot.

—SWAHILI PROVERB

23

TEACHING IN UGANDA

In 2002 I have the opportunity to take
veterinary students from Saskatoon to Uganda.
The undertaking proves to be both challenging
and rewarding.

WHEN WE LEFT KENYA IN 1975 and I joined the faculty at Saskatoon's Western College of Veterinary Medicine (WCVM), both to teach and conduct research in the field of zoo and wildlife medicine, I did not sever my links with Africa. And during my time in Canada I lectured to, and chatted in the canteen with, students about my particular interest in the relationship between people, their livestock and the wildlife around them. In 2002 I had the opportunity to put the talking and slides into action and actually take students to Africa, so that I could show and not just tell. The opportunity to teach on the ground would take the students' education to a whole new level and of course provide an interesting challenge for me.

Credit for the idea goes to a Ugandan graduate student, Edward Bagu, whom I met during a seminar series in Saskatoon in 2001. We had been discussing conservation issues when he told me of a program run by the Department of Wildlife and Animal Resource Management (WARM) at the vet school in Kampala that had folded but was ripe for resurrection. That very name of the department at Makerere University clued me in to the fact that in Uganda, thinking and teaching about wildlife, livestock and people were closely linked. The conversation tripped a switch in my head, and I was soon in touch with the head of the department, Dr. Christine Dranzoa. It was with pleasure and a smile that I read her letter ending with the phrase "WARM regards." What a useful acronym.

I soon found out that the first barrier I had to pass was right at home. When I proposed the trip to the WCVM dean, the idea was almost dismissed out of hand because someone in the university's insurance office had checked the Canadian government's travel advisory website and noted that travel to Uganda was not recommended. This was mainly because the rebel group known as the Lord's Resistance Army had been conducting a long-running series of atrocities in the country's north; atrocities that included kidnapping, mutilation, murder and the use of children as soldiers or sex-slaves. A few years earlier there had also been the well-publicized kidnapping and murder of gorilla-tracking tourists, including a Canadian, by invading rebels from the Congo.

Determined to go ahead, if I could, I pointed out that I was not planning to take the students anywhere near the northern regions of the country. I also advised them that I was not planning to take them to the downtown core of any large North American city where violence and murder were common currency, or to Vancouver's notorious drug capital of East Hastings Street, where I would never go after dark. There are even streets in Saskatoon where it would be most unwise for a woman to walk alone late at night.

The vet college administration finally gave me a provisional go-ahead after I proposed to go to Uganda on my own, take a look at what was on offer and report back.

I had first been to Uganda in 1965, when I travelled over a long weekend with men's and women's teams from Nairobi's Parklands Sports

Club to Kampala for a seemingly crazy weekend devoted almost entirely to the striking of various sizes of ball with one of several different mechanical devices. We had started off with field hockey and then moved on to tennis, squash, and then, after suitable lubrication on the Saturday night, we had played a round of rather indifferent, and only hazily recalled, Sunday morning golf at Entebbe, overlooking Lake Victoria.

I set off for the teaching program investigation just before Christmas in 2001. Dr. Dranzoa came to meet me at Entebbe airport, and as there were only two other adult unaccompanied male Europeans on the flight it was not too difficult for her to guess my identity, especially with the bald head. The photo I had attached to the e-mail no doubt helped a bit as well.

"Welcome to Uganda, Prof," she said, with her radiant smile.

"It's good to be here again."

"Again?"

As we drove from the airport I told her about my previous visits, and she did something of a double take as I made comment about the traffic in a mix of English and Swahili.

"You speak Swahili?" she said with an upward inflexion on the last word in her voice.

"No problem." I told her more of my Kenya birth and East African history as she explained that Swahili had fallen into disuse in Uganda because of its association with the ugly days of Idi Amin and soldiers, policemen and wars.

We headed back to Kampala and the Makerere campus using a borrowed car. I was soon out cold in a friend's house, as I had travelled for something over 28 hours, with two exhausting airport changes. Next day we began to meet people, and it soon transpired that the Ugandan atmosphere was much more formal than that in North America. Dr. Dranzoa used my full title, Professor Haigh, all the time, even when addressing me directly. After a couple of days, I felt I had to break the cycle, as I had been using the informal "Christine," in Canadian fashion. Only when I threatened to call her "Head of Department Dranzoa" did she begin to relent.

As I got to know her I found out that Christine has an interesting history. She is a member of the Madi tribe, from the West Nile region,

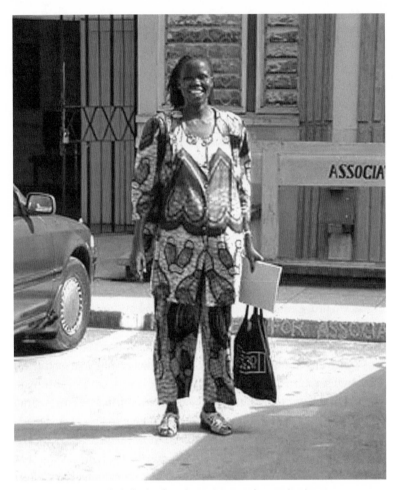

Dr. Christine Dranzoa outside the faculty of veterinary science at Makerere University.

and had to flee for her life when the despot Amin, whose father was a Kakwa, also from west of the Nile river, was ousted from power. Amin's ghastly reign had been enough to make all people from that region the targets of revenge as he had recruited many of his soldiers, including Madi men, from the area. Christine had fled with her family to the Sudan and for the next few years lived in a refugee camp. She told me very little about those dark days, even as I got to know her much better over the next few years, but I guess that she had been through everything that a young female refugee would suffer.

Showing both the tenacity that would make her a young head of department in a male-dominated system, and academic smarts, she had managed to get out of a difficult situation and finish high school before going on to university and ending up with a Ph.D., her topic being the effects of logging on the bird populations of Kibale Forest in western Uganda. While still a student she had dreamed of a department within the veterinary college at Makerere that would take on the mandate of linking studies in all forms of animal wildlife—fish, insects, birds and mammals—as well as the role of wildlife in human society and the potential for wise utilization of wildlife as a resource. She was able to persuade the dean of the college, Dr. Eli Katanguka, of the merits of her idea and soon found herself, in her early thirties, head of the fledgling department, with its own building and staff.

Not only had she escaped the morale-sapping environment of the refugee camp to obtain her degrees, but also she had taken on the care-giving role for a large family. The children of two of her siblings and their spouses who had died occupied her small home. One couple had been killed during fighting in the north; the other had both died of AIDS. Over and above these children, the youngest being Fiona (Fifi), aged only six, Christine gave house-room to one of her less fortunate sisters and an adult niece named Alice, who would become one of the most popular Ugandans when she cooked for the Canadians. I can not count the numbers of dependants accurately, but it seems as if at least a dozen people rely upon her, not only for food and shelter, but in many cases for school fees, as well. No wonder she had met me at the airport in a borrowed car: she did not have one of her own.

The business of looking after a gaggle of kids is not unusual in Africa. Many families across the continent find themselves in situations like Christine's. Taking in less fortunate relations is a standard practice, and the support is often a two-way street. When a family member makes good, perhaps after going to a big city or earning an overseas degree, they usually send funds back home to contribute to the support of others.

After a night's rest, Christine took me down to the WARM office where, still jet-lagged, I met Dr. John-Bosco Nizeyi, whose receding hairline would soon match my own. He would be my guide for the next week as we headed out on the scouting trip. JB, as he is known to just about everyone, is on staff with the Mountain Gorilla Program and was in the throes of completing the class work portion of his Ph.D. studies into human x primate disease interactions at Colorado State University. I knew immediately that he would be an integral member of the teaching staff, if I were to come back with students.

Because they took their own students on what they called "field training," every year, Christine and JB already had in place the elements of a course that would work for Canadians. I needed to see what would work for my own students in terms of learning. I wanted to find out what mix of species we might see. It would be important to offer the Canadians a chance to see the charismatic species such as chimpanzees, lions and elephants, because teaching and learning need to be fun, but I also wanted to be sure that we experienced as many aspects of the wildlife equation as possible. I also needed to be sure that we would be able to work with cattle and meet farmers and herders so as to learn what problems they had to deal with from day to day. Then, I had also to see what sort of transport, accommodation, meals and other experiences would be available. I needed to see and feel any potential negative elements, as I did not want to go to the trouble of organizing a big and expensive overseas outing that might not be worthwhile.

Back in Saskatoon I put together a guardedly optimistic report. I emphasized that there was no shortage of experienced faculty to teach the course and that other elements, especially accommodation and food, would vary from excellent to adequate, with a few days under canvas near the end of the trip.

With support from Dr. Jeremy Bailey, associate dean in charge of academic programs at wcvm, we decided to go ahead on a one-year trial basis. Jeremy is an expatriate South African who graduated from the veterinary school at Ondesterpoort, so he well understands some of the issues of travel and work on the continent. It is Jeremy who is ultimately responsible for student safety. Although it did not appear in any official documents, the fact that Jo would travel with me for the entire trip and be able to act as an unofficial physician, with years of tropical experience, probably helped to allay concerns about heath risks.

With the go ahead, I now had to organize the trip at the Saskatoon end.

Preparation for the first trip took months and has continued to do so in every year since, as it has to fit into the veterinary students' busy work schedule. I meet each new batch of students in late March, almost eleven months before they will travel. We have a series of meetings, with particular emphasis on travel safety. For this element, bearded Merv Dahl, a senior member of the university's Risk Management and Insurance Office, spends over an hour giving a seminar on safety that covers behaviour—especially relationship behaviour in a country struggling with AIDS—and other disease-prevention measures, particularly regarding malaria, the world's second biggest killer. He then administers a battery of written tests to make them aware of what to avoid, how to manage contacts and how to deal with emergencies.

Jo and I provide as much help as we can, down to even the seemingly mundane matter of packing: the kinds of clothes to take, the importance of having some string to use as a make-shift washing line, as well as the need for a roll of toilet paper in your day pack, ready for use at any time. Each student on the trip takes on at least one task in preparation for what will, for almost all of them, be an adventure into the unknown. We need a recording secretary, a treasurer, a phone manager, a tip master, a menu boss and even someone to make sure that everyone wakes up bright and early in the morning. It usually takes at least two students to organize the fundraising and gift collection for the little primary schools with whom we have established a relationship, of which more on pages 385-93. One student takes on the task of organizing flights, and another contacts the local Health Region office, as vaccinations have to be administered months in advance. Some students have never had a passport, so obviously that has to be dealt with. I also assign students a variety of readings and essays, and I give a talk that prepares them for the wildlife, the diseases and the challenges that they will face. The written and source materials created by the students goes into a "text book" that becomes a much-thumbed resource during the trip. We leave a copy behind at WARM, as well as providing one for our own WCVM library.

Of all these tasks, the one that initially appears to be the simplest, but always turns out to be the most vital for both students and their families, has been the cell phone management. The student who takes this on must make sure that there is enough "air time" on the card and be quite certain that the batteries are charged at any time of day or night.

The cell phone helps the students, who have no African experience, to keep in touch with the more familiar reality of home. Lovers, spouses, parents and friends have all been sent our two mobile numbers via e-mail. They can then phone in, at no cost in Uganda, and keep in touch.

The cell phone has been a personal benefit for Jo and me, as well, as we had news of the arrival of Rachael, our second granddaughter in Minneapolis, as we were having a glass of beer and a soda at the Lake Mburo canteen, many kilometres from the nearest town.

One student found out what happens when the phones are not properly managed. Her colleagues briefly placed her in Coventry, refusing to speak with her, when calls could neither be made nor received for almost twenty-four hours because the batteries were flat and she had mislaid the chargers.

The cell-phone system in Uganda is superb. Of course the land-line system is not well developed, which may have something to do with the fact that all that overhead wire has proved enormously tempting to locals who find it a most useful commodity. It can be turned into all sorts of items, from bracelets to toy model cars and fences.

The sight of a young woman silhouetted against the water-rippled reflection of the setting sun, hippos surfacing and snorting not twenty metres away, phone more or less glued to her ear as she talks sweet nothings to her boyfriend in Saskatoon, remains an indelible image.

Of course, the unexpected importance of the cell phone was all in the future when I planned that first trip. The preparations seem endless every year, and near our departure, they seem to accelerate. Finally we are ready to go, leaving in February each year, not least because that is usually a bitterly cold month on the Canadian prairies, and the temperatures in Uganda will be from warm to hot (18 to 35°c). With a mixture of excitement and trepidation, the students set out for the Saskatoon airport, happy to leave behind, depending on the year, a mass of packed snow on the streets or a blizzard.

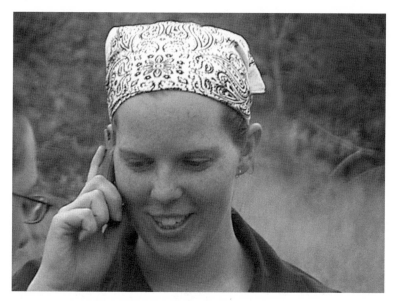

Hi there! Jen Currah chats with her brother and sister in Manitoba.

Our flight schedule involves a stop-over in Amsterdam followed by the last leg of the thirty-hour trip to Entebbe, Uganda's international airport. For Jo and me it is all fairly routine stuff, but for the students it is obviously quite different. How different had not occurred to me until petite raven-haired Amanda, asked, on our first full day of the first trip, "Don't you find this all a bit strange?"

Without hesitation I replied, "No, it's pretty routine." I paused and thought for a moment. "I imagine that's not the case for you. Don't worry, you'll get used to it." Of course she probably wouldn't in four short weeks, but my "white lie" was made with the good intention of helping her with the transition and the flood of new sensory input she would soon be dealing with on an almost daily basis. I knew Amanda and most of the other students would not be familiar with the masses of people, virtually none of whom have white skins; the lush and varied vegetation, such a contrast from the very limited range of plant species on the prairies; not to mention the traffic, city pollution, strange (to Canadian ears) accents, and general atmosphere of organized chaos. Of course, the very first change the students always notice is the temperature, as we have come out of the deep-freeze and

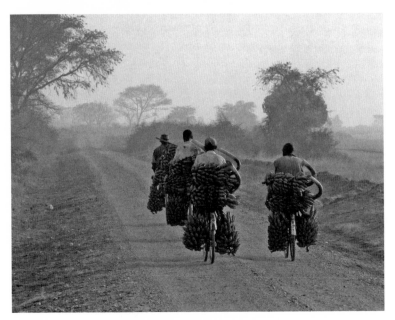

Plantains, a.k.a. *matoke*, on their way to market. (Photo by Karen Kemp)

the temperature at our arrival point is forty degrees warmer, at least. Even at night the temperature in Kampala does not drop below 20°C.

After greetings from one of the local colleagues, who change from year to year, we pile into the waiting bus. Then come the roads and traffic and the hour-long drive to Kampala, the capital. We were not fifteen minutes from the airport when tall skinny Ross, with his quick wit and instant repartee, said, "I see that they have the same road engineers here as we do in Saskatchewan."

He is referring to the myriad potholes, separated by varying, but not very long, stretches of good road.

"Yup," I replied. "We've got only two seasons at home, winter and road repair."

When we arrive in daytime there is a universal reaction, voiced first by lanky Brigid, hair all in a muss after the long journey, of wonderment at all the traffic. First it is the herds of bicycles being used as workhorses.

"That looks heavy, and really, really awkward," she exclaimed as we came up behind half a dozen huge branches of green bananas, each at least a metre long and sixty centimetres across, all stacked on the cross-bar, saddle and pannier of a bicycle. One can only just see the man leaning forward and straining with all his might as he climbs a steep slope, pushing his goods to market.

"That's called *matoke*," I tell them. "It provides the most important staple carbohydrate of the diet for most of the country. The other important carbs are potatoes, which they call 'Irish' here, sweet potatoes (which they call potatoes) and cassava."

We pass an entire bike almost hidden in brushes, shovels and other bits and pieces, making up a mobile hardware store, and another bearing a mass of little girl's dresses on hangers, in every colour of the paint box. Then into view looms a huge open-air clothes market, with hundreds of three-metre-wide stalls, packed like sardines and being examined by a seething horde of people. Most of the bus ride takes place in silence as the students are too exhausted to think much and are dealing with sensory overload every kilometre of the way.

We come to the first of several roundabouts or traffic circles. I can still see Jenna, eyes wide, clasping the sides of her seat as we charged up to a seeming logjam of Toyota vans-turned-taxis that inched forward, only a skin of paint apart, to cut across each other's lanes and emerge unscathed to head off to their destinations. As if this wasn't enough, the roving herds of small motorcycles, like gnats, buzz around the cities and towns carrying passengers who risk their lives, or at least their knee caps, every time they book a ride and are threaded between all the other traffic. At least these two-wheeled taxis, known as *boda-bodas*, are cheap to hire. With the all-day rush hour and vast traffic jam that is Kampala, *boda-bodas* provide the quickest way to get around—you need only remember to keep your knees clamped firmly in.

While the crowds are no surprise—the city has 1.5 million people—and the traffic is bedlam, there is a wildlife surprise in the city that most students could never have anticipated. There are marabou storks everywhere in Kampala, standing like Father Time clones at every rubbish tip and roosting in the tall eucalyptus trees. One soon learns not to walk in places where the tarmac has been marked with white from above. The marabou may well qualify as the ugliest bird in

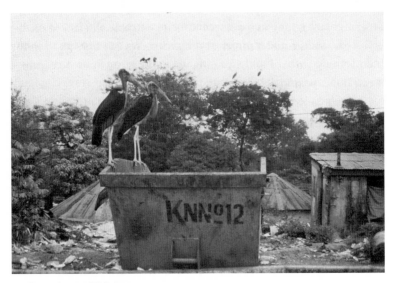

Marabou storks at a rubbish tip.

creation (except to another marabou), but they perform an admirable service. Away from human settlement they are scavengers, picking up bits and pieces of carcasses left by predators, or whatever else they can find. In the towns and cities of Uganda they have parlayed this activity into being garbage men. There is a direct relationship between the numbers of marabou and the human population of Kampala. While the human population booms, in the space of forty years the bird numbers have risen from a few dozen to almost one thousand.

Finally we arrive at the faculty of veterinary medicine, part of Makerere, the oldest university in East Africa, and an exhausted party crashes into bed in the dormitories at the Spartan, but clean and quite adequate, visitor's apartments. Most of them are sleeping under mosquito nets for the first time in their lives.

Tired as everyone is, there is really no time to waste, and certainly none to hang about and recover from jet lag. A packed program is ready for us, and we are here to study something new about veterinary medicine, not to lollygag in bed. Next morning we head into the city to do three important things. We visit the Canadian consular office, where long-time Ugandan resident Mr. Don Campbell, with his refreshing Scots accent, takes copies of our passports, in case anything should go awry, and warns us once again about being "too friendly" with Ugandans, for fear of contracting AIDS. We head to one of many Internet cafés to let family and friends know of our safe arrival, and we change our money. Everyone is promptly a millionaire, changing his or her US money—the most readily accepted international currency—into Uganda shillings. We will need money for park entrance, food, accommodation and so on, so US$600 becomes a million shillings and quickly gives everyone a bulge in the money belt.

The students are at once plunged into new experiences as we walk from place to place. Beggars, many with horribly bent limbs, probably a result of contracting polio, sit every few metres along all the major shopping streets. Street vendors, mostly women, all offering similar arrays of newspapers, ball-point pens and a variety of trinkets, sit under umbrellas everywhere that pedestrian traffic is heavy. Many of them have infants snuggled up to them, some asleep, others grubbing and idly scratching patterns in the dust. We meet the boda-bodas, all tended by young men gathered like small herds of antelope at most intersections, waiting for fares.

Then it's back to the vet college and time to meet our colleagues and the Ugandan students who will join us for the full month, which, from the first trip, has been one of the most important parts of the entire experience. The exchanges, at both the professional and social level have been invaluable.

First, however, the Canadians must meet Christine and other members of her department, and we usually have a formal greeting from the dean. Christine gives us a heartfelt talk about her country and its history. She is a fiercely proud Ugandan who tells us about the challenges her kinsfolk face and quotes Winston Churchill in saying that Uganda is the pearl of Africa. She closes with her trademark WARM welcome, slightly emphasizing the pun and gaining smiles from the Canadians as they realize that they are among friends.

Cultural differences soon become apparent. On our first trip, on the first full day in the country, during a laboratory session when we were learning about some tropical diseases, a smartly coiffed young Ugandan woman, dressed in a white lab coat, approached me at the back of the room and furtively asked a favour.

"My brother is not married and is looking for a wife. Would any of those girls be interested? Would you check for me?"

Over a lunch of chapattis and fish in ground-nut sauce—served by Angela, Christine's sister, who runs the college canteen—I passed this request on to our group of nine young women, knowing that it would surprise them, but also to show them some of the culture.

"We've never even met the guy," said Karen, her eyebrows rising just before she grinned.

A memorable scene, a tiny moment, also highlighted differences in attitudes to political correctness. One of the Canadian women, solidly built, was browsing the clothes stores in town when a young man approached with a broad smile and a thumbs-up signal, saying, "Man, you're big!"

She laughed as she told us the tale, "I didn't know whether it was an insult or a compliment." I was able to reassure her that the "hip to waist ratio" method of judging a woman's potential as a mate was different in Uganda than in Canada. Moreover, the records of early English explorers like John Hanning Speke and Sir Richard Burton tell how in some cultures in the region girls were force-fed cream and not allowed to exercise in order to increase their beauty quotients.

It has not usually taken long for the initial cultural barriers between Canadian and Ugandan students to be breached, although some students have taken longer to become comfortable than others. One student in particular sticks in my mind. Ugandan Jesca (whom we christened Jesca N. to distinguish her from our own Jessica P.) seemed unusually quiet, and at first I put this down to shyness and perhaps a feeling of being dominated by my older male and professorial status. However, she did not come out of her shell during our seven-hour bus ride to the first field station where the wildlife studies would begin. Jesca did not really merge into the group until we began our fieldwork and everyone slept in dormitory accommodation. Over the next three days, Jesca began to get to know and chat with the Canadian girls, who soon found out that part of her reticence probably had something to do with experiences that we could hardly imagine. At twenty-four years of age, Jesca was one of oldest people in her village and so was responsible for several younger siblings. All the

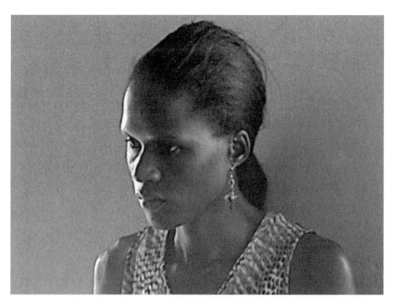

Jesca N. in a pensive mood.

parents and grandparents in the community had died of AIDS. All of them.

Another of the Ugandan graduate students in that first year was Celsus Senhte, a short stocky man of the Banyaruguru tribe who played rugby as a prop forward when he attended Uganda's oldest secondary school (Namilyango College, founded in 1902). Celsus's story is another interesting example of how extended families in Africa work. He is one of eleven children, five of whom are no longer alive. His people come from areas around Queen Elizabeth National Park, which was on our itinerary, and it was here as a child that he began to develop his steel. As an eight-year-old lad, he became a fish trader, purchasing each morning as many fish as he could carry (about thirty on average) from the fish landing in the village of Kasenyi, which lies deep inside the park on the shores of Lake George. He would haul them home over several kilometres on his shoulder. At this age he had no shoes or shirt, but his entrepreneurial success with the fish soon fixed that. With the financial help of his older brother, Nkakyekorera, who was already practicing as a doctor, he moved to Nairobi and finished primary school. Then it was back to Uganda and on to Namilyango, where his final marks were not enough to get him into medical school but good enough for the veterinary program.

Other graduate students have also travelled with us. One year, two veterinarians from the Democratic Republic of Congo, Jacques Iyanya and Eddie Kambale, who had recently been employed by the Morris Animal Foundation to work on gorillas in that country, joined us. This presented an interesting teaching challenge for everyone because of the language mix. Jacques and Eddie speak their native tongues, which no one else knew. They also speak excellent French, Kinyarwanda (the main language in Rwanda) and Swahili, but not quite the same Swahili as that spoken in Kenya and Tanzania. Both could also converse to some extent in English. As two of our Canadian party were fluent in French, and one of our Ugandan colleagues, Innocent Rwego, was fluent in Kinyarwanda, Swahili and English, we were able to make do, even if the Babel-like mix of sounds tended to be a bit confusing at times.

My final impression of the new status of Uganda at the end of my exploratory trip occurred when I picked up the daily newspaper and read about a novel scheme to try to get the AIDS situation under control. The banner headline read "TV SETS FOR VIRGIN BRIDES." The story itself stated how an award of a TV set was to be given to women who could prove that they were virgins when they married. The idea was sound and certainly fitted with the US- and church-led drive to get away from condom promotion to encourage abstinence. Then came the kicker. The judge of the bride's condition was to be the new husband. Talk about setting the fox to guard the hen house!

I describe many components of our times together in Uganda in the chapters that follow. Another view can be seen on the University of Saskatchewan website, where a search for "Uganda rotation" will bring the reader to descriptions and to the blog written in 2007. The whole experience of the Uganda rotation, the people, the wildlife, the environment and the learning, will stay with the students for the rest of their lives. ✻

24

—

FOREST
WALKS

*We start our animal work on the ground. Visits to
dairy farms around Kampala, a six-hour bus trip
through the countryside, rain forest experiences,
chimpanzee politics and wildlife encounters.*

THE FIRST STEP IN THE ACTUAL VETERINARY, as opposed to cultural, teaching starts right near Kampala. Right away the students begin
to learn about differences between the practice of their intended profession in the wealthy environment of Canada and the very different
tone in Uganda. An important element of this part of the program is
for students to see how agriculture differs between the tropics and the
temperate prairies of home.

On the second day in the country we visit a smallholder's dairy farm.
Dr. Benon Kanyima is our teaching and tour guide to the local dairy
farm just outside the city. Kanyima is a tall robust veterinarian with a
winning gap-toothed smile. He is also another member of the vet fac-

ulty teaching team, whose main interest is reproductive management of dairy cattle. He studied in Michigan for two years, so he knows about the weather we have left behind and can join in the happy feelings when within ten minutes of boarding the bus a phone call from Canada is relayed to us with the news that it is-35°C, with a high wind chill.

Treating cows for sleeping sickness is something very new for the North Americans, and students must adjust their expectations from what they know of high-end dairy practices in Canada to the reality of a Ugandan smallholding, with ten cows on half as many hectares. The animals are fed grass and sweet potato vines that have been run through a hand-cranked mechanical chopper, and the students' cameras click away as they note how simple the system is and so different than the one Canadians are used to. Other management methods of the herd are similar to those at home, and we are soon donning coveralls and plastic sleeves to check animals for pregnancy.

After a day around Kampala and an evening meal in a local hotel that is brimming with life and also serves several local brews such as Nile Special and Bell, we head almost due west to Kibale National Park, the first of the national parks that we will stay in. Our activities there centre on primates, birds, small forest rodents, an amazing variety of plant life and wide-ranging discussions of how all these elements mesh together. We also discuss how the people who cultivate their small farms around the park fit into the ecology of the area

The bus is piled high with gear and masses of gifts that have been collecting, as well as the ones we purchased in Kampala with the cash that has been sent to us by generous donors in Saskatoon.

As we leave the city we crawl in a seemingly never-ending stream of traffic, and we stare wide-eyed at the bustle around us. There are shops of every variety, selling anything from yellow plastic jerry cans to gaily coloured mattresses to heavy wooden furniture with dark upholstery. Often stores with similar merchandise have set up along side each other, in a sort of flock mentality, so that every now and again, alongside the furniture stores, a stack of wooden coffins sit at the roadside ready to be sold. The little ones, only a metre long, tell a sad story. Every sixth storefront is a bar, advertising one of the local brews, and, almost as frequently, rival mobile phone companies have anything from whole

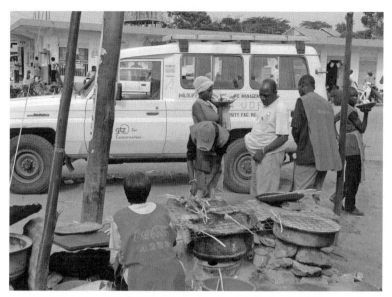

Dr. JB Nizeyi at the Mubende road-side chicken-on-a-stick stall as he checks that the kebab is properly cooked. A vendor offers some grilled matooke.

buildings to tiny stalls, each seemingly more garishly painted than the rest, in the colours of their particular line. A red so bright it almost hurts for Celtel, the yellow and blue of the Finnish flag for Celtel's rival, MTN.

At last we escape the city's clutches and are in the countryside. Small farms flash by. Banana trees dominate the landscape, but other plants are interlaced, sometimes straggly coffee bushes, sometimes maize standing dry above sweet potatoes or yams. In each valley bottom, where the clay soil has been dug and turned into bricks, kilns, some of them smoking as they bake the building materials, vie for space with the bush and papyrus stalks. People stand and dig in the muddy pits that contain the raw material for the bricks.

In every village along the way, speed bumps slow the traffic, and we get another chance to see the array of produce and the bicycles stacked high with just about anything you could imagine.

After three hours the bus stops in the small market town of Mubende, where the hungry will have their first chance to try the delicious chicken kebabs grilled on charcoal burners made from the top sections of old oil drums. A seething mass of vendors mobs any open window, holding up their various wares for inspection and trying to sell the chicken-on-a-stick or the alternative meat product: goat kebab. Bottled water, chapattis, grilled matooke or peanuts are also available.

Another three hours brings us through many hectares of pale green, almost billiard-table-flat tea estates to the gates of Kibale National Park at the Makerere University Biological Field Station at Kanyawara. What a contrast to everything that has gone before, and what a delightful place. The field station is a research facility, as well as a well-appointed centre, with hot showers, a library, video facilities and a solar-powered electrical back-up system. While the dormitory accommodations are not a problem for the Canadians, some are a bit taken aback the first time they see pit latrines, built as concrete slabs with rectangular holes in the middle and known colloquially as "long-drops." The station lies on the park edge, but right away we know we are somewhere special.

By the time we reach the station, Jo and I know we can start to cut back on the mother-henning of our Canadians as they begin to fit into the Ugandan scene, accepting the slow pace, enjoying the new diet that includes plenty of avocado and roasted peanuts (ground nuts as they are known locally), as well as the scenery, with the spectacular bright red flowers of the Nandi flame trees (*Spathodea*) growing right outside the dining room. They watch sunbirds flitting from flower to flower in the red bottlebrush tree near the concrete path. If the students want to watch a scene with more drama, they can also easily view the male black weavers racing back and forth to their nest projects in nearby trees, determined to show the females that they have the know-how to be the best guy on the block, and so be allowed to pass their genes on to the next generation. Most students however, are much more enthusiastic when the local, somewhat habituated, baboon troupe tries to creep into compound, check out the garbage cans and maybe raid their rooms if they have not heeded the warnings about locking up whenever they leave.

As we arrive there is a welcoming cup of tea and an even more welcoming smile from Innocent Kato, the field station manager. Almost before the students have their backpacks into their dormitory-type rooms, the student cameras are burning disk-space or film—there are still a few purists who prefer the old-fashioned techniques—as the camp's almost resident troupe of habituated black-and-white colobus monkeys, long hair blowing in the breeze or flying out behind their tails as they leap from branch to branch, complete the transition from the lecture theatres and clinics of Saskatoon to Uganda.

At this point in the trip, we know that Jo can begin to enjoy making her sketches of the many beautiful plants, and I can begin to watch out for opportunities to do some bird photography.

Kibale National Park is a smallholding- and tea-estate-surrounded tropical rainforest island of under eight hundred square kilometres that is home to thirteen species of primates, including groups of human-habituated chimps, which are second only to gorillas as revenue earners for Uganda's tourist industry.

Our walks in the forest are almost ethereal. Having been wakened before first light by the territorial calls of the dominant male black-and-white colobus, and then having enjoyed a welcome cup of something hot swilled down with a sweet and delicious finger banana, we set out just after dawn. The overnight mist shrouds the treetops towering above us and noises of cracking branches intermingle with a chorus of bird song. Occasionally we hear chimps or monkeys calling in the distance, and we are constantly on the alert for the more worrying sounds of elephants trumpeting, feeding or simply breaking branches for the hell of it. We heard them once, all too close. We know that they can move much faster than us, especially through the thick underbrush, and may well be aggressive. As there was really no chance of getting away if we should have encountered one around the next corner, we took the sensible option and retreated.

For the first two years of the Saskatoon–Uganda program we worked with Christine, whose thesis work was on the nesting ecology at the farm/forest fringes in this very place. Indeed we are walking the very trails that she walked to study the birds. In order for the students to gain a broader understanding of wildlife research methods, and especially to allow them to study diseases of wild species in their natural habitats, we set mist nets and examine the small birds that fly into them, just as Christine used to do. We take blood samples to check for the bird version of malaria and fecal samples to see if there are any

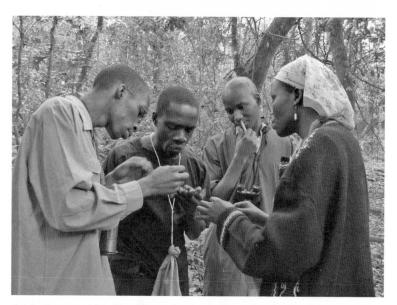

Christine Dranzoa, at right, with students Denis Muhangi and Bernard Ssebide flanking wildlife technician Eric Sunday.

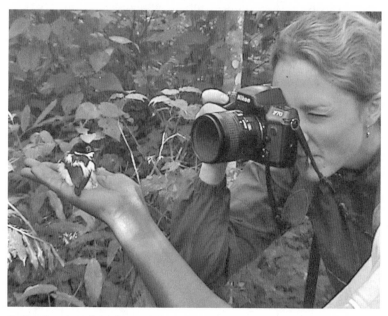

The biter bit. Catharine being photographed as she photographs a bird in the hand (a male black-throated wattle eye).

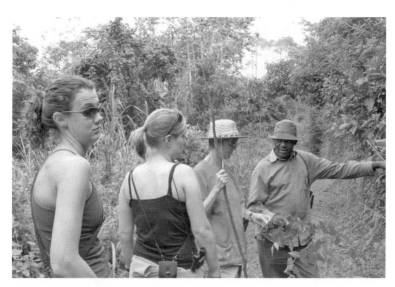

A forest walk with John Kasenene. From the left: Erica Anderson, Anna Wallace, and Jo.

other parasites. When Christine obtained her well-deserved promotion to the graduate college of the entire university and no longer had the time or luxury of an escape to her favourite spot, her former graduate students ably replaced her.

The chief forest ecologist at Kibale is also part of our teaching team. John Kasenene is a powerfully built extrovert whose home village is only about seven kilometres from the park gate. He has an encyclopedic knowledge of vegetation and a fascination, which he can transmit with great enthusiasm, with the field of ethnobotany, the study of medicinal plants. Not a student who has met him has failed to be turned on by his wit, style and vast knowledge as he tells us about well-known cures for diseases from prostate cancer (from wild *Prunus* trees) to malaria (from plants too numerous for me to take in).

We also meet Professor Dr. Gil Basuta, whose bald head, fringed with white close-cropped hair, matches my own style. With him we work on forest rodents, again taking tiny blood samples that we will examine in the station's laboratory to check for disease, this time for the rodent form of sleeping sickness. As we walk in the forest and look for monkeys in the canopy, it is Gil who introduces us to the concept of chimpanzee politics. With an infectious laugh and the use of grunts,

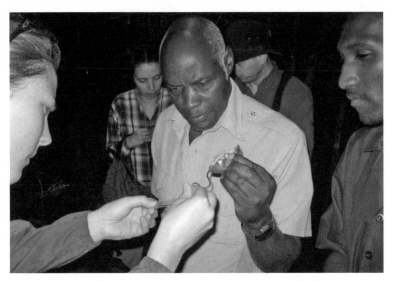

Dr. Gil Basuta, surrounded by students, holds a Jackson's forest rat for a blood sample. Dr. Eddie Kambale of the DRC is on the right.

grimaces and sideways looks, he is able to transport us into the head of an adult male chimp.

"Just as in human politics," he says, "the alpha male has his allies, like his ministers, and he will gang up with others to form temporary alliances to gain control of social groups." He points upwards and continues as a troupe of monkeys skitters through the trees, moving constantly, the odd tail dangling down, a head poking around a trunk, a body half-suspended in midair as it leaps from one tree to the next. "Those are red colobus, and they are the chimp's favourite prey. When they decide to catch one of these monkeys they surround it and attack.

"The adult male chimps are too heavy to be agile in the canopy, so they wait on the ground." He hunches his shoulders, stares straight ahead with his lips pouted out, just like a chimp, and continues, "They stand like a group of NFL linemen, where they know that, as group leaders, they will get the spoils of the hunt. The captured colobus is given to the alpha male, who usually kills it like this."

Holding his hands like a cradle, he brings them up to his face and makes several chewing motions. "They eat out the belly button or sometimes hold it by the legs and swing it against a tree."

Even veterinary students used to the post-mortem room and many aspects of animal behaviour have trouble with these images, especially as they must realize that the death by the first method will not be instantaneous.

Gil continues, "They then dish out some of the meat either to male allies, who are current close supporters in the dominance structure, or to compliant females in exchange for sexual favours."

He tells the students to take a look at the little text in the field station library.

"It's by a man named de Waal and is called *Chimpanzee Politics*. Although it was published in 1982 and is set in a Dutch zoo it fits the situation here exactly," he says.

Politics indeed. As all of our party come from a university and read newspapers about the goings on of elected people running many a government, we did not need Gil to draw further parallels.

The grisly account of chimp predation on monkeys is only an introduction to a much more dramatic story that really gets the students thinking each year as they begin to realize how close the park boundary and the farms really are to one another.

The smallholder farmers along the porous boundary at Kibale wage a constant battle against several primates, especially baboons turned crop-raiders. It is the women, as in most parts of Africa, who do the bulk of the cultivation, and they spend considerable time ground-breaking, planting, weeding and harvesting the crops that feed their families and perhaps generate a few shillings. When these farmers come to do their work they may well have infants with them in the usual cloth sling on their backs. In order to do their work they often put their children down, and as Gil tells it, "Five times in the last seven years a single male chimp has emerged from the forest and taken a child to eat. There have been other attacks, some just sheer aggression. In all there have been fifteen attacks in the last seven years."

This account is gruesome enough, but when, in 2004, *Swara*, the magazine arm of the East African Wild Life Society, ran the story and showed a picture of Beatrice Wambari whose two-year-old son had been seized and disembowelled, we could all relate personally to the tragedy.

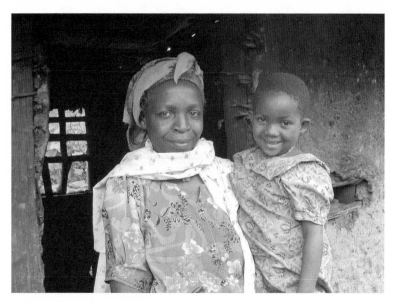

Beatrice Wambari and an older daughter at their home near Kibale National Park. (Photo © Paula Kahumbu, used with permission. Courtesy Gordon Boy and *Swara* magazine)

In 2006, as we sat in the little lecture theatre at Kanyawara with the various faculty and opened this subject up again, we learned that the problem had not gone away. It had escalated. Tiny forest fragments, now isolated from the park, still hold chimps, which inevitably get into conflicts with the smallholders all around. Forceful John Kasenene joined in the debate with even more that his usual vigour, on the side of the smallholders. At first, I did not know why. Gil plainly knew what was coming however, and he cleverly shifted his position, role-playing with great subtlety, to become a chimp protagonist.

"Just put yourself in my shoes," said John as the discussion wound up. "Last year my seven-year-old nephew was caught and emasculated by a male chimp. He bled to death."

No wonder John's words had been strong. The students emerged from our workshop with a whole new level of understanding of the human-wildlife matrix. They were silenced for a while, trying to absorb the account. Later, over a beer at the Obbligato bar, dark-haired Kristin said, "Boy that story of John's puts things in a whole new light. I can't imagine being in his shoes, let alone the boy's parents.'"

There is other dangerous wildlife in the park, and one does not always need to give verbal warnings about them to make the point. During our first trip the students had seen a seemingly never-ending stream of safari ants, *siafu*, crossing a track. They knew my own story of the effects of these little terrors when clamped to the "family jewels" inside a man's shorts, and they had been careful to avoid stepping on their moving columns. But in the dark shade of the forest, with precious little direct sunlight, and a carpet of greenery, the odd mistake was bound to occur. Eventually the inevitable very close encounter with these ants came.

As we walked along a narrow trail, several of the students started to squawk and leap about, pulling at various bits of clothing under which lay numerous ants. Charlene, herself a victim, took time to record the impromptu dances on film as Mike, Chantelle and Catharine partially disrobed and removed the attackers. No wonder the footage is a bit wobbly.

As Gil and I, who were walking with the group, pointed out, we had all been lucky. Safari ants will sometimes climb up into the trees and fall like rain upon potential victims. They have been known to consume an entire coop-full of chickens that have been locked up for the night, leaving only bones and feathers. Tethered dogs can be turned into glove puppets in the same way. Those who have been victims will attest that there must be some sort of communication among a group of *siafu*. When a sufficient number of them have clambered over a person they all seem to bite at once.

IN OUR WRAP-UP AT KIBALE we hold a small workshop and not only de-brief what we have seen but also take a look at the wider issues surrounding primate conservation. In particular, we look at diseases that may move back and forth between gorillas and chimps, monkeys and people, a subject of growing concern as human populations expand and primates are constantly exposed to a battery of human pathogens. What with John Kasenene and Gil Basuta to cover eco-

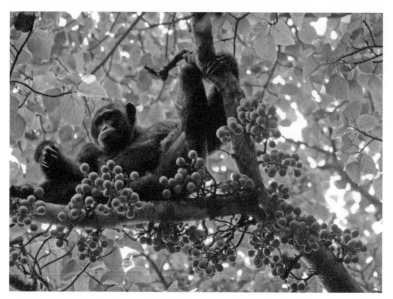
On a forest walk. A chimp feasting on wild figs in Kibale.

logical ground, and my first-year guide and mountain gorilla expert JB Nizeyi, who has travelled with us, we have the ideal facilitators to guide us in probing the material we have covered.

Then there is slim sharp-minded Innocent Rwego, whom we met on our first trip when he was a new graduate student. He has continued to study and understand these issues and is working right at Kanyawara toward his Ph.D. as he manages the Kibale Ecohealth Project. We could hardly have a better group of instructors.

After the wrap-up, everyone has some time off. The students are able to go on a guided chimp-tracking walk, which is pretty special.

"We were lucky," said Maryanne, our slim brunette group secretary. "The guides knew almost exactly where the chimps were and we found them inside thirty minutes. We spent almost an hour with them, and they were mostly in the trees above us. However, one female came down onto the path just in front of us with her infant. I was able to get some great pictures. It was amazing."

Evenings, after supper, we retire to the Obbligato bar, which is only fifty metres from the dining room. It is conveniently located about two metres from the other side of the road that comes into the station and is technically outside the park boundary, so we can have a beer or two without breaking any field-station or park rules.

When it is time to move on, we say our farewells and head to the nearby town of Fort Portal, where we can get Internet access—albeit only through an agonizingly slow and unreliable dial-up connection that from time to time fails right in the middle of a transmission. This important market town, sited in the heart of the kingdom of Toro, was named for Sir Gerald Portal, who died in 1894 after a brilliant career in the British diplomatic service during which he was appointed special commissioner for Uganda. His statue still stands in the middle of the town roundabout.

After a fuel stop, pit stop and brief foray to a small but well-stocked supermarket, we are on our way again; next stop Queen Elizabeth National Park. ✳

25

QUEEN ELIZABETH NATIONAL PARK

At Queen Elizabeth National Park we come face to face with problem animals, unusual animal interactions, injured lions, poaching and witchcraft.

OUR NEXT DESTINATION IS QUEEN ELIZABETH NATIONAL PARK, conveniently known as QEP. Our focus will shift, both in terms of the people–wildlife relationship, which is in some ways even more complex here than it is in Kibale, and in the species that we will encounter.

The species mix at QEP include lions, hyaenas, leopards, elephants, hippos, shaggy grey waterbuck (about the size of a large pony) and Uganda kob, as well as a wonderful variety of bird species. Here, we assist with a long-running project on large predators, as well as a small research project on a nasty zoonotic disease called brucellosis. The students see lots of new things.

There are eleven villages in the park, which have been there since before the area was gazetted, and the inhabitants cling to their ancestral rights.

The 130-kilometre drive to the community of Mweya, where the park headquarters is located, should only take a couple of hours, but we have yet to travel this road when it is not undergoing extensive repair, with potholes, diversions and other delays the order of the day. We live in hope. There is a steady elevation drop from the 1,500 metres at Fort Portal to nine hundred metres at Mweya. As we go down, the ambient temperature rises about ten degrees from the pleasant 20°C or so at Kanyawara. The roadside agriculture changes steadily from small plots of tea, through matooke or other banana types, which are evident almost all the way, to cassava and cotton at the lower elevation. All the while we have the foothills of the Ruwenzori Mountains on our right.

"The Ruwenzoris may be the Mountains Of The Moon that the ancient Greek merchant Diogenes reported on after he travelled inland from the East African coast. He said that the natives called the range by this name because of their snowcapped whiteness. When we see them they are usually a bit hazy, what with all the deliberate burning that goes on at the end of the dry season. Some people believe that the smoke brings the rain," I tell the crew. "Farther down the road one can sometimes see snow on the tops as they rise to over five thousand metres. There are other mountains in the world that vie for that lunar title, but in Uganda it's not even debated."

As we get nearer to QEP, and if we are lucky, we can pick up some delicious pineapples at a road-side stall. A few kilometres later there is a shout from redhead Jeni as the bus approaches a giant, white-painted, three-metre-tall concrete ring standing on its side with a line bisecting the centre of its base.

"Can we stop please," she asks the William, our diminutive and charming driver—everybody's favourite Ugandan. Of course, as he has been here before, he is already slowing down and pulling into the lay-by that must have been specifically built for tourists. "I don't know about anyone else, but I'd like a group picture inside that thing. I want to have a picture with one foot on either side of the line for my mom. Come on, who doesn't want a picture of themselves at the equator?"

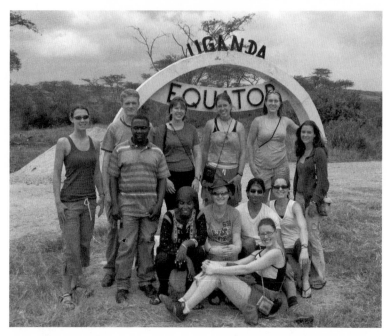

Obligatory pose at the equator sign near the border of Queen Elizabeth National Park. The 2007 student group, standing left to right: Erica Anderson, Ross Hawkes, Celsus Senhte, Jeni Liggett, Barb Weselowski, Anna Wallace, Kelti Kachur. Seated: Elizabeth Kebirungie, Rayna Gunvaldsen, Kevin Oomah, Maryanne Spady. In front: Julie Bulman-Fleming.

It is about time for a leg-stretch anyway, so everyone piles out and the cameras get clicking again.

Soon afterwards we turn right onto a rough dirt road and I resume my position as tour guide. "There are some kob—Uganda kob—those beautiful antelope, about the size of the white-tailed deer you see at home. It's common to see groups of females and young like these, and we may yet see some males today. They're a bit bigger and have lyre-shaped horns, about forty-five centimetres long. We will definitely see them when we start work, as we will be going to their breeding grounds the day after tomorrow."

We are soon inside the heart of the park at Mweya, disembarking at the hostel where we will spend the next several days. Before we move off to our various double rooms, I call the group together for a brief moment.

"I just wanted to remind you that we are not in Saskatoon. No jogging. No walking anywhere after dark. There may be any one of the big carnivores right in camp. We have seen elephants and hippos close up, as well, and remember that hippos are reputed to kill more people than any other single species in Africa. When we go to the canteen at night, even though it's only about three hundred metres down there," I gesture with my chin, "we go in the bus or the Land Cruiser. The lab is closer, just fifty metres straight back down the track, so if you go in pairs or larger groups you will probably be okay."

Several of the students have been keen athletes, wanting to keep up their exercise regimes, and at first it is a trifle difficult to persuade them that I am not engaged in an elaborate leg-pull about the wildlife. Direct experiences have always made the point more strongly than words, and as each year has brought its own real version of the verbal warning the reminder speech has become less theoretical and more vivid.

"You're back quickly," I said to two of the young women in our very first group, a week after we arrived at the park, when they reappeared at the hostel no more than two minutes after leaving.

"Yes," replied Karen. "We were going to process blood samples at the lab, but we suddenly heard branches cracking. In the dark we could just make out the silhouettes of several elephants that were feeding on that big tree with yellow flowers on the path. We figured that the samples were not that urgent." The next year my message about the dangers of the local fauna was reinforced as we drove into camp after dark. The entire group became committed converts to caution when a leopard emerged from the bushes right beside the filling station, about one hundred metres from the hostel.

In 2006 Nick and Holly, who were walking hand-in-hand to the canteen at night, were rescued by the driver of a small truck who had been within five metres of a lion that was chasing a member of a different research team. The chase had taken place no more than fifty metres from them.

A really close encounter occurred the year after that. Before we had unpacked, the hostel manager told us, "Be careful! A lion killed a hyaena right here in the compound just the night before last."

Just a day after the hostel manager's warning, Jo witnessed a very scary moment when one of the hostel's staff had a narrow escape as he crossed the airstrip just behind the hostel compound. When I got back from our day in the field she at once told me, "You missed a scary moment. A lion chased one of the waiters through the hedge. The visitors drinking coffee saw what was happening and started to scream. Luckily, the lion gave up and turned and ran off."

One particular elephant also created novel problems. Imagine Donna's surprise when she opened her room's door to answer the call of nature in the early morning and found a 2.5-metre-tall elephant standing no more than 1.2 metres away. As she put it, "The only solution was to shut the door, cross my legs, and wait."

The elephant in question was ex-bottle-fed baby Maria, now fourteen years old, who had been looking for handouts and was, as usual, being a nuisance. She became even more of a pest once she caught the scent of the bananas we had brought from the market. She obviously thought they were for her. As Innocent, our Ugandan graduate student and friend put it, "She tried repeatedly to get her one-metre-wide frame through the seventy-five-centimetre-wide door of the dining room."

On another occasion, Kendra, who had just finished doing her laundry, was talking on the cell phone to her mother in Canada, standing outside for better reception. She let out a squawk as she saw Maria emerge from under the washing line with shirts dragging across her muddy back. There was nothing for it but to start the wash again. A snapshot of Maria drinking the soapy wash water eventually helped to convince a no-doubt-skeptical mother in Regina about the incident. Shirts caked in mud that has lately been on an elephant's back are not a laundry hazard in southern Saskatchewan.

Maria distinguished herself again when she emptied the Land Cruiser of nineteen packed breakfasts, omelettes wrapped in chapattis, which I had stored there overnight in order to be ready for a pre-dawn start. She had used her trunk, aptly called *mkono* (hand) in Swahili, to slide the side window open and delve in the cardboard box. Luckily the manager of the Mweya Lodge, the beautiful tourist spot only a short distance from our hostel overlooking the Kasinga Channel, rescued us by proving a couple of loaves of bread and a tin of jam.

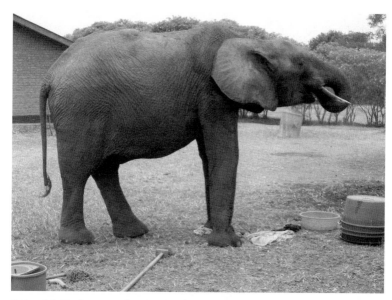

Maria and the laundry water at the Mweya Hostel.

Maria's trust in humans eventually got her into trouble. A couple of years after the breakfast theft, she turned up at the fishing village of Kasenyi, about forty kilometres away, a mere walk in the park for her, and began to enjoy the rewards of a banana from residents when tourists wanted a photo of the animal and her "friends." Of course it was too good to last. Maria became an utter nuisance, demanding fruit and raiding the village shops. One enraged housewife, trying to save her meagre food supplies, threw a pan of near-boiling water over the elephant's leg, which is now badly scarred and causes her to limp. One can only see a grim end to Maria's story.

While Maria only turns up now and again, and predators are happily very infrequent invaders, there are two species of wildlife that are frequent visitors to the hostel. Warthogs love to graze the short grass of the lawn, almost vacuuming it up as they slowly progress. To do so they bend their front "knees" (actually equivalent to human wrists) and snuffle along. They also like to raid the rubbish bins, and one must be extra careful not to carry food items that they think they can steal. Their razor-sharp tusks are deadly weapons, used to good effect in self-defence, and a human is no match for an aggressive warthog.

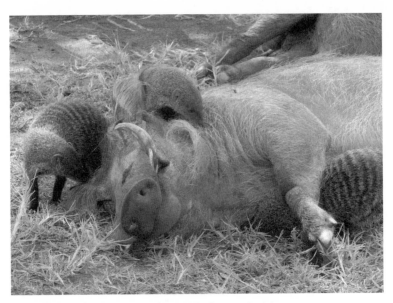

Seventh heaven for a warthog as it gets a free grooming from some banded mongoose.

The other frequent guests are banded mongoose, roving in groups as constantly questing, dark grey, black-striped bundles of energy, shaped a bit like torpedoes with short muscular legs and tails about as long as their bodies. There has been a very long-term study of these amazing little creatures by scientists from Cambridge, who have several of them wearing radio collars and know each adult individually. The study has been going on for so long that the mongoose have become utterly blasé about people and are completely habituated. One large group is a frequent visitor to the hostel, and the members will wander in and out of rooms, if you let them, and even beg for food at the canteen.

Most remarkably, and very unusual in the animal kingdom, a symbiotic bond has developed between the two species, warthog and mongoose. When the troupe appears any nearby warthog is likely to lie down and offer itself for grooming. One can often see two or three, or maybe even half a dozen inquisitive little mongoose exploring every nook and cranny of the warthog's body, even sticking their pointed snouts into an ear canal, no doubt searching for parasites and other edible goodies. The warthogs grunt contentedly, with eyes closed, and seem to be in seventh heaven.

While the students are seeing a whole range of new species they are also receiving formal and informal instruction. Our main Ugandan faculty member in QEP is Dr. Ludwig Siefert, a slim sharp-faced man who is virtually never seen without his leather hat, chin strap loosely knotted under his chin. His main interest is the park's predators. Originally from Germany, he obtained his veterinary degree from Munich and then headed straight to Uganda, where he has been for over thirty years. His monotonous speech pattern is a trifle difficult to get used to, but once one tunes into it, the information flow is spellbinding. The students—and I—have learned a great deal from him over the years.

We are able to lean on Ludwig as an instructor for subjects as diverse as his encyclopedic all-round knowledge of many aspects of wildlife medicine and much more related to the ecology of the country, the effects of fire on the grass and shrubs, the changing face of the park and the impact of cattle and human activities on the park.

He also seems to need almost no sleep and, as a result, has little concern about time.

Once the day's fieldwork is done Ludwig is the first to set up equipment for laboratory examination of specimens. After dinner, usually quite late, when everyone else is exhausted, he will announce, "I am going off with some baits to check hyaenas. I'll leave at nine o'clock. There's lots of room for students if anyone wants to come."

This simple invitation has buried implications because in order to see the animals, or especially for the students to get pictures, one has to be where the animals are, and hyaenas are most active at night.

After the first two of these nighttime forays, I had to put the brakes on. The students were coming in at 2 and 3 A.M., having had eventful trips, watching animals and listening to Ludwig recount stories of his work, which was no doubt a wonderful experience. But it was easy to discern which students had been out on patrol, as they alone among the group looked like anemic cauliflowers when asked to get up at 6 A.M. and be ready for another day's work.

The nighttime activities with Ludwig were not confined to all-night surveys, however. On one occasion there was considerable excitement, and some nervous fear, as the students treated an injured lioness. She

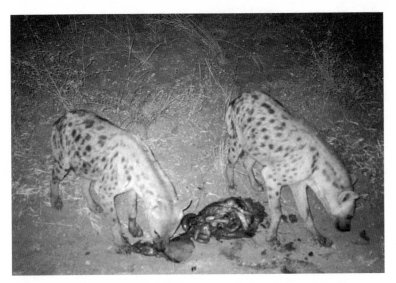

Hyaenas come to the bait and can be identified by unique coat patterns.

had taken a severe beating in a fight and had several deep bite wounds in her legs. Working entirely by flashlight and the headlights of the vehicle, the students had cleaned out the wounds and given her antibiotics as the pride hung around not more than two hundred metres away.

Rekha, who was involved at every turn in this event, relayed the account to me when the team got back to the hostel.

"We darted her just as dusk closed in. Siefert said that he really didn't like to do it that late, but that there was no choice, because she might be difficult to find in the morning. We had to chase the rest of the pride off, and it was a bit spooky, as we really didn't know how far they had moved off. When Siefert turned his flashlight toward them we could just see eyes glinting in the dark. The armed guard, with his AK-47, was most welcome."

"How long did it all take?" I asked.

"I'm not sure, as we sort of lost track of time, what with all the things we had to do. Anyway, we christened her Canada in honour of the red and white maple leaf bandana that we used to cover her eyes while she was out cold."

Ludwig later sent us an e-mail, telling us that she had not only reintegrated into the pride but had also delivered a litter of cubs.

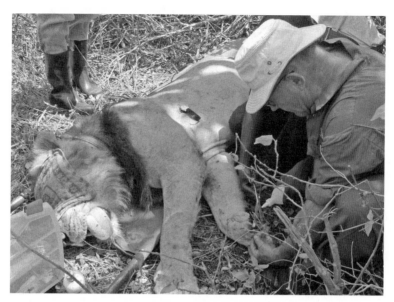

Checking an injured foot. Treatment consisted of cleansing the wound and administering antibiotics. (Photo by Karen Kemp)

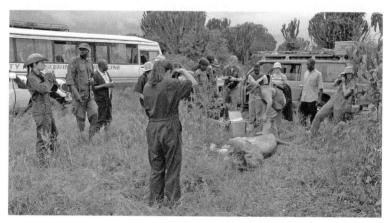

As Dr. Siefert (middle, near cooler box) works on a lion, the students look on. Park Ranger Charles (second from left) is looking around to ensure our safety. Dr. JB Nizeyi is standing next to Charles.

Virtually every student has had a chance to work with an immobilized lion, either to treat an injury or to change a radio collar. There is no single animal event that causes so much excitement and interest for them.

Of course, the lions are also a constant threat to those villagers who keep cattle. Just like the stories of chimp interactions that we heard in Kibale, we see first-hand what some of the local villagers think of the wild animals in their midst.

In most of the villages in QEP there are cattle, and as the human population grows so do the numbers of cattle. In dry times the cattle are likely to finish the good grazing around the villages, and then comes trouble, because, as the stock stray farther into the rest of the park they come into conflict with lions.

In 2005, as we boarded the bus for our next destination at Lake Mburo National Park, Ludwig, who was to join us, stopped by, leaned out of the cab of his green Nissan Pathfinder and said, "I am going to be late joining you, maybe even not today. I have just had a call from the ranger at Hamukungu. Two lions that had killed a cow near there have been poisoned. I must go and see."

When he did eventually rejoin us, late the next day, the story was even worse than we had imagined.

"When we got to the site the two lions were lying no more than five metres apart," he said. "Within a short distance we counted forty-eight dead vultures that must have also consumed the poisoned carcass. I have taken samples and sent them to the lab in Kampala."

Of course, the people don't only kill lions and not always in revenge. Every time we have travelled to Uganda we have seen the carcasses of other animals that have been poached, usually for meat.

Through the years kob have probably taken the biggest hit from poaching in the country. Queen Elizabeth National Park was once home to many thousands of them, but the numbers have declined sharply there, as they have throughout their once-extensive range. As Jonathan Kingdon has pointed out, kob were once very widely distributed in a swath all the way from the coast of West Africa to Uganda. By 1990 the range had been reduced by 89 per cent, and it has continued to decrease. The kob have not only suffered in Uganda because of the bushmeat trade but also because of the desire of the Acholi people of the north to wear kob-skin cloaks when dancing.

The clearest evidence of kob decline comes when we travel through the park with Ludwig and his research assistant, Moses Mzee. Moses

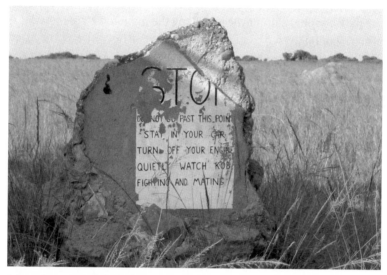
Kob monument, Queen Elizabeth National Park.

is sitting atop the Pathfinder with an antenna in his hand as he tries to pick up signals from a radio-collared lion, something that he does every day as Ludwig continues to gather information about the prides. At the edge of a grassy plain dotted with termite mounds, we stop to look at what amounts to a memorial. Inscribed upon a rough-edged block of concrete, a trifle worn with age, are the following words:

STOP
Do not go past this point
Stay in your car
Turn off your engine
Quietly watch kob
Fighting and mating

There is not a kob in sight.

"Twenty years ago this was the best area to see kob in the whole park, but they have long since been poached out, probably for meat," Ludwig tells us. "One of the techniques used by poachers is to set fire to the grass. Naturally, on windy days the fire moves relentlessly across the savannah, and the kob move out ahead of it. Waiting at the park boundary, or maybe just along the main road, are the AK-47-armed shooters."

Kob are not the only victims of poaching in the area. We had been returning from the little fishing village of Kasenyi, where Celsus did his fish-buying as an eight-year-old, which is located on the shores of Lake George, when Ludwig suddenly pulled off the track as he had seen a stack of vultures careening down to a vortex point just over the next hill. Of course they were centred on a carcass, and as we arrived we saw that the carcass was not the result of an accident. The old bachelor buffalo had not been taken out by a lion, either, but by a hail of bullets. The previous day he had stood there for us to photograph, as calm as calm could be, clearly identifiable by the small plastic ear tag that had been placed there a couple of years previously during a government tuberculosis-testing campaign. Today, the meat had been stripped off his body by a sharp instrument; the hide lay to one side, the telltale neat cuts proving how he met his end. Even the ear tip had been cut off, thus removing the tag, although there was no doubt which animal it was, as old bachelor bulls do not stray far from day to day.

Our park ranger, with whom, for safety reasons, we have to travel at all times when working, is a tall grizzled Acholi named Charles Okwanga. We have come to rely on his sharp eye—and his AK-47—for security from possible buffalo, elephant and lion alarums as we are working outside the security of our vehicles. Most worrisome are these same old bachelor buffalo that could be hiding in any one of the hundreds of small thickets scattered about the plains. It would be a nasty shock, definitely bad for the system, if one were to step around a bush to answer a call of nature or check the view and disturb a tonne of angry and frightened buffalo.

Charles pointed with the barrel of his gun at a smashed rib on the left-hand side of the skeleton.

"See the bullet injury," he said.

"I suppose that he was killed for meat," said one of the group.

"Almost certainly, it would be worth hundreds of thousands of shillings," responded Charles.

We left the buffalo, after taking pictures to show to the park authorities, and headed back toward the headquarters at Mweya. Suddenly, not two kilometres from our destination I saw another spiral of vultures, just to our right.

"Let's see what that is about," I said, turning the wheel of the Land Cruiser that I was driving sharply and crawling over the roadside embankment between two of the giant euphorbias that dot the park. Not fifty metres from the track lay the neatly skinned and trimmed carcass of a hippo, covered in a seething mass of vultures. We stopped not far away and the cameras went to work again as Ludwig, in his four-wheel drive, came up alongside. We waited for a few minutes until everyone, including Ludwig and me, had the pictures they wanted. As we walked over the vultures took off, some struggling a bit because of full bellies.

"See the straight cuts on the hide, and the feet neatly severed and cast aside. This was another poaching case," said Ludwig as he pointed first a handy stick and then his camera, at the various body parts. There was probably no more than a couple of kilos of meat left on the entire skeleton.

"This must be quite a problem. How much poaching goes on?" asked blonde curly-haired Charlene.

Ludwig replied, "We don't really know, but it is widespread. As you have seen, the kob get hammered, and we know that numbers of all hoofstock are declining." The hippo carcass, however, was quite possibly the result of a belief in witchcraft and magic.

Hippo meat is seen by some people, especially the Banyaruguru people who live in and near the park, as more than just a source of food. For generations they have known—yes, known—that a bride must have a meal of hippo meat on her wedding night. Traditionally, the hunting of hippo with spears was an extremely hazardous undertaking, not helped by the fact that it can only be done at night when the animals are out of the water. Some would-be grooms did not get to their weddings, or if their fathers-in-law-to-be undertook the hunt, they might well be bitten in half by what at first would appear to be a slow-moving lump of walking lard. In fact hippos move with astonishing speed, going from standstill to full tilt (about forty kilometres per hour) in a couple of strides. No human on foot would stand a chance, and in fact hippos are reputed to kill more people in Africa than all other wildlife species combined, not so much because they are being hunted, but probably because the unfortunate people have the misfortune to stumble upon a grazing two-tonne tank in the dark. It is no joke to step outside in the middle of the night for a pee and see a hippo chomping away at the short grass a few metres away—something that plenty of our students have experienced.

Of course today there is another motive for taking hippos, which are much easier to hunt with a gun than they had been by more traditional methods. That almost two-tonne carcass can generate hundreds of thousands of shillings on the retail market, just like that of the buffalo, far more than the average Ugandan's yearly income.

Veterinarian Celsus Senhte who was with us as one of the Ugandan graduate students in 2002 on the afternoon when we saw the poached buffalo and hippo, is himself a member of the Banyaruguru and of course knows the hippo story well. He has said, "When they need hippo meat they link up with a ranger who has a gun, or an army deserter who has one, or even use snares. They go into the park late at night. As soon as the animal is dead the men cut it up, put the meat on their bicycle cross-bars and saddles and leave again, of course avoiding the roads and gates, and secretly get back to the village."

There is another important element about hippo that also affects humans, and we see this in Kasenyi. At one time in the late 1960s and early 1970s, the villagers had a thriving fishing industry and were major exporters of dried fish to several neighbouring countries from the TUFMAC (The Uganda Fish Marketing Corporation) Fish Factory. The factory now lies as a pile of rubble half hidden among the acacia trees and giant euphorbias about five hundred metres along the shore from the village boat launch.

The collapse of this thriving industry can be put down to two factors. The villagers used undersized gill nets, and hippos were an easy target to provide a mountain of meat. As human numbers increased in the village, the people became caught up in the endless pressure to obtain food. Hippos have no doubt been hunted for many years, and when human population numbers were low, and hippos plentiful, the off-take may not have made an impact upon overall animal numbers. The Kalashnikov revolution has changed that, so the hippo population has tumbled. This may sound inconsequential, but students of ecology know only too well that the hippo is the engine that drives a successful fishery in the lakes of Africa's heartland. Every night they come out to graze. During the day they return to the water and spend the next twelve hours or so passing on the digested grass—the perfect food for many species of fish. When the hippo population goes, so do the fish numbers.

Celsus has been able to give us many other fascinating insights into the part played by wildlife in Uganda's rural life. By 2007 he had parlayed his veterinary and wildlife master's degrees into a career in the wildlife field. Together with partners, he has formed an NGO (non-government organization) working in conservation, and he has used his questing mind to survey the use of animal parts in traditional medicine and witchcraft in his homeland. He has produced a series of reports from various regions of the country.

Of course, being a member of the Banyaruguru tribe, albeit one who has left home and made a success, he knows their customs best of all and tells us that they do not just rely upon hippo meat. His own people—those who have remained in the village at the southern boundary of the park—are renowned and feared as the most active users of witchcraft in Uganda. I found this out when I referred to some of their activities to a group in Kampala and at once got a collective nod of recognition. They believe that the teeth of a male hippo help in increasing conception rates and they use the tails for various sex-related problems.

Another species reputed by the Banyaruguru to have magic properties is the chameleon. They are widely used for magic purposes across the continent, and for the Banyaruguru they can be used to target enemies. A captured chameleon should be covered with pipe ash when the target enemy is named. The chameleon will change through all its twelve colours and then die. At the last colour the victim also dies. Others believe that chameleon saliva is seriously bad news and that if some of this fluid gets onto your skin you will get sick and die.

Then there is the universal challenge for women the world over who try to keep their unfaithful men at home. Ugandan women who smoke pipes are sometimes doing so for this purpose, and lizard tails or dried toads are also supposed to keep a man around if used correctly—placed under his pillow or mattress.

One of Celsus's most detailed studies involved owls—his favourite bird—and the way people think about them. They are detested in the communities where he gathered his data in eastern Uganda. There, an owl call is believed to be a bad omen and to bring misfortune. If an owl roosts in a house, the building will be abandoned. It is therefore not surprising that some medicine men or women used their parts— feathers, eyes and ears—to bring curses upon enemies.

Our conversations and e-mail exchanges with Celsus have moved beyond the wildlife elements in witchcraft. He admits that the almost impenetrable pea-soup-dense miasma of the subject makes it difficult to study.

Among other beliefs among the Banyaruguru include one that demands that a human head from a child that has been killed should be placed under a building at the time of ground-breaking to keep away evil spirits and ensure that the house stands for a long time. A child sacrifice will lead to prosperity for the perpetrator of the killing.

Another strange (to my ears) belief related to me by Celsus is that if anyone who was susceptible to Banyaruguru beliefs were foolish or unfortunate enough to step over or into feces, particularly human feces, deposited across their path or in front of their doorsteps or compound by a Banyaruguru witch, death would certainly ensue.

I CORRESPONDED WITH CELSUS IN MARCH 2007, when I was checking for the exactness of these accounts. He added some very personal insights:

As a result of the high prevalence of witchcraft, there is a high level of uncertainty amongst the locals. When a child is born, certain rituals have to be performed to protect it from any unforeseen trouble that could emanate as a consequence of hate and envy from other locals. All my brothers and sisters went through these rituals except me and for that matter, I try as much as possible to avoid going to my home area. Usually my father has to come to town to see me and not vice versa. It's been approximately eight years since I went to Bunyaruguru. The deaths of some of my brothers and sisters a few years ago were associated with witchcraft as no postmortem was performed to confirm the cause of death. Most of these evil deeds are done as a result of hate and envy by another—often a neighbour, relative or even a close friend—to punish a family that appears to be successful and peaceful.

He went further, with a positive spin, as he wrote:

Interesting, though, is the way that some of the cultural beliefs have significantly contributed to wildlife conservation. The highly feared and revered animals—especially those that act as totems to the rural clans—are not normally touched or disturbed. Their local extinction is rarely a result of human activity. There is therefore a greater need for conservationists to work closely with the rural communities, especially those adjacent to protected areas and those living amongst wildlife, if communities are to be completely integrated with wildlife conservation.

During our time in QEP we are learning constantly. Our discussions and hands-on activities cover the gamut, from strange (to us) cultural practices to ecology, from geography to the taste of soft drinks, such as Jo's favourite, Tangawese ginger beer, known as Stoney, that we cannot get in Canada.

Sometimes one may briefly forget that we are a group of veterinarians and near-vets (only three months to go until graduation for the Canadian students), so it is my task to make sure that we keep something of a focus on disease- and management-related issues while also ensuring that everyone is comfortable and having a good time. The veterinary side of the challenge is not difficult to find, and the mixture of cattle and wildlife allows for some important questions to be asked. One of these, about a disease that can affect both livestock and wildlife, and cause serious symptoms in people, is discussed in the next chapter. ✳

26

KOB RESEARCH AND A NASTY DISEASE

Disease research in cattle, wildlife and humans involves students in some new experiences. We discover that a raunchy sense of humour can be an international trait.

ON MY FIRST SCOUTING TRIP to Queen Elizabeth National Park in 2000 I had been surprised to see cattle near several villages. Their huge metre-long horns and dark chocolate colour were distinctive.

I had said to JB Nizeyi, "Those must be Ankole. I saw them in Rwanda in 1975, but I didn't really expect to see them in a national park. They're beautiful."

"Yes," he had replied. "There are several villages in this park. Some concentrate on fishing, but there are also many cattle."

As I thought of the implications, I asked, "Where do all the people at Mweya get their milk?"

"I think it all comes from Katwe, the village just across the lake from headquarters. You can see it easily from just below the entrance gate. A milkman delivers it daily on his *pikipiki* [motor bike]."

As I asked the questions and looked at the cattle, I was thinking of an infectious disease called brucellosis, which causes abortion, sterility and swollen joints in its animal victims. Humans who become infected can develop an unpleasant condition called undulant fever or suffer damage to the reproductive system and eventually severe arthritis. The most common way for people to become infected is via the drinking of unpasteurized milk.

Cattle spread the disease to other animals in their birthing fluids, so almost any species that shares grazing with them may be at risk before the sun kills off the hardy bacteria. I knew from reading the scientific literature that the disease had been detected in cattle in Uganda.

In QEP the main species that graze where cattle also live are buffalo and kob. I knew, again from my reading, that brucellosis had been found in buffalo in the park. The question forming in my mind was: Do kob get brucellosis?

"I wonder if anyone has ever studied the kob here to see if they, too, have the disease," I asked JB.

"I don't know, but I don't think so."

I let that stew in my mind. But once home in Canada again, and beginning to plan the entirety of that first trip with my students, I decided that a small research project to study the dynamics of the disease in the park would be worthwhile. There were three closely related questions. Were the cattle infected; were the kob and other wild animals involved; and most important, were people getting infected?

These questions were relevant because the symptoms of undulant fever, as its name implies, mean that those who have it get intermittently sick over long periods of time with high fever and the associated chills, general malaise and pain. The symptoms exactly match those of malaria. Malaria is so common in Africa that almost no one goes to a doctor for treatment, unless things get really bad. They simply go to any one of myriad little shops that sell one form or another of the "right" pills and then self-medicate. If a person misdiagnoses herself and actually has brucellosis, then these pills will be entirely ineffective.

For anyone suffering recurrent bouts of fever that would not respond to the anti-malarial drugs, it would be important to know if something else were causing the condition.

I have a special interest in the cattle and human brucellosis part of the story for two reasons. One, because an aunt of mine had the disease and lost three babies in midterm and with late miscarriages, quite probably because of this nasty infection, as she had lived on a farm in England and drank unpasteurized milk for most of her life. The second because veterinarians are at extra risk, especially when they have to assist a cow that is having difficulty delivering a calf, as the birthing fluids may be full of the bacteria. The bacteria can enter the body through cuts and small abrasions in the skin (and most large animal vets have at least one of these most of the time) or through the delicate membranes of the nose, mouth and eyes. It is not possible to assist a birthing cow without having hands, arms and face "up close and personal" with the patient during the process.

Other people who are at risk of getting brucellosis are legitimate butchers or poachers, when handling infected animals.

If we were to make a proper study of the brucellosis situation in QEP, I knew we needed to get blood samples from the cattle, and this part of our activities has given Canadian students a chance at something quite new. It has also served to let our Ugandan student colleagues show their colours, as they have plenty of both theoretical and practical experience with the native cattle. In the villages, we arrange, after lengthy negotiations that are themselves part of the cultural milieu of Africa, to collect blood from herders' animals. The negotiations have had their dramatic and engaging moments, particularly for the students.

On one occasion, three of our female students joined me and our colleague and translator, Denis Muhangi, the newest member on the WARM faculty, as we visited the home of Yonah Matojo. Yonah had agreed to let us continue the work left over from the previous year and examine another forty-three head of his cattle. Yonah was away, but two of his wives, both suckling small infants in the shade of the small mud-and-wattle home that is the main house in the compound, were present as we arrived. After some introductions, I asked if we might bring the Canadians from the vehicle and of course

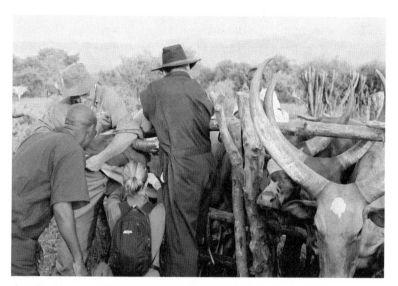
The author holds a cow by the head as students collect blood samples.

the senior wife, Beatrice, concurred at once and was most welcoming. We sat for a while and chatted about this and that before getting down to the cattle business. Beatrice looked at the young women, all of them in their mid-twenties, and I could tell by the slight tilt of her head, and the small furrows in her brow, that she was wondering about their relationship to me. She left the room and returned a couple of minutes later dressed up in her beautiful traditional print dress and handed Jennifer the gift of a necklace that she had made. She then asked Denis a question, and before he could translate or reply I picked up enough to answer.

"No, no, these are not my wives, or my daughters, just my students."

Either of the former was of course possible, as Yonah's number two wife was in much the same age bracket as the three white girls.

Quick as a wink, with a grin and a wicked gleam in her eye, Beatrice responded, "Come back tomorrow—alone—and I'll give you a daughter." Thus proving that a raunchy sense of humour is an international trait.

My response? "Can I bring my wife?"

Another huge grin from Beatrice.

The blood sampling is done early in the morning, before the cattle leave to their grazing grounds for the day. We use the huge horns as convenient levers to twist the heads and make the task fairly simple.

Ugandans are quite used to women having serious roles in society, so there is no particular cultural shock to see our crew getting to work. One large cow, with horns over a metre long, escaped from the crush—the construction was a trifle flimsy. Before she could make a break for freedom, Rory, a powerful redhead and one of two males in the group, had grabbed her in true steer-wrestling style and brought her to a halt.

It was obvious from the murmurs and wide-eyed reactions of the many small boys standing around that this had impressed the audience like nothing else. Three of the village women who were standing, watching, put their hands to their mouths and uttered the universal "Ai ai ai" expression of wonder, but no one took up my suggestion of renaming the animal in Rory's honour.

We have continued to study the brucellosis story in various areas of the park each year, and I am particularly interested in the cattle near Katwe, as the milk everyone, including me, is drinking, comes from that village. Two years after Rory's heroics, just west of Katwe, some regional history, as perceived by local Basongora tribesmen, caught up with us. Like the Maasai and the Tutsi, the Basongora are cattle herders above all else. In 2006 they began to return to the park in large numbers, bringing something between eight and ten thousand head of their Ankole cattle with them from the DRC, where they had lived for many years after fleeing from the troubled times of the 1970s and 1980s and even earlier catastrophes. Before we even arrived, I had received an e-mail telling me of the "invasion," as the park authorities put it. The new settlers, who claimed that they were merely returning to their ancestral lands after an absence of sixty years, were met by the president of Uganda, who dealt with this unexpected political crisis by facing the problem, rather than hiding from it. But nothing seemed to happen, and as he went to the meeting alone, no information reached us. The cattle certainly had not moved out at the time (although, as the reader will see, positive changes did eventually occur).

In 2007 Ludwig had made arrangements with the village chairman for us to collect blood from fifty or so head of cattle in order to take a look at the brucellosis situation there. We left the hostel good and early, some students grumbling a bit after being out late on hyaena work, and drove for an hour on a rough track into the northwest area of the park to the tiny settlement of Nyakatunge. It was obvious that cattle had been using the area hard. The grass was grazed right down, despite the recent good rains, and patties were evident everywhere. We stopped the bus by a desolate pair of shops standing like lost sentinels in the grass, and waited for our contact man. JB and I stepped down from the vehicle, as did our ranger, Charles.

There was no sign of the chairman but an older man, about my age, with grey hair, walked slowly and purposefully toward us from a homestead about four hundred metres away to the west. We greeted each other cordially in traditional African style with an exchange of questions about the news and the two-phase handshake. He did not want to use Swahili, although he clearly understood it well, and it was plain to see that he also spoke some English. It was also clear that he was a, or the, local opinion leader, a fact brought home to us a few minutes later when the village chairman came past on his motorcycle and did not even stop to pass the time of day—an almost unheard of action in a rural environment and in African culture.

Of course, multilingual JB was able to translate, but with the added advantage of being a vet himself he was able both to provide the rationale for our presence and to know the technical terms.

It soon transpired that we were not going to be able to get anywhere near any cattle.

"You have brought the two worst enemies of the Basongora people here today," said the old man, "a white man, and a park ranger."

He went on to explain. "In 1933 the white man began to poison our cattle, and by 1940 they were nearly finished. The tails of the cows dropped off and many of them died. Then in 1943, they declared this area to be a national park and we could not return. We do not like the park rangers because they protect the game and persecute us if we kill it, although it gives us much trouble."

The man was my own age, so he had not been alive in 1933, but a collective memory had been built up and condensed, as much history is all over the world. It is highly unlikely that any poisoning took place.

What did happen was a severe outbreak of lethal Rinderpest in the early 1930s, which is both highly infectious and can kill 90 per cent of the animals that contract it. It is aptly co-named cattle plague. This was followed by another scourge, Contagious Bovine Pleuropneumonia. The vaccine for the former was effective, but it could only offer protection if used in a timely fashion, and for the latter, the only protocol at the time was to pass a needle and thread that had been dipped into the diseased and abscessed lung of a dead cow just above the tip of the tail of the animal to be protected. Indeed, the end of the tail did then drop off, but the animal was protected, probably because its limited exposure to the pathogen in an unusual body part had acted like a vaccine. As if these two diseases were not enough, tsetse flies spread a massive outbreak of sleeping sickness (*ndagana,* as it is known in cattle) and killed both cattle and people. The humans fled the area, which had become unlivable, and that was when the park was gazetted.

Given the uneasy atmosphere there was absolutely no point in arguing or giving him the real versions of events, so we left, sampleless, after a frustrating forty-five minutes.

We went back to headquarters where JB told us about the discussion and the confrontation.

"He told me that he wished he could speak more English," said JB. "He said 'I would have told this white man where to go, and would have given him a blow that he would remember for the rest of his life.'"

By July of 2007 the situation had deteriorated even further. An estimated 40,000 head of cattle now grazed in the park. The problem was naturally on the agenda at a wildlife disease conference held in the nearby town of Kasese. Unfortunately none of the government ministers scheduled to attend were able to make it. The Uganda Wild Life Authority (UWA), whose mandate it is to protect the park, were in a real bind and could only hope that negotiations would stop the desecration. Their prayers seem to have been answered, at least for now. In late September I received an e-mail from Dr. Gladys Kalema-Zikusoka, a Ugandan vet who, with her husband has started an NGO, the name of which reflects its admirable goals—Conservation Through Public Health—in which she told me that according to the *New Vision* newspaper a ministerial directive has been issued and that the cattle keepers have started to leave. By late October 2007 they had gone, to be relocated on ground belonging to the Uganda Prison Service a few kilometres north of the park.

Despite the set-backs we have gathered enough blood samples from cattle in previous years and other areas of the park, to show that the infection is indeed present there, and other reports by other veterinary researchers studying cattle diseases in nearby areas of Uganda have shown that the disease is fairly widespread in the country.

The wildlife part of our study involves the buffalo and the kob, and possibly other animals that may consume those cattle birthing fluids as they graze.

The answers about the presence of brucellosis in the buffalo have come from two sources, one direct, the second from an observation when I had students with me. In 2005 Dr. Kalema-Zikusoka reported on several diseases in the park and found brucellosis cases in buffalo. The evidence of my observation was much less certain, but certainly interesting. We saw a mature buffalo cow with a swelling almost as big as a honeydew melon, on her front leg, right over the carpal joint. We could not get near enough to immobilize her to make a closer examination, but the swelling certainly made me suspicious that she was infected with the disease.

As for the kob, it was, and still is, an open question regarding their susceptibility to the disease. Luckily, the now-empty area by the old monument that Ludwig showed us is not the only part of the park in which kob congregate, as there are other areas not far away, still well inside the park, where we can see them. Within three kilometres of the village of Kasenyi lies a major breeding area, and here we can stop to show the students something new about African wildlife, as well as to conduct our study. We can expand their knowledge of biology in general and watch the interesting reproductive strategy of kob. It is here that the animals use defined breeding grounds, at which the mature males gather in large numbers. Just a kilometre or two across, the breeding ground has within it small territories, known as leks, sometimes as little as twenty or thirty metres across, and one male takes up residence in each, displaying and sometimes fighting fiercely with his neighbours for sole possession.

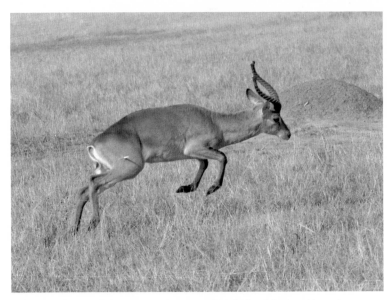

On the lekking grounds. All the action is at the centre, and it is hard work for the resident male.

Numerous scientists, starting with Hans Buechner in 1961, have examined this unusual system in which each male knows his own boundaries, although there are no lines drawn on the soil.

The females then try to get to the most desirable male to garner his genes for the next generation. There is nothing new in this among mammals, but the interesting thing is that the most desirable male takes up his stance right in the middle of the breeding grounds. When you watch kob in these areas, you can soon find the centre, as the occupant may have up to thirty females in attendance and is in a frenzy of sniffing, mounting and displaying to would-be neighbours who want his spot. Some nearby territories may hold a few females, perhaps half a dozen, but the real action is in the middle. These leks, which Jonathan Kingdon dubs "hot-spots," have recently been shown to be attractive to both male and female kob because of the estrogen-charged urine of females in estrus. Sounds to me like a self-perpetuating phenomenon.

Worldwide there are only seven species of antelope or deer that lek. Among these, kob are unique in that males continue to interact and display with the female after copulation. It might be that this serves to make the lekking ground more attractive to the female, thus keeping her nearby during the time that she is in estrus and thereby ensuring that her consort actually fertilizes her.

Not surprisingly, the attendant male soon gets exhausted, and a waiting rival, usually the male that shows the most impressive behaviour among those nearby, takes over as tenant while the exhausted lover goes off to recuperate. He will then have to fight his way back into the middle, using body language when he can, resorting to his impressively sharp horns when he has to. The activity in these central leks is so intense that an individual's tenancy may only last a few hours.

Real fights usually occur only between younger males that have not yet sorted out their position in society, but woe betide the male that turns sideways in a fight. He is likely to get skewered in some vulnerable part of his body. Not surprisingly, the entire breeding grounds are littered with the bones of losers.

The bones are not there just because of horn injuries. Lions and leopards are no fools, and they can easily lie in wait in any one of the small patches of bush that have sprung up on the fertilizer-rich termite mounds that are scattered throughout the area.

In order to get blood samples and examine the kob for other possible signs of brucellosis—such as hard, very swollen testicles, one way that males of any infected species can suffer—we have to catch them, and the best method of catching them is to dart them on the lekking grounds, where they do not run off at the vehicle's approach.

My previous experience with the capture of numerous African species led me to propose a research program to the Uganda Wildlife Authority that the students and I can conduct in QEP each year. In the written application I have included the names of Christine Dranzoa, as head of the WARM department, and Ludwig, who also has lots of experience with immobilization. I made the point that we would be helping in the education of students, both Canadians and Ugandans. UWA quickly approved of the protocols.

Since those early days of my work immobilizing wildlife in the 1970s, new drugs have appeared on the scene, and it is one of these, a more powerful and more rapidly acting version of the fentanyl with which I had grown comfortable, that I have chosen to use, again with a sedative to smooth out the process. Its name is Thiafentanyl, and it is the result of some clever chemist adding and subtracting bits of the morphine-like molecule until he found something worthwhile. It has not been used in kob before, but little by little, research reports are coming in from wildlife scientists that show how effective, and especially how fast-acting, it is.

The first step in the process of the kob research project is each year to teach the students about safety, both with the dart guns and with the potent drugs. Almost none of them have ever fired a weapon of any sort before, and none of them are familiar with immobilizing drugs. I do not want any of them misusing the equipment or failing to act quickly if an accidental injection were to occur. For these reasons, we always spend an entire morning simply putting them through their paces on the airstrip behind the hostel.

Now comes the acid test. We get the students to break into small teams, providing an opportunity for them to integrate with the Africans and to take responsibility for an entire procedure. Both Ludwig and I have lots of experience with the process, and when my former student, friend, colleague and then professor Nigel Caulkett, a veterinary anesthesiologist at wcvm, was able to join us, we were able to expand our faculty base and so give even more attention to the students. With Nigel along, we were also able to expand our research by examining the physiological effects of the drugs themselves on the animals, studies that require expensive and sophisticated equipment that Nigel uses like most people use a toothbrush—just a routine part of his job. Nigel was joined in 2005 and 2006 by one of the bright sparks who had been with us on our very first trip. Dark-haired Jessica Paterson took an anaesthesia–wildlife career path after her graduation in 2002, and so she came back to Africa, as she had sworn to do after the experience of her trip that year.

The immobilization protocol works like a charm. We are able to approach the lekking kob with surprising ease. They are more interested in keeping potential rivals off their little piece of hard-won territory than in the slowly circling four-wheel drive vehicle.

As Ludwig or I act as coach and whisper the range, twenty-four or twenty-five metres on the range finder, the student sitting in the passenger seat fires a dart into the hind leg when the chosen animal is

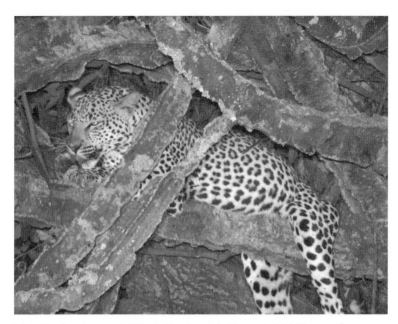

Is he waiting for a chance at a kob? Leopard in a giant euphorbia near the kob lekking grounds.

standing perfectly still. We have taught the students to try to ensure that we do not hit anything other than good solid muscle, where damage would be minimal, and drug absorption rapid. In five years, and seventy-plus kob, we have only ever recorded three misses and two misplaced darts. The inaccurate shots were usually associated with sudden gusts of wind that would blow the light plastic projectiles very slightly off course.

Within a minute of being darted, the kob start to wag their tails and then show some apparent loss of control of their hind legs. That loss turns into a full-blown stagger and then they might high-step for half a minute, or run in an uncontrolled canter for one hundred metres or so before falling down. It is during this period that a kob could be at some risk from neighbouring kob who think he is invading their space. In one amazing case, a leopard shot out in blur of spots and went after a kob that had just been darted and was looking wobbly. He was easily deterred when Ludwig gunned his engine and gave chase. The students who were in his vehicle and saw it happen were full of the story and excitement, allayed by concern for their newly darted patient and the fact that they might have caused its demise. While this was happening, the group with me in the Land Cruiser was in another area, only a couple of hundred metres away, but shielded by the bushes, and we missed out on the spectacle.

When the kob we have darted have fallen down, Ludwig and I demonstrate the next step in the process of handling the animals to our respective teams: a careful approach and the placing of a damp towel over the recumbent animal's eyes to protect them from dust and glare. The students, by now working really well in their teams, take over. They all very soon realize that a kob is an animal just like any other, requiring similar care.

One student in the team records everything we do and marks the check-list as the procedures are completed. The team leader, the shooter, has directed the other tasks. A very important one that has to be maintained throughout the twelve-minute procedure, is to have a strong person holding up the kob's head so that if any stomach contents are regurgitated they will not go down into the lungs. Other vital tasks involve frequent checks of heart-rate and breathing; blood sample collection, for later brucellosis testing in the lab; checking the body temperature and pouring water over the animal to cool it if need be; measuring the size of the testicles with a tape; and, of course, weighing the patient on the scale that Ludwig carries at all times in his vehicle in order that we might exactly calculate our drug doses for future reference.

Then comes the finale. An antidote to the immobilizing drug is injected as the head-holder keeps the damp towel in place. In under a minute, the kob's body tension suddenly changes. The ears flick once or twice and the animal gathers its legs underneath it. Seconds later, as the student lets go of the towel, the kob bounds to his feet and runs off about twenty metres. He stops to look at us for a moment, and his expression, if it were human, seems to say, "What the hell happened there?" He then moves off in a more sedate manner, and we gather up our bits and pieces before going on to the next animal.

A segment of adhesive tape has been fixed to each animal's horns so that we can check its status over the next few days and also ensure that we do not immobilize the same animal twice.

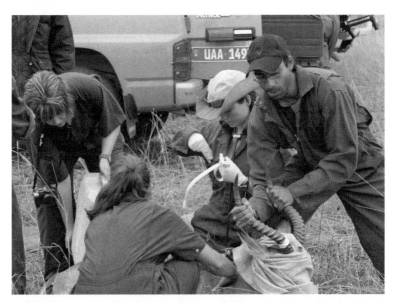

Kevin Oomah controls those sharp horns as (from left) Jeni Liggett pours on cooling water, Kelti Kachur holds the kob, and Maryanne Spady collects some data.

The final leg of the brucellosis study involves a visit to the health centre at Mweya. Tom Okello, the dapper and friendly chief park warden is very interested in the study, and he encourages us to liaise with the medical staff. As a result, we have linked up with the clinical officer, Mr. Basiimwa Godfrey, and found out in 2007 that there have indeed been cases of the disease at Mweya, twelve of them diagnosed in the last year. He is very interested in our work, particularly in how the disease is spread from animals to humans.

OUR WORK WITH LEKKING KOB occupies over half of our time in Queen Elizabeth Park. Of course, as we drive to and from the lekking grounds we are very likely to see a variety of other species and animal interactions. Four that stick in the mind include a huge martial eagle tearing at the carcass of a python; dozens of marabou storks, a single saddle-billed stork and at least fifty vultures all gathered within an area not

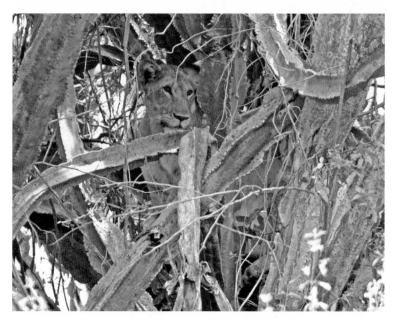

A lioness watches us as we watch her resting and "roosting" in a giant euphorbia.

more than two hundred metres across, the storks in feeding frenzy on grasshoppers, and vultures just hanging out (I'm not sure why); a pride of lions, all draped in various postures up a euphorbia tree; and buffalo wallowing in the numerous mud pools. ✳

TIME OFF AND REALITY CHECKS

*We take a day to relax at a beautiful lodge,
celebrate birthday parties and experience school
visits that make an emotional impact.*

THE QUEEN ELIZABETH NATIONAL PARK HEADQUARTERS COMPLEX
lies on the Mweya Peninsula that juts into Lake Edward and has its
own small community, with staff accommodation for all the rangers
and workers, two churches, two canteens, our hostel, campgrounds
for tourists and one meticulously maintained, up-market tourist
lodge—aptly named Mweya Lodge—that is beyond the pocketbooks
of our students. The lodge setting was chosen by someone with a real
eye for scenery and designed by someone with tremendous panache.
The ceilings are high, at least five metres at the peak, and therefore
allow cool air to flow under the thatched roof. The open design gives

a feeling of spaciousness, and many of the dining tables are set on the verandah that overlooks the Kasinga Channel, sixty or so metres below. The channel is a thirty-six-kilometre-long body of water, about three hundred metres wide near Mweya, and it meanders along between Lake Edward and Lake George.

The lodge was sited directly opposite a right-angle bend in the channel that has a gently shelving beach, almost devoid of vegetation, which is favourite watering point for the buffalo and elephant that wander down daily and hang out on the flat inside bend. In addition, there are always pods of hippo in view in the channel, and one can see that many species of bird use the beach as a daytime roosting spot. The opposite bank is too far away for detailed bird observation, but the overall scene is enthralling, a lot like watching a fire or a waterfall.

The lodge also has Internet access, which gives everyone a chance to catch up with home, check the latest hockey, rugby or cricket scores, and update the blog that the students run.

We cannot get up early and work in the heat every day, and everyone deserves a break. I try to organize for this to occur on a Sunday, so that churchgoers can take in a new environment in which to worship. For others, it is a dawn arrival at the lodge and, for a ten-dollar entry fee, a poolside day that normally runs from dawn to dusk. We usually enjoy an excellent dinner at the lodge that same evening.

While the students hang out sunning and dipping, I spend hours trying to get the perfect photo of a sunbird or some other brightly coloured jewel that flits from flower to flower and has become quite blasé about human presence. The most rewarding outdoor studio is a large flame (*Erythrina*) tree, covered in hundreds of red flowers, and with almost no leaves. I have counted up to nine species of bird using it in the space of an hour. Jo relaxes, reads and gets out her watercolour paints if she sees a flower or plant that she wants to record.

On at least one day, we board the tour boat that leaves regularly from just below the lodge and chugs slowly down the Kasinga Channel to be greeted by pods of snorting and grunting hippo. Hundreds of photos are taken, many of them attempts to catch a hippo with its head stretched back and its mouth wide open. There are pods of hippos every couple of hundred metres all along the banks.

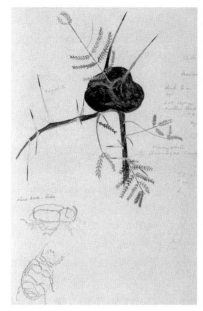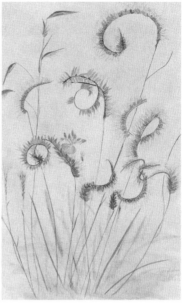

Two of Jo's studies from nature. Left: *Acacia drepanolobium* (whistling thorn) near Mount Kenya. The tree seems to whistle when the wind blows across the tiny openings made by the ants that enter the swollen black galls that they create on the tips of the branches. Right: *Sporobolus panicoides*, a common grass in Africa.

"I really want a picture of one with his mouth open," said Rekha in 2002. We had discovered that she had developed a real fascination with these watery monsters.

"Do you know why they open up so often?" I asked.

"I thought it was a challenge thing," she replied.

"No. It's like this. Legend has it that a long time ago hippos lived on land, only coming to water for a drink and a bath. They wanted to change this, mainly because they got so badly sunburnt and kept asking the great god *Ngai*, who lives on the top of the mountains, if they could dwell in the water. He denied them many times because he was worried about his fish and the number of them that the big hippos would eat.

"They kept asking until at last he agreed to their plea but only under three rigid conditions. Ngai said, 'You must first of all promise never to eat fish again, but only grass. You will have to leave the water every night to do this, and then you can return by day, when the sun is

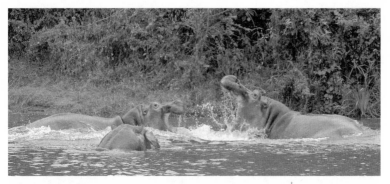
Hippo fights are usually about dominance and access to breeding opportunities. They can be vicious.

out. Second, you must scatter your dung with your tails so that I can check it for bones. And third, you must open your mouths very wide every now and again so that I can check that there are no little fish trapped inside.'"

Just as I finished relating the folk tale there was a huge swirl in the water, not fifteen metres from the boat, and all attention turned to the ensuing spectacle. For the next couple of minutes a pair of bulls were engaged in a vicious brawl, mouths wide open, snapping at each other, chasing and being chased through and around a large pod of about twenty females and young, until one of them began to spend all his time trying to get away from the other, which continued to relentlessly chase and bite with his huge fangs at the shoulders and sides of the loser. All the while loud grunts, wheezes and snorts accompanied the scene and loud splashes preceded mini tidal waves as bodies rose and crashed back into the water. I did not have a movie camera with me, but my Nikon continued to fire off several frames a second as the drama unfolded.

The cruise, however, is most often a calm one. We watch buffalo wallowing in the shallows and once saw a single elephant, framed in the ball of the setting sun, cross the skyline on the slopes above. At several points along the shore there are crowds of water birds—at least ten species all jumbled together. We have seen the evening light glinting off the feathers of a pink-backed pelican and heard the raucous screams of fish eagles that soar majestically above us or perch every few hundred metres along the banks. We have watched mobs of cormo-

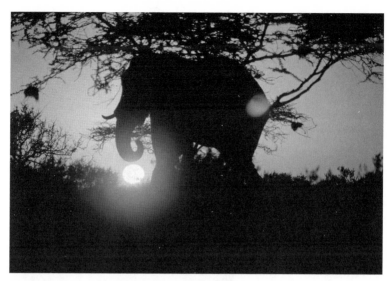

A lone elephant against the setting sun. (Photo by Karl Ammann)

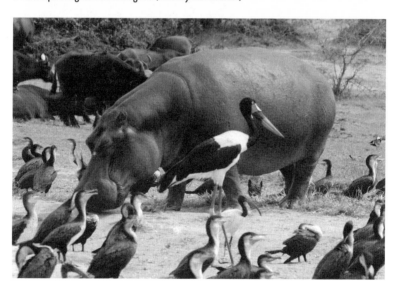

Hippo and friends on the banks of the Kasinga Channel.

rants, some standing with outstretched wings like aircraft on a packed runway, others with heads stretched out, throats vibrating as if in silent ululation, a technique they use to cool themselves. Special moments have included watching a tiny young elephant struggle up an embank-

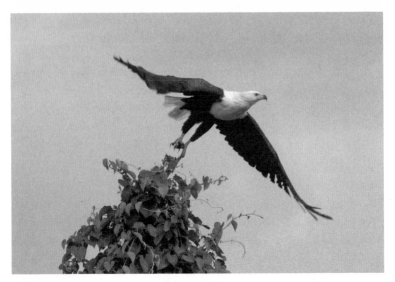

Take off! An African fish eagle. (Photo by Karen Kemp)

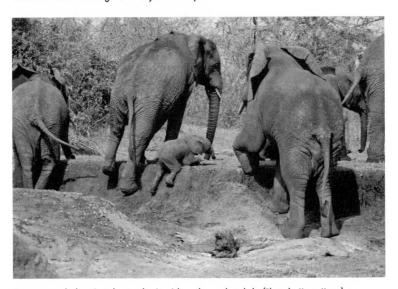

A very young elephant just about makes it, with mother ready to help. (Photo by Karen Kemp)

ment as its mother stood by ready to help, and a leopard lapping at the water not ten metres from the boat. This last was somewhat spoiled when an obnoxious group of a dozen people on board refused to keep quiet.

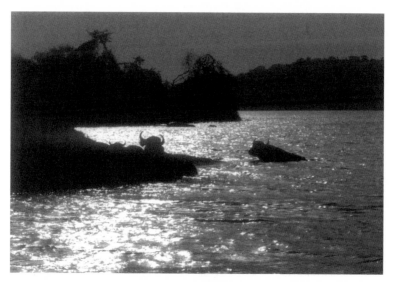

Kasinga Channel sunset with buffalos. (Photo by Charlene Olson)

The idyll of the cruise can be broken, however. On our first trip we spotted the upside-down carcass of a marabou stalk hanging in a thorn tree, a length of heavy fishing line emerging from its throat and suspending it from the branches above. As we rounded a bend in the shore, we understood why: there were half a dozen fishing boats drawn up on the bank. The village above that bank is one of the eleven in the park, and fishing is the only source of income for the community. The unfortunate bird must have picked up a baited hook, swallowed it, and flown off to roost, the dangling line becoming snared in the branches with lethal consequences.

Other evenings are usually spent at the Tembo canteen, three hundred metres south of the lodge, which also overlooks the channel, where we can watch the hippos and buffalos wallowing, spot the odd crocodile and of course try to identify the many birds that flit among the euphorbia, lantana and other bushes and trees nearby. There are pied kingfishers everywhere, climbing up above the water surface, hovering briefly and then closing their wings to dive-bomb after some food item. The weavers buzz, almost like bees, in the nearby bushes. When our meals arrive, the weavers waste no time in joining us at the serving table, doing their level best to steal a few grains of rice or whatever takes their fancy.

We all eat together each evening, often enjoying one of the brands of local beer. My favourite is Nile Special, which has a tangy flavour. Others prefer the sweeter touch of Bell.

By now, all of us are comfortable in each other's company, and one can never tell which way the conversation will go. I enjoy African folk stories and use them when I change hats from that of the teacher/vet to that of the storyteller. The chance to use a favourite comes up most years, usually after we have been out to the kob lekking grounds.

"You saw those kob all leaving their manure at one location today?" I ask. A few heads turn, thinking that I am off again on some sort of seminar or teaching rant, which they plainly do not need at 8:30 at night. "Well, the tiny dik-dik, the smallest antelope of all, no more than about thirty centimetres at the shoulder, is another one of the animals that always does its business in one spot and for a good reason.

"It's like this. Many years ago, the king of the dik-dik was walking along, minding his own business, when he had the misfortune to trip over a big elephant turd. He was so cross that he called all the dik-diks together to a *baraza*, or meeting. 'We can't allow this to happen again,' he said. 'From now on I want all of you to use the same place when you have to go. I know that we only have tiny pellets to pass, but if we do this properly, then one day an elephant will come along and trip over the midden. In that way we will get our revenge.'"

Denis Muhangi, who is usually very quiet, but enjoys a laugh and has a ready smile, is a very useful contributor to our seminar sessions. Sitting just a couple of places down the long communal table that is set up each evening by the canteen staff, he puts on a straight face and joins in. "I've never heard that story before, but here's another one that may interest you. You know why it is that those sheep we saw at Kasenyi yesterday walk along with their tails covering their rear ends, while the goats hold their tails in the air?"

For a brief moment, some of the students think he, too, is being serious, but of course, seeing which way the conversation has headed, an extrovert in the group, Marie, a Métis from Manitoba, takes her prompt and says, "No, tell us."

"Well," says Denis, "in the beginning the sheep and goat were sisters, walking along the road to a wedding. The sheep, who was the shy one, said to her sister, 'Why do you always walk with your tail in the air, showing your private parts to everyone. You should behave with more decorum and carry your tail down over the back, so as to hide everything.' 'Phooey,' said the goat, 'I will do as I want.' From that day forward, the sheep and the goat went their separate ways. All sheep carry their tails downwards, while goats walk along with their tails in the air, showing everything off." Everyone seems to enjoy the folk tales, and I can add Denis's to my collection.

I have emphasized the importance of time off and the need for personal space on the trip, as we are all more or less living in one another's pockets. I have never before found myself teaching from dawn until suppertime, every day for almost a month, and it is a sometimes difficult and always challenging task. I am also conscious of the need to help the students deal with the unusual environment in which they find themselves, and I try to create an environment that allows for positive group dynamics and bonding. Of course the kob immobilizations, above everything else, have helped create the team atmosphere, but other parts of the overall program have also played a role in team-building.

One important morale builder that has been effective each year are the surprise birthday parties I spring for anyone who qualifies. I do some sleuthing at home and discover what flavour of cakes are favourite. The cook at Tembo makes up the mix that I have secreted in my luggage from Canada, and we stick a single candle on top. Of course, there can be mix-ups! For example, I spoke to Julie's husband, who had suggested that chocolate was the very thing. Meanwhile, Karen, one of her classmates, had surreptitiously found out directly from Julie that carrot cake with cream cheese icing was the cat's meow. When I asked about the husband's suggestion of chocolate, Julie had replied, "Oh! That's his favourite, not mine."

One year I discovered that not one member of the group, not even any of the Ugandan students, had a birthday to celebrate during our time together. I puzzled for a few days and then found out that William, our diminutive driver, did not know the actual day of his birth.

"I was an orphan," he told me, "and I never did know. In fact I have never had a birthday party." Here was my solution. I laid on the usual

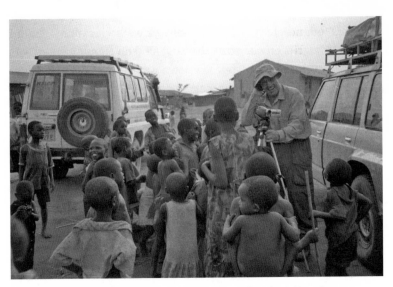

The author shares a laugh with children at Kasenyi Village as they see themselves in his movie camera. (Photo by Jessica Paterson)

cake and made sure that he was going to be with us at supper. As we finished up our dessert I tapped on my glass with a spoon.

"Guys," I announced, "we need to have a meeting. We have a problem." Some student faces looked glum, some inquisitive. "The problem goes back twenty-five years or more and is really your parents' fault, because they did not get it on at the right time and none of you were conceived in May." The puzzled, but smiling, looks were now on every face. "If you had been, we could have had a birthday party for you. As it is we have decided to have an honorary birthday party for William."

At this moment Jo, who was in on the scheme, emerged from the kitchen carrying two cakes, one a lemon sponge the other chocolate. In the absence of candles, each cake was crowned with a single sizzling sparkler. The faces broke into wide smiles and then laughs and within seconds someone had started up the standard "Happy Birthday" that the occasion demanded. William was visibly moved and later found me to offer very personal and private thanks.

At an entirely different emotional level are the visits to two primary schools in the park that we conduct, not as veterinary activities, definitely not as time off but certainly as an important element in the overall experience. Judging by the student feedback about our month together in Africa, these visits are undoubtedly some of the most memorable things we do.

The first visit is to the children at Kasenyi, where Celsus started on his business career.

The school buildings are set in an L shape. The older longer one has been plastered and painted blue, and the newer one has no finish, just dull red bricks. Both roofs are clad with corrugated iron sheeting. Facing the dusty road are four classrooms each about six metres square, two either side of a tiny three-by-four teacher's office. The wooden doors and window shutters are painted grey. The short arm of the L has just three classrooms, none of which has either door or window. Set back from the road about one hundred metres, the approach is across an open patch of dirt that has a few once-painted stones that someone once set in line to indicate a road.

On our first visit to the village, the mantra from the kids, of almost any size, was: "Give me my water bottle." We soon figured out that for them the single biggest possible present was an empty plastic water bottle, to use either as a toy or to drink from. These were not the fancy Nalgene ones carried by backpackers, but the clear thin ones sold everywhere that contain pure mineral water of one brand or another. The kids were not asking for the water. They wanted the empty bottles as something in which to carry water. In Canadian terms—some gift!

Our early contact with the school was almost by chance. I met the principal, Beatrice Nyakasiki, a matronly woman with a shy sunshine smile, in the village square just by the fish landing, when a gaggle of inquisitive children surrounded the Land Cruiser asking for their bottles. Finding none, but obviously curious to be close to a white man, they started laughing, giggling and shoving each other, when I turned my digital camera around and showed them the results of the snaps I had taken. Much the same scene was going on around each Canadian.

Beatrice tried, half-heartedly, with no discernible results, to drive the children away, but I excused them, as she was speaking in English, and introduced myself. Before long we were in the vehicle and heading up the road a kilometre to the school, where I asked her if we could bring some gifts on our next trip, the following year.

From that small beginning, things have escalated and have developed into annual school visits. Jo spotted at once that there were no hand-washing facilities near the pit latrines. The latrines are four joined brick and concrete cubicles set behind the school buildings, with a sloping roof and a low wall in front to offer some small measure of privacy. We have dealt with the hygiene issue by providing the standard equipment, available in any decent-sized market: a twenty-litre can, fitted with a tap at the bottom, custom-built to sit on top of a galvanized metal four-legged stand just over a metre tall. The more up-market hand-washing stations have an attached soldered ring just below the bottom of the can, into which a plastic bowl can be set. The really fancy ones also have an attached soap dish.

We have taken exercise books, textbooks, pencils, crayons, chalk and sports equipment. The first year we came with a few small gifts, crayons and exercise books, was 2004. In 2005 we had more of an idea of the needs. Within minutes of the soccer balls appearing from the case, we were challenged to a game against the school first eleven team, all boys. Girls, we found out, do not play soccer. The pitch was a ten-by-fifty-metre strip of dirt right beside the classrooms. If the ball went into a room, a throw-in ensued. The kids were adept at using the walls to carom the ball past an opponent and leave one high and dry. Luckily a couple of Canadians were used to indoor soccer—if you play at all you had better be, given the prairie winters—and two WARM students had obviously played before. The ten-minute each-way game fortunately ended in a 1–1 tie, which of course meant a rematch for the next year.

When I asked what gifts she would like us to bring for the children the next year, Beatrice's immediate response was "soccer uniforms."

"I'll see what I can do."

"We have another problem. When it rains, the children get thorns in their feet and we cannot play football."

This was certainly not something I had ever thought of as a hazard of playing sports, but back at home it has taken no time for generous donors in Saskatoon to offer us uniforms and shoes, or even cleats, for the school. The following year, in 2006 we arrive with a full set of smart white uniforms, donated by the Saskatoon East Soccer Association. Boys vanished into a classroom to change, and five minutes later

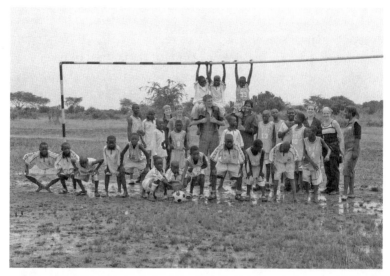

Soccer teams after the rain at Kasenyi in 2007.

they emerged for a group photo, pleased as punch, seeming to have grown at least five centimetres.

Since that first match in 2005, the game has been played on a full-sized pitch. In 2006, the boys made us look pretty foolish but only managed two goals in the thirty minutes played. Our excuse: most of our students had never played the game before. One year, with injuries limiting our side to only ten students, a sixty-four-year-old bald vet had to be drafted. The inevitable pulled hamstring did not help, so in the second half I had to play in goal.

In 2007 a bigger challenge came. We had acquired some donated volleyball uniforms so that girls could join in the fun, and again we were instantly challenged by the children. There was only one problem. It had been raining, in true tropical fashion, for two solid hours. By the time we had been narrowly beaten at volleyball and once again thrashed at soccer, all of it played on a mud surface covered in an inch or more of standing water, we were all completely filthy.

The most emotional moments at the school occurred in 2007, when, before the soccer and volleyball games, we were ushered into a classroom to view all the bits and pieces that the school had purchased with the money we had brought in previous years. There were desks with

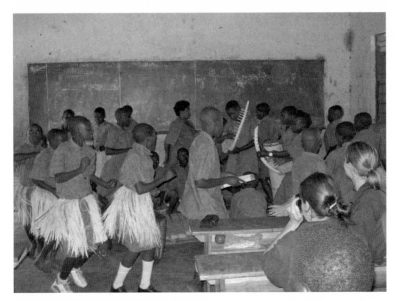

A concert in the classroom at Kasenyi.

carved acknowledgements to the WCVM (Western College of Veterinary Medicine), sports gear, plastic jerry cans for water and a bicycle for carrying them up from the lake, and a stack of musical instruments in the corner. Kiiza George, the robust and smiling new headmaster, explained to everyone what was on show and then said, "What we have developed is a program of full integration. We hope that each child will reach his or her full potential, so we now have, with your generosity, acquired many things. We have academic materials, although we would like to improve the ratio of textbooks to one for two children. We also have sports equipment for boys and girls, and a music program. With this range of programs we are now considered a model school."

As he spoke I looked around at the small room, with wooden shutters for windows and badly in need of a lick of paint. I thought of the other classrooms in the school that had no plaster, let alone paint, no blackboards, and no doors or windows, just those holes in the brickwork. What an interesting thought, that this would be considered a model school.

I returned from my reflections to hear George say, "If you will remain seated the children have prepared a small concert."

At this, the door opened and Beatrice ushered in a group of twenty kids, all in matching uniforms, who went straight to the instrument pile and then formed up. In the middle was a large wooden xylophone, its base no more than ten centimetres off the floor. There were several different drums and three hand harps. Half the kids formed a ring around the musicians and then the singing and dancing began.

For half an hour we sat and listened to the pulsing drums in perfect beat and the words of songs that mixed joy and thanks or bemoaned the fate of the impoverished. The rhythm of the children's feet pounding the floor as they danced in a circle around the instrumentalists matched the drums to perfection. A boy with an ancient bell-covered leather anklet that was obviously not something we had provided, and was most probably an item of a traditional costume, led the dancers.

There was hardly a dry eye in the room. Mine certainly weren't.

The sheer lack of facilities and the basic needs of the kids in no way prepared us for the other school we visited in 2007. It is run by the same Kiiza George in his home village, not far from Kasenyi, and is specifically for AIDS orphans. If Kasenyi had little, the Equator Primary School had nothing. Built of mud and sticks, it has just three rooms, no bigger than about four metres on a side, covered with thatch. Jo took one picture of about thirty kids crammed into one classroom, all sitting at ancient narrow desks. As soon as we arrived the older children put on a beautiful musical play.

Each child wore a purple dress or shirt. They stood in a semi-circle near the building, rhythmically stepping back and forth as they sang beautifully, in a native tongue I did not know. One small girl stepped out of the line and performed simple hand actions, mostly rubbing her wrists and wrapping her arms around her slim little body as the song progressed. The lead singer, another young girl who was next to the acting star, was a true canary, with a lovely voice. The language used during the performance was almost irrelevant, the overall effect was so poignant. At one point all the girls in the line put their hands to their mouths and let out high-pitched joyful ululations.

After it was over, George told us what it had been about. "This song is about AIDS and its effect upon the children. Its poetry describes a child with AIDS who leaves the shelter of friends in her village and becomes

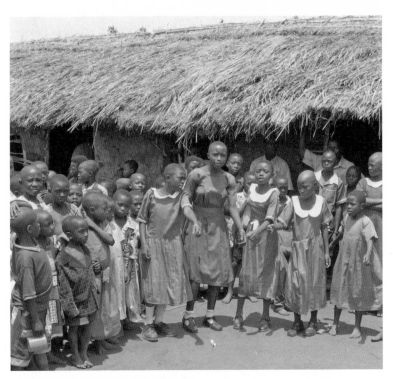

The children at Equator Primary School perform their AIDS poem.

sick and emaciated. She finally returns—that is when you saw the children greet her like this," he put his hand to his mouth and waved his palm back and forth. "She recovers with the help of the antiretroviral drugs she can get there, and the song ends on a cheerful note."

Again it was impossible to remain detached. Even writing or telling this story is emotionally draining.

Gifts were again handed out, especially sports equipment, exercise books and crayons. The biggest cheer went up when an Arsenal banner was unfurled—we had given the Kasenyi kids a Manchester United banner in case the two schools ever played against one another. It was interesting that we had needed to offer no explanation about either banner. The brand recognition was instant.

Each child received a new T-shirt and a small stuffed toy. They had never had either in their entire lives. All knew about the shirts but some were quite frightened of the strange fluffy objects. The fright quickly

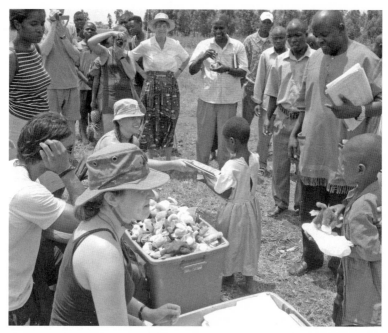
Gifts for the children. Kiiza George at right.

turned to giggles when they were shown that the magnetic hands of the toy monkeys would stick to the metal parts of our bus.

Unbelievably, with twelve cameras around, we somehow failed to get *the* picture of fifty monkeys festooned on every available metal part, while some children with puzzled expressions tried to stick their toys to the plastic parts of the bus's body.

We asked George what the kids might need in future and made up a list, which included hand-wash stands, cash for metal roofing for the store and three sewing machines that could be used to start the kids on the path to learning a trade.

To provide funds for our support of the schools, some of my bird pictures have been turned into money-raising calendars, and the students have raised enough funds with simple schemes like bake sales, so that every year we can leave well over $1,000 for each group of children. The craziest money-making scheme—so far, who knows what students will come up with—has been the self-sacrifice of red-haired Ross and dark-skinned Kevin, whose parents immigrated from Mauritius, who both lay down in the public arena of the wcvm buffeteria and had all their above-the-waist body hair waxed and yanked. This alone raised over $1,800 from the wcvm community, who have supported our efforts to the hilt.

In addition to our school visits, we also visit a couple of the salt-mining lakes in the park, which both owe their properties to the active volcanic activity that brings up a mixture of salts from deep down. The one near Kasenyi has no high-tech equipment. The villagers simply walk out into the shallow water and make small pans, building up walls that divide each ten-metre-square plot. As the water evaporates the salt is collected.

At the village of Katwe, not far from Mweya, the salt is also mined by men who wade out into the metre-deep water and, using iron bars, break the five-centimetre-thick salt crust that forms on the bottom of the lake. The salt floats up and is then carried to shore on rafts made of *ambach* logs, which have similar properties to balsa wood. There is only one little problem. The water is so corrosive that the men have tried to find protection by wearing condoms. Unfortunately, these do not really protect a flaccid penis, so some other solution, such as waders, which would also protect skin on other parts of their bodies, is being sought.

Katwe also provides an example of the blindness of some aid programs. In the late 1970s, a high-tech salt-extraction plant was built on the shores of Lake Edward. It had lots of pipes, including one over the hill to the source of the salt about a kilometre away, as well as concrete and brick offices, houses for expatriate managers and so on. Seemingly everything had been thought of. Only one little mistake. All the pipes that were designed to carry water were made of iron. Someone forgot their basic chemistry. Over time rust has become the predominant colour on the outside, and no doubt the predominant chemical inside as the pipes clogged up within two years, producing yet another aid white elephant, much like the unfinished highway I saw in Cameroon and mention earlier in this book. Parts of the structure are used for student accommodation, but the factory is useless.

The villagers have gone back to their traditional methods, and the hundreds of pans, all privately owned and once passed on to family members, are nowadays often traded for large sums of money. About 70 per cent of the village's income is derived from the salt, the rest being from the fishing activities in Lake Edward and from the cattle that some villagers own. The salt industry supports about ten thousand people in this community alone.

The defunct salt mine in Katwe is not the only African aid program that fulfils the saying, "The road to hell is paved with good intentions." As Ian Parker has succinctly put it, in his 2004 *Jua Kali's Voyage on the Jade Sea*, the fish plant at Kalokol on the shores of Kenya's Lake Turkana is the "world's only fish plant that never produced a fish." It was built with Norwegian aid money and was "a technological marvel of glass, steel and neat layout that must have cost millions." It was never used because the builders did not check one important fact. They failed to find out about the fluctuating levels of the lake, which was at its highest level ever during construction. As a result, the never-used plant is now about three kilometres from the water's edge. Adjacent to the plant, Italian aid organizations built a fish farm that was equally non-productive. Fortunately, there is no record that either of these projects actually did any harm to anyone, which is in contrast to the camel abattoir built by Food and Agriculture Organization of the United Nations (FAO) at Mogadishu in Somalia. The blood and offal from this plant discharged straight into the sea nearby, making it unsafe for swimming as it attracted sharks, which not only feasted on the freebies but also killed twenty-three unfortunate swimmers in eighteen months.

FROM THE SALT PANS, we head back to the lodge and wrap up this part of our program. The next park visit will be to Lake Mburo, an entirely different setting that will provide new learning, as well as reinforce experiences and insights already covered.

We debrief, discussing what we have seen, and hold formal and informal sessions that cover ecology, diseases and, of course, the now well-understood and very complex issue of the human–wildlife–livestock interface. At the schools and the villages, the students have seen a real face of Africa up close, not really a part of their veterinary education, but providing them with a bigger world picture that will stay with them for the rest of their lives. ❋

28

CONTINUOUS LEARNING

We wrap up in Uganda with a camping trip and a finale at a chimp sanctuary. Reflections on learning.

AFTER MY FIRST SOLO TRIP TO UGANDA IN 2000, and the guided tour with JB Nizeyi, I realized that the time spent in Lake Mburo National Park is a core component of the WARM department program. WARM has its own permanent campsite away from the tourist centres, and every Ugandan veterinary student spends a few days there during their five-year sojourn at the school. Here, the interface between people and wildlife really comes home for veterinary students, and they see in more detail than at QEP how fishing fits into the scheme. They also learn a lot more about cattle management and diseases and wrap up the presentations that they had prepared in Canada. The trip to the park takes us through the bustling market town of Mbarara, with its large hospital, university and crowded centre.

Because we will be camping for five nights at Lake Mburo, we have to buy rations for the entire party, and the Canadians learn some new lessons about pricing, bargaining and team work, as they get involved in menu selection with much help and guidance from our Ugandan colleagues, who know what is available, affordable and appropriate. Our white skins relegate us to supermarkets where prices for things like peanut butter, water, milk, flour, maize meal and cooking oil are fixed.

We do not normally go to the open-air market for other items because, on the one occasion when we did so, the price of eggs, vegetables and fruit rose sharply. However, this one trip did provide some amusing moments because our friend and fellow vet Innocent Rwego was the guide and buyer. The three Canadians with him watched with awe as he managed the traders. The first large lot of bananas was brought over for inspection. With no words, just a glare and a head shake, they were rejected, so also the second. Finally Innocent accepted a much less ripe bunch, with no rotten ones hidden in the middle. The performance was repeated with other perishables. At this point the students left, as the prices were beginning to rise, but it had only taken them that short time watching him work in the market for them to laughingly liken Innocent to the Marlon Brando character in *The Godfather*. They nicknamed him Don Innocenti.

After a lunch and an Internet stop in town, we fuel up and head out for the two-hour trip to the park, picking up charcoal along the way. We are all under canvas, and for the students there are two large tents at the campsite, each able to accommodate about twenty people, set up for when the Makerere students visit later in the year. At my insistence, Jo and I get our own tent.

As a conservation area, Lake Mburo has had a roller-coaster history. Before 1935 the region was part of the Nkole Kingdom, where the Banyankole people lived and were ruled over by the Omugate, their king. The valleys around the lake itself were the king's private hunting reserve.

As with so many interesting places all over the world, there is a legend about Lake Mburo. Long ago, two brothers, Kigarama and Mburo, lived in a large valley. One night, Kigarama dreamt that they were in danger. The next morning, he recounted his dream to Mburo and urged that they should leave the valley. Mburo disregarded his brother, so Kigarama moved up to the hills alone. The valley flooded, drowning Mburo.

The lake is named for Mburo, and the hills are called Kigarama after his brother.

At the end of the nineteenth century, the region was swept up in the continent-wide Rinderpest outbreak that devastated populations of all the even-toed animals, domestic cattle and wild animals alike. Added to this catastrophe was the smallpox epidemic that arrived with European explorers. People, livestock and wildlife died in incalculable numbers. The numbers bounced back and between 1935 and 1964 a controlled hunting area was available for the wealthy and influential, and grazing, fishing and farming was permitted for the local people. However, in the 1940s, a second disease epidemic created further havoc. This time it was sleeping sickness in both people and cattle. Many people left the area, and a massive slaughter of wildlife took place in an attempt to get things under control as they were considered to be the main reservoir of the disease.

Uganda became an independent country in 1962, and a year later the Lake Mburo area was officially gazetted as a game reserve. Although pastoralists also occupied the area, it was teeming with game and had an amazing variety of bird species.

Because of the wildlife diversity, the reserve designation was changed to that of national park in 1983, but within a couple of years the government was overthrown. The locals took revenge after years of oppression, murder and warfare and moved into the area to settle and graze their cattle in droves.

Soon afterwards there were moves to eliminate the park entirely, but after lengthy debate, 40 per cent of the original was left as park and the rest given over to settlement. With the decline in browsing species—elephants had long since vanished—and the massive intru-

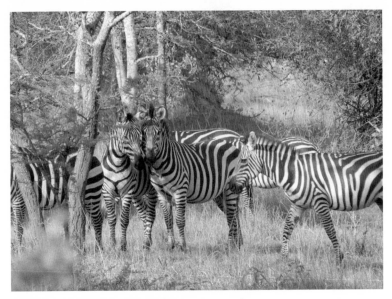

Zebra secrets at Lake Mburo National Park. (Photo by Karen Kemp)

sion of cattle from nearby ranches, the park has become overrun with
acacia thickets (mainly *Acacia hockii* with its mass of pretty little yellow button-ball flowers), and game viewing is now somewhat limited,
although bird viewing, especially from a boat, is spectacular.

Among the mammals there are zebras, known to almost any western child because they appear in just about every alphabet learning
book; graceful impala, the most northerly population in Africa; and
small groups of topi, a 150-kilogram antelope whose sloping shoulder
profile, rust colour, and blue-black, hip-hugging trouser-like rear end
make them so distinctive, especially when the males stand atop termite mounds declaring their territories. Another large bovid we have
not seen in our first two park visits, but known to be in the park, is the
dun-coloured eland, with its spiralling horns, massive in the bulls,
which weigh as much as nine hundred kilograms.

Several species that were once seen in the park are no longer present. Among them are elephants; patchwork-coloured Cape hunting
dogs; giant forest hogs, which are basically big black hairy pigs; and
grey coloured roan antelope, with their distinctive large ears. Lions
were poisoned out and have not been seen in the park since 1997.

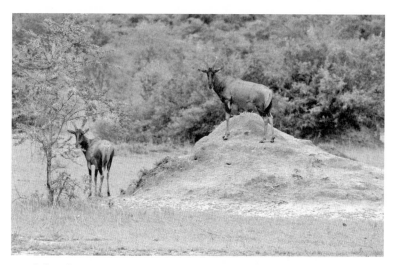
A topi bull stands atop a termite mound, declaring his territory for all to see.

One of the reasons for the diminishing variety of species lies with the cattle situation. It is a puzzle, at least if you come at it from the point of view of the wildlife conservationist or park visitor. On my first trip to the park, as we planned future student experiences with JB Nizeyi, I saw the puzzle first hand. Within two hundred metres of the park gate, but inside the boundary, we found a large herd of Ankole cattle, their enormous horns glinting in the evening sun. The herder was nearby, and JB called him over.

"What are you doing inside the park?" JB asked.

The herder, somewhat the worse for drink, promptly produced a piece of paper that showed the official Uganda Wildlife Authority green and yellow crest at the top. Written with a ballpoint pen on the dotted line were the words "Illegal Grazing Permit." It took me a moment to absorb the implications of this statement.

As I later found out, an agreement had been reached that would allow the numerous cattle owners to use designated corridors to get their animals to the lake water by going through the park. Of course, there was no suggestion that the cattle hurry through, drink and return to their home ranches. Next year, we found a huge mob, probably over one thousand animals strong, grazing at the remote eastern end of the park. The herder was nowhere to be seen, but Ludwig told us that he was no doubt crouching in the very middle of the herd, which was all bunched together. By February 2006 the situation seemed to be more or less out of control. The grass in many areas was almost shaved off. Cattle patties lay everywhere; where we had once seen zebras, eland and topi in abundance, there were no more than twenty-five head in a twelve-kilometre drive.

The explanation was soon forthcoming. We were in Lake Mburo only a week before the national elections. At the park headquarters, I asked the deputy head warden what had been happening.

"We tried to get them to move out," he said. "Then a big delegation came and threatened us. They said that if we did not allow them to bring their cattle to graze, not just for water, they would not vote, and would go and complain to the president."

I knew, without having to voice it and embarrass him, that the owners of these cattle included very senior military officers and well-connected government ministers. I was told that one owner was the president's brother. The abiding culture in which cattle numbers are a sign of wealth and stature played a central role in this situation.

The cattle conundrum is not new. In a Swedish report penned in 1993 the authors wrote: "The greatest current threat to mammal diversity in the park is the existence of very high numbers of cattle within the park."

Putting it another way, in 2007 Ludwig said, "Why would tourists come to the park when they mostly see only cattle?"

As if this was not bad enough, in 2006 a major change occurred when the Ruizi River, which is the main water source for the park and Lake Mburo itself, was entirely diverted to supply an irrigation scheme. The consequences of this action have not yet been seen, as a prolonged and heavy rainy season followed almost at once, masking the fall in lake levels that would have occurred, but it is bound to create major changes once the next dry season comes around.

We not only see cattle everywhere inside the park but we also visit a government cattle breeding station just north of the exit gate, where we have a chance to learn more about the wildlife–livestock interface, watch the cattle go through a dip for tick control and hear from the manager how wild animals are viewed by many people.

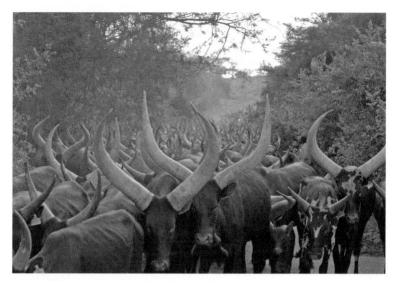
Ankole cattle at the government breeding station. Lake Mburo.

The manager of the station is charming slim Nathan, and he is set in his views that the wildlife coming from the park, bringing diseases with them and eating off all the ranch grass, are his main problem. Most of the diseases are transmitted from the host animal through one or more of several species of tick, and the most lethal one, East Coast Fever, is transmitted by one particular species of tick. The so-called brown ear-tick can move between buffalo and cattle, and the disease it carries is lethal to the latter, or very expensive to treat, while causing no apparent signs of disease in the buffalo.

To prevent the ticks from latching onto the cattle long enough to transmit any of these diseases, a poisonous fluid, an acaricide (from the Latin name for the tick family *Acarinae*) must be applied regularly. As long as it remains on the skin, it is poisonous only to the ticks, so once a week, the cattle, instead of being let out to graze at dawn, are brought into a corral and then driven into a narrow chute at the end of which they have no choice but to jump into a four-metre-deep dip tank full of tick-killing chemical. The morning sounds are a mix of some bellowing, shouts from the herders, the odd thwack as a stick is applied to the rumps of the reluctant slowcoaches, and a series of loud splashes as cow after cow leaps out as far as it can into the fluid. We

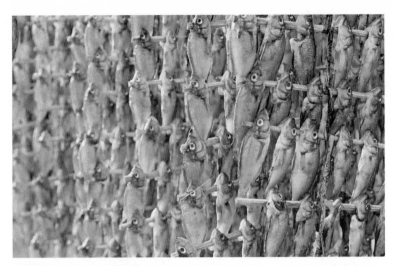
Cichlids on the rack. Each rack sells for less than a dollar.

watch as bodies of the beasts submerge briefly, which ensures that the ticks inside the ears are exposed to the chemicals. The long beautifully curved horns are, for a moment, the only evidence that the animals are on the move as they swim the short distance to the exit ramp. There they stand, coats glistening wet in the morning sunlight, until they are let out to graze.

However, our activities in Mburo are more centred on community conservation than animal contact. During a visit to the conservation centre, we learn how the local villagers are able to benefit from park income, as 10 per cent of all entrance fees are allocated each year to community projects, such as schools or health centres within parishes. We watch videos, with equipment powered from solar panels, and admire the way in which the complex has been designed to make the most of water availability via drainage off the hill above and storage in large tanks. The centre takes in groups of students from across Uganda.

Unfortunately the 10 per cent cut of the entrance fees is not enough to counterbalance the herder's imperative to water their cattle and to acquire ever more of them. Moreover the money goes to group projects, usually within parishes, and not to individuals, so the wealthy cattle owners have little incentive to cherish the park.

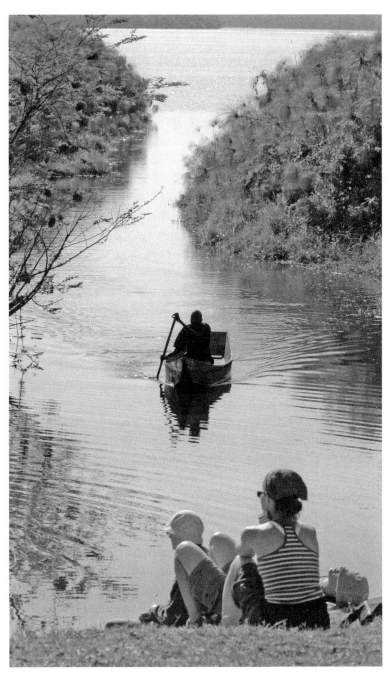

A fisherman returns with his catch. Lake Mburo.

We visit the fishing village in the park where ten-centimetre cich-lids, spiked on a rack by the hundred, each rack selling for a very few Ugandan shillings, are a major commodity. Someone pointed out that in Canadian pet stores a single cichlid would sell for several dollars (roughly fifteen hundred shillings to the dollar). I'm not sure how much this was believed by the fishermen; I think it went into the same box as moon-walking or extra-terrestrials.

Another really enjoyable learning experience in Mburo has been to go on early morning walks, with either Christine or Ludwig, and be shown tracks, bedding sites and salt licks in the park. At the extensive salt licks it is even possible to distinguish which species have been visiting, as the gouges in the vertical salt walls show that an eland has been by and done his digging at almost two metres, while a warthog has been at work just above ground level.

Each time an armed ranger, usually himself an accomplished track-er and bird enthusiast, accompanies us. On a couple of trips we learned first-hand that the ranger's presence is a good thing. Once we nearly walked into a thicket where a couple of bull buffalos had been resting and the dung they had left was still steaming, and another time we came face to face, or nose to smell, with the pungent and recently de-posited odour of a very recent leopard marking around a small clump of grass. Those whose own tom cats have taken to peeing on carpets would have recognized the smell at once.

Camping "rough" has its special moments. The showers we enjoy at Kibale and Mweya are here replaced by a three-sided corrugate iron enclosure, about a metre across and two metres tall, with an unin-terrupted view of the bush on the open side. Charlene, an attractive vivacious member of one of the groups, who was always able to boost everyone's morale with her amazing smile and infectious laugh, had been taking a shower and returned to the table area with an account of how she had been convinced, while standing in her birthday suit, sluicing water over herself from a bowl and cup, that she was being watched.

"I was certain that there was a peeping Tom around until I looked up and saw, in the branches above me, a male vervet monkey, blue testicles and all, examining me."

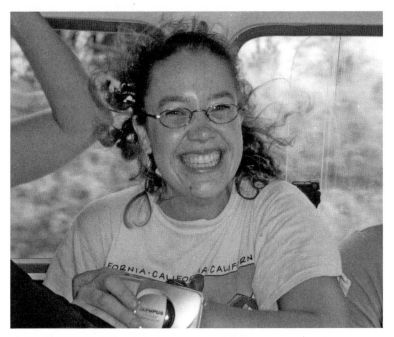

Charlene and a happy moment—one of many. (Photo by Jen Currah)

One party member, knowing something of primate biology, promptly remarked, "He was probably just checking you out for his harem."

As the trip nears its end, Jo and I have been pleasantly surprised at the very few medical emergencies that have arisen. Her vast experience with tropical medicine, which started at medical school in India and was followed by a year in Zambia and eight years in Kenya, was almost never put to the test. Only twice has anything arisen. One student suddenly developed a violent allergic coughing fit that needed Jo's expert attention, and the other medical situation was more of a learning experience for us all.

Upon Jo's advice, we make sure that we are all equipped with a small armoury of medications when we set out for Uganda. First and foremost are antimalarials, but antibiotics, antiallergy and antidiarrhoea drugs, and others besides, are also included in our kit. However, we had not allowed for the completely unexpected. One student began to look increasingly uncomfortable at Lake Mburo over the first three days of our stay. As I headed one morning to answer a call of nature

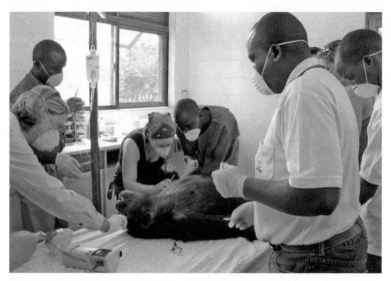

Chimp health check on Ngamba Island. Dr. Lawrence Mushiga, in white shirt, at right, supervises the student team.

after breakfast, I asked after her well-being and received an unexpected reply, "Not so good, Dr. H. I'd give anything for a fleet enema right now."

For all subsequent trips, we have added a laxative to Jo's list of suggested medications.

On the last morning at Mburo, as everyone pitches in to breaking camp and tidying up, I cook up the remaining eggs and transform the by-now rather stale bread into French toast, having remembered to secrete a bottle of maple syrup in my luggage before we left home. Most students come back for seconds, and even thirds. I get the best bits, the crusty brown chips that have fallen off the edges, as cook's privilege.

From Mburo it is back to Kampala, where we set out on our last veterinary visit to the chimp sanctuary on the one- kilometre-square island of Ngamba that lies out in Lake Victoria, a two-hour boat ride from Entebbe. The management is rather different than that at the sanctuary that Annie Olivecrona ran at Sweetwaters, but the rationale is identical. Debbie Cox, the driving force behind this one, is in frequent touch with Jane Goodall, Annie and all the other members of the Pan African Sanctuary Association.

There is no pretence that one square kilometre is enough for the forty-eight chimps in residence. This might be enough territory for one chimp, so the management is fairly intense. For instance, the animals are fed four times daily and all the females have contraceptive implants. Students are given the chance to work hands-on with the chimps as they undergo their annual health checks, which include blood tests for a variety of diseases and routine Tb tests.

The declining level of Lake Victoria has had interesting consequences at the sanctuary. Chimps do not swim and will only go into water up to mid-chest, so the island shore has not had to be fenced, except, of course for the small portion of the island that holds the accommodations, offices, dining area and hospital. This area is kept separate from the apes by a very high-tech electric fence, as the chimps know, even before they are five years old, that puny humans are no match for them.

As Lawrence Mushiga, the sanctuary vet, put it to us, "One chimp is about as strong as five humans." He told us about one interesting event. "A group of young fishermen got too close to the island, and a wading adult male chimp climbed into the boat. The men wisely jumped out. Luckily some of our staff were returning from a neighbouring island and saw this boat, full of fishing gear, about two hundred metres from shore, being sailed by a lone chimp." They took the craft in tow and all ended well.

We also learned that the chief of a nearby fishing village, located on one of the myriad islands in the lake, came calling a few days after a couple of young men had tried to hide on the island to avoid paying their taxes. The men had obviously not known that chimps can be dangerous and aggressive. They were attacked, which must have been a terrifying experience, but fortunately one of them managed to escape into his boat and paddle for help round to the management camp, safe behind those many strands of high-voltage wire.

When the rescue party of chimp handlers arrived, the other truant had been stripped of all his clothing and was being mobbed. He was incredibly lucky not to have been emasculated, as might have happened in a chimp-to-chimp fight. As far as the chief was concerned, the chimp island is an excellent deterrent to tax dodgers. I doubt Revenue Canada would try it, but you never know.

THE FINAL DAY OF OUR TRIP is spent in a frenzy of souvenir buying, and then, after a farewell party at WARM we are on our way. Naturally speeches make up an important part of that final gathering, and the Canadians sometimes have trouble expressing everything that they feel. The briefest, and somehow the most apt expression came from super-fit Rekha, who started out describing some of her emotional responses to what she had seen and learned, before she stumbled, stopped and simply said, "All I can really say is, we are ecstatic!"

Three years after she joined us on the trip, blonde slim Catharine Shankel, working in a Vancouver small animal emergency clinic, wrote to tell me, out of the blue, how the experience had affected her:

> *I see that the Uganda rotation is still running, which is wonderful. I thought you might appreciate some comments about the effect this rotation had on me, even three years later...The more patients that I see and clients that I meet, the more I realize that most of my veterinary education had very little to do with what I deal with on an average shift. What the Uganda rotation provided me with is an appreciation for veterinary medicine on a broader scale, and an understanding that although a diagnosis sometimes hinges on the most minute of details, the wellness of the client, the patient, and myself rely on something much greater than that. A sense of perspective is important, and having had the opportunity to participate in veterinary medicine in another country (with a foreign culture and unique wildlife and domestic animals) has given me a greater sense of what this field can offer. Medicine changes and quickly becomes obsolete and outdated, but an experience like the Uganda rotation will last forever, literally. Thanks so much for the opportunity! I'm sure this year's students will appreciate it as much as I did.*

By 2007 I, and several students, had become members of the Canadian branch of Vets Without Borders/Vétérinaires Sans Frontières, and Julie Bulman-Fleming prepared a detailed report for them. The last paragraph of her report summarized the experience this way:

All of us left Africa slightly darker (mostly red dust!), much closer to our classmates and each somehow different than when we left. None of us will ever forget the challenges and adventures of our trip, and can't help but view veterinary medicine and actually, the world, differently. There was so much spirit, hope and passion from the veterinarians and professors we worked with, the children we visited and the culture.

There is almost twelve months of preparation and teamwork among all the Canadians before departure, and each emerges from the four-week trip with life-long memories. Some have already returned to Uganda, and others have vowed to do so. They have become used to the minor inconveniences, which at the time seemed major but soon morphed as everyone got used to "Uganda time," which has been likened to the Spanish *mañana* but lacks even its sense of urgency.

The entire Uganda exposure has been my most rewarding teaching experience in a thirty-odd-year career, but it is not just the teaching there that has made it so. The mantra of all professional schools ought to be a preparation for continuous learning. Aeschylus, the earliest of the three great Greek tragedians, phrased it slightly differently when he wrote: "Learning is ever in the freshness of its youth, even for the old." For me, the Uganda rotation fits, whichever way things are worded. ✽

EPILOGUE

I do not believe conservation can or will work.
Perhaps it would be more accurate to say that
the African megafauna is beyond conserving.

—IAN PARKER, FROM *What I Tell You Three Times is True*

I am absolutely certain that in Kenya wildlife will
ultimately be confined to national parks...wildlife
everywhere as we know it is disappearing fast and
will be gone in a decade.

—RICHARD LEAKEY, IN MIRELLA RICCIARDI'S *African Visions*

THE STATUS OF THE LION, as a symbol of what is happening to wildlife in Africa, is like a giant whirlpool. Whirlpools tend to suck everything down with them, and the state of the wildlife on the entire continent, represented by the lion, is in that vortex.

Among those who have written about large predators is David Quammen, who has a gloomy vision of the year 2150, when the world's human population may be 10.8 billion. His vision: "When I look into that future, I don't see any lion, tigers or bears."

Another perspective comes from Luke Hunter, of the Wildlife Conservation Society:

For television viewers who watch film after film of tourist-friendly lions in the Serengeti National Park or the Masai Mara, it is difficult to imagine that lions require any conservation effort at all. But as the number of lions continues to decline outside the parks and reserves—and in some cases, within their borders—we can no longer ignore the warning signs. Today the power balance is overwhelmingly against the lion, and the decisions we make now will decide the big cats' fate. We hold the future of the lion in our hands.

If Africa's lions and other large predators are under such enormous pressure, what of other species?

Ian Parker and Stan Bleazard have gathered seventeen stories by former members of Kenya's Game Department. They called the collection *An Impossible Dream*. The dedication in the book sums up much that has happened on the continent: "We dedicate this book to a Pleistocene Africa, which we so enjoyed and sought to preserve, but which is gone. It was an impossible dream."

It would be naïve to suggest that wildlife utilization and declining numbers is something new, or that it never took place on a large scale. Witness the recent discovery of ancient trading records from the Egyptian city of Alexandria. One ship alone in the third century BCE carried one hundred tonnes of elephant tusks and 135 tonnes of ebony in a single voyage. Acquiring so much stuff must have been a massive undertaking. We will never know how much of the ivory was "found" from carcasses, but the wood will surely have been logged.

A rapid growth rate of the human population in Africa—the fastest of any continent—is putting all wilderness areas under relentless pressure. The pressure comes from a wide spectrum. At one end there are the poor and needy, living on a dollar a day or less, trying to scratch out few more metres of forest or scrub to cultivate a few more beans or a couple of dozen more maize plants. At the other end, there are the powerful and the greedy wanting ever more cattle on ever more land so as to further enhance their own prestige. A new term for them has come into the lexicon. They are known as megapastoralists.

Our trips to Uganda provide a nice example of the wildlife situation across Africa. Wildlife now exists in island settings across the country, and a small number of dedicated people are trying to preserve what remains. Everywhere else, however, people abound and cultivation is widespread. Elephants, baboons and chimpanzees invade cultivated areas and endanger human lives.

It is not just smallholders who struggle with wildlife. Long-time Kenya friends wrote, in a Christmas letter: "Our love for wild animals gets a bit thin what with elephant (breaking fences), leopard (eating sheep), wild dog, jackal, monkeys (eating all the vegetables), pigs, and masses of bucks eating all the crops!"

It is all very well for people from the so-called "First World" to decry the disappearance of wildlife and wild places in Africa or other "Third World" areas, such as India, Indonesia and Malaysia, where wild places and wildlife are disappearing under cultivation or unbridled logging. First, though, they should look to their own history and continued desecration of the environment and all that is in it, from the highly visible large mammals to the very smallest microbe, all of which have been more or less irrevocably altered in so many ways. As "The Gospel According to Matthew" has it: "Why do you see the spec in your neighbour's eye, but you don't see the log in your own eye?"

While television viewers who see the massive wildebeest migrations of the Serengeti–Masai Mara would have trouble believing hoofed animal numbers are in decline, there is no doubt that it is happening and probably happening at an increasing rate. All wildlife numbers continue to tumble as hunting pressure for bushmeat continues, with ever-smaller species, such as small birds and ground squirrels being targeted.

The occasional poaching of a hippo for a new bride's feast, or meat for a family is one thing. The wholesale slaughter of huge numbers of these barrel-shaped creatures is a different matter. Such a slaughter took place in late 2006 in Democratic Republic of Congo's Virunga National Park, on the western shores of Lake Edward. This was just another incident in the ongoing carnage in which hippo numbers have plummeted from 22,875 to a mere 315 head over twenty years. The killers were the same Mai Mai rebels who achieved worldwide media attention in 2007 by attacking rangers in the park, killing one and wounding others, and then threatening to kill off all the mountain gorillas there if the authorities came after them.

There is no reason to think that the bushmeat situation will change anytime soon, at least until population numbers of wild animals become so low that hunters become frustrated with their lack of success. It will be equivalent to the attitude of more prosperous people of other nations who plunder forests, fish or whale stocks until to do so is "no longer a commercially viable proposition." A chilling phrase.

Those by-products of the bushmeat trade and the logging industry, the orphan apes in one of the twelve sanctuaries across Africa devoted to their care, certainly give the humans involved in that care many rewards, but the cost of maintaining the animals, which comes from the donations of a well-meaning public, is enormous. There is no doubt that the sight of so many orphan chimps is captivating, but a deeper question about conservation funding arises. The chance that any of these animals, all of them psychologically scarred, will have of ever getting back into the wild are virtually nil. A better way to spend the money would be to take a leaf out of the Kilimanjaro Lion Conservation Project's book and use the funds for primate conservation in some other way, perhaps in making a film with which to educate the people who live among primates. However, it would be a hard sell, as doleful orphan chimps are a sure-fire attention grabber, and sophisticated fundraisers know it.

Raymond Bonner's book *At the Hand of Man: Peril and Hope for Africa's Wildlife* is a sometimes-scathing examination of how the West has interfered with and abused the African continent, its people and the wildlife there. His summary is pretty straightforward: "All we have to do to preserve Africa's wildlife heritage is care about the people as much as we care about the wildlife. Both are in the hands of man."

The trouble is that in every situation, in every country, there are powerful people who do not see things from the conservation perspective. The challenge is to change that view.

An example of this challenge comes direct from Uganda, where in 2007 President Museveni approved the excision of 23 per cent of the Mabira Forest Reserve, a beautiful pristine area of tropical rain forest, to the Mehta Group, which is headed by an Asian-Ugandan sugar baron. Hidden in the initial press reports was the little matter of a possible income of at least US$50 million from the hardwood sales that would have followed. The decision, vigorously opposed by many people, led to riots in the streets of Kampala, the death of three people and multiple arrests. Under pressure from several quarters, the president backed down, but he has not revealed a change of heart. He may yet win his way after a comprehensive environmental impact assessment has been conducted. Given the record of many another politician in almost any country, I cannot help wondering how much of that $50 million would be channelled into powerful pockets and Swiss bank accounts.

A recent deeply perceptive view of the likely future of Africa's fauna comes from Tim Caro of the University of California, Davis, and his co-author Paul Scholte of Leiden University in Holland. Writing in the *African Journal of Ecology* in 2007, they have taken a long look at wildlife populations across the continent, building on the works of people like Jonathan Kingdon and Ian Parker, as well as many others. They discuss the historical records from long ago, as well as the much more recent history of the last fifteen years.

As they show, we have moved beyond the point at which wildlife populations (ranging well beyond just large mammals) have more or less vanished outside protected areas, and we are now seeing destruction at a different level. They write: "now a raft of studies are showing that...we are losing species from many of Africa's national parks." Many such studies "generally focus on antelopes, which are easy to count from the air" or in other ways. They end this paragraph with a telling phrase: "Most are delicious to eat."

As Caro and Scholte point out, there are some exceptions. Elephants are doing well in some regions, partially because they are such a high-profile species and therefore attract significant resources, but this is not the case in central Africa, as I pointed out in the second section of this book.

There are a few parks, most notably Kruger National Park in South Africa, that are well-funded and where human impact is not the major problem, but even here populations of some species are in decline because of lack of dry-season rainfall.

The final paragraph in the Caro–Scholte report ends with an interesting view: "In the final analysis, we may have to get used to faunal relaxation in Africa's network of famous reserves leaving a continent containing isolated pockets of large mammal diversity living at low population sizes. Just like Europe."

There are a few star-glimmers of hope in this dark firmament. One can hope that the initiatives taken by the Maasai people of the Mbirikani Group Ranch will spread rapidly to other parts of Kenya, and indeed the rest of Africa, so that the downward-spiralling whirlpool may stop. One can find other glimmers up and down the African continent, and they come from several countries.

The very name of the veterinary school department that Christine Dranzoa co-founded in Uganda, "Wildlife and Animal Resource Management," makes one realize that there are people across the continent who continue to struggle against land encroachment, widespread poaching with gun and snare and the indiscriminate poisoning.

In Kenya wildlife forums have been established. Ian Parker has reported in *Swara* about each of them. Some are obvious successes as people recognize the value of the wild animals around them.

One of the longest-running conservation programs that involves all members of a community is in Zimbabwe and has the lengthy acronym of CAMPFIRE. The letters stand for Community Areas Management Program for Indigenous Resources, and the program has managed to stay afloat through the collapse of so much of that country's society. It was originally set up so that villagers would have a stake in every aspect of wildlife resource management in their own communities, thus ensuring their continued interest in preserving the wildlife around them. As every single householder in a village has a stake in the program, they all have an interest in policing the communal lands and ensuring that not only is the income derived—mostly from hunting—channelled back to them directly but also that wildlife numbers are maintained at sustainable levels.

On another brighter note, consulting ecologist Rowan Martin, who was the lead architect of CAMPFIRE twenty years ago and is still involved, has also been working with a group of people in the Mudumu North Complex (MNC) of Namibia's Caprivi Strip. He has written: "I regard what is happening in MNC as the most significant and enlightened development in wildlife conservation to have happened in southern Africa in the past half-century."

The initiative entails the co-management of some 4,500 square kilometres of land laying either side of the Kwando River, which is right where I worked with Mike Briggs and Kallie Venske in 1997. Martin further wrote: "The stakeholders have already established a preliminary joint management structure, formed a Management Committee, developed a work programme, are in the process of zoning their land for wildlife and have set themselves *the goal of increasing the numbers and diversity of wildlife within the Complex.*"

In an e-mail sent to me on March 26, 2007, Martin was slightly less enthused: "I wrote the paragraph which you quote in the middle of last year when the mood of all participants (including the State) was extremely buoyant. Since then it would appear that the State is becoming a more difficult bride to bring to the altar."

The problem is a semantic one with considerable implications. Martin uses the term "co-management" in his report. Some government official had a problem with this term and wanted him to change it to "collaborative management." There is quite a difference, as the latter does not actually commit anyone to anything.

Another more encouraging new development lies with AHEAD, the Animal Health for the Environment And Development Program, which was founded in South Africa in late 2003. It focuses on the interface between wildlife, livestock and human health and has been able to draw in a diverse range of institutions and disciplines—veterinarians, ecologists, economists, medical doctors, social scientists, agriculture specialists, wildlife managers and other stakeholders. One of its most exciting initiatives has been the first steps in the development of a transfrontier conservation area that involves South Africa, Mozambique and Zimbabwe. The members of AHEAD are working to persuade governments to embrace issues related to health, conservation and development in a way that could become a model for Africa, and beyond.

Perhaps the most striking new finding with a positive spin has been the observation, reported by the Wildlife Conservation Society (WCS) in June 2007, of a massive migration of antelope and other species in southern Sudan. The team of which Paul Elkan, with whom I had worked in Cameroon, was a part, counted about a quarter of a million animals.

Over half (800,000) were kob, like the ones we work on in Uganda. Of the other hoofstock species, four thousand were Nile lechwe, which are found nowhere else on Earth.

On the wcs web report appears the statement: "This could represent the biggest migration of large mammals on Earth." The team leader was another wcs scientist, Michael Fay. He stated, "I have never seen wildlife in such numbers, not even when flying over the mass migrations of the Serengeti."

Another bright spot that concerns the environment in general, rather than wildlife specifically, was the announcement in June 2007 of a ban on lightweight plastic bags in both Kenya and Uganda. These countries join Rwanda, South Africa and Tanzania in making positive steps to deal with the pervasive menace of fly-away plastic bags. A follow-up report from the bbc in October that year stated that the ban in Uganda had had no visible effect. The police were taking no action, and vendors everywhere were still using the bags. The interval was only four months, so perhaps the bbc reporter was expecting more than could reasonably be delivered.

All over the world members of my own profession are becoming increasingly active in the field of conservation and teaming up with ecologists with a wide variety of backgrounds. It is encouraging that many of them are newer "in-country" graduates like the ones in Uganda with whom we spent time.

Students who have been to Uganda with me have asked, "Is there any point in choosing wildlife medicine as a career path? What chance does wildlife have?"

My reply has always been, "Yes to your first question, and, to your second question, just think, if we didn't get involved, along with the hundreds of other conservation biologists and wildlife professionals everywhere, then things would be really grim."

Just after I had sent the intended final draft of this manuscript to the publishers I learned from Dr. Siefert that an entire clan of twelve hyaenas had been poisoned "right next door" to the village of Kanesyi. Perhaps we are reaching the children at some level, but we have obviously not reached at least one adult.

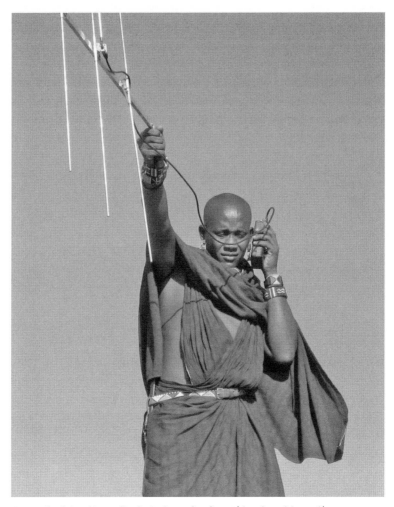

Lion Guard Mokoi tracking a collared animal. Hope for a future? (Photo by Leelah Hazzah)

And what of the future for those children in Kasenyi and Equator schools, as well as that of my own grandchildren and the children yet to come of the Canadians who went to Uganda with Jo and me?

Our Canadian children will be brought up in an atmosphere that gives them a chance to become fascinated by, and concerned for, both the people and animals of foreign lands. The Ugandan children and their teachers well know that the only reason they have met us is because we came to the park to work with wild animals. If we have affected their lives, it is through that avenue. Have we sown tiny seeds of hope? Perhaps not as prolific of those sown by Jane Goodall and her Roots & Shoots organization, but maybe the little seeds we have scattered will also establish their own roots. Will the Ugandan children whose lives we've touched be like Celsus and cherish the wildlife around them?

Time will tell. ✽

APPENDIX 1
GLOSSARY
OF PLANT AND
ANIMAL SPECIES

COMMON NAME	TAXONOMIC NAME
MAMMALS	
Carnivores	
African lion	*Panthera leo*
African wild dog (cape hunting dog)	*Lycaon pictus*
Asiatic (Gir) lion	*Panthera leo persica*
Banded mongoose	*Mungos mungo*
Black-backed jackal	*Canis mesomelas*
Cheetah	*Acinonyx jubatus*
Leopard	*Panthera pardus*
Ocelot	*Leopardus pardalis*
Spotted hyaena	*Crocuta crocuta*
Spot-necked otter	*Lutra maculicollis*
Tiger	*Panthera tigris*
Primates	
Black-and-white colobus	*Colobus guereza*
Central African red colobus	*Piliocolobus oustaleti*

COMMON NAME	TAXONOMIC NAME
Chimpanzee	Pan troglodytes
Gorilla	Gorilla gorilla
White-nosed monkey (greater)	Cercopithecus nictitans
Zanzibar red colobus	Piliocolobus kirkii
Elephants	
Elephant (forest)	Loxodonta cyclotis
Elephant (Indian)	Elephas maximus
Elephant (savannah)	Loxodonta africana
Odd-toed ungulates	
Rhinoceros	
Black rhino	Diceros bicornis
White rhino (northern)	Ceratotherium simum cottoni
White rhino (southern)	Ceratotherium simum simum
Zebras	
Common zebra	Equus quagga
Grevy's zebra	Equus grevyi
Mountain zebra	Equus zebra
Even-toed ungulates	
African buffalo	Syncerus caffer
Bongo	Tragelaphus euryceros
Dik-dik	Madoqua kirkii
Gemsbok	Oryx gazella
Giraffe	Giraffa camelopardalis
Hippopotamus	Hippopotamus amphibius
Jentink's duiker	Cephalophus jentinki
Kudu	Tragelaphus strepsiceros
Nile lechwe	Kobus megaceros
Oribi	Ourebia ourebi
Red lechwe	Kobus leche

COMMON NAME	TAXONOMIC NAME
Roan antelope	*Hippotragus equinus*
Sable antelope	*Hippotragus niger*
Sitatunga	*Tragelaphus spekei*
Thomson's gazelle	*Gazella thomsoni*
Topi	*Damaliscus lunatus*
Uganda kob	*Kobus kob thomasi*
Warthog	*Phacochoerus africanus*
Waterbuck	*Kobus ellipsimprymnus*
Wildebeest	*Connochaetes taurinus*
Other species	
Cane rat (pidgin—cutting grass)	*Thryonomys* spp. (2 species)
Fruit bat	*Rousettus aegyptiacus*
Fruit bat in Ebola study	*Hypsignathus monstrosus*
Fruit bat in Ebola study	*Epomops franqueti*
Fruit bat in Ebola study	*Myonycteris torquata*
REPTILES	
Dwarf crocodile	*Osteolaemus tetraspis*
Nile crocodile	*Crocodilus niloticus*
BIRDS	
African fish eagle	*Haliaeetus vocifer*
African golden weaver	*Ploceus subaureus*
Brown-hooded kingfisher	*Halcyon albiventris*
Cassowary	*Casuarius casuarius*
Collared sunbird	*Hedydipna collaris*
Crimsonbreasted shrike/gonolek	*Laniarius atrococccineus*
Drongo (Fork-tailed)	*Dicrurus adsimilis*
Egyptian goose	*Alopochen aegyptiacus*
Fischer's turaco	*Tauraco fischeri*
Greater blue-eared starling	*Lamprotornis chalybaeus*

COMMON NAME	TAXONOMIC NAME
Grey heron	Ardrea cinerea
Hadeda ibis	Bostrychia hagedash
Helmeted guineafowl	Numida meleagris
Long-tailed cormorant	Phalacrocorax africanus
Marabou stork	Leptoptilos crumeniferus
Ostrich	Struthio camelus
Pelican	Pelicanus onocrotalus
Pied kingfisher	Ceryle rudis
Red-billed teal	Anas erythrorhyncha
Red-chested sunbird	Cinnyris erythrocerca
Sacred ibis	Threskiornis aethiopicus
Saddle-billed stork	Ephippiorhynchus senegalensis
Sarus crane	Grus antigone
Scaly francolin	Francolinus squamatus
Vulture guineafowl	Acryllium vulturinum
Yellow-billed stork	Mycteria ibis
Yellow-necked spur fowl	Francolinus leucoscepus
INSECTS	
Safari ant	Dorylus spp.
PLANTS	
Alligator pepper	Amomum melegueta
Bottlebrush	Callistemon citrinus
Candelabra euphorbia	Euphorbia candelabrum
Fever tree	Acacia xanthophloea
Flame tree (also Lucky Bean)	Erythrina abbyssinica
Flat-topped acacia	Acacia abyssinica / Acacia hockii
Nandi flame	Spathodea campanulata
Sickle bush	Dichrostachys cinerea
Wait-a-bit thorn	Acacia brevispica

APPENDIX 2
GLOSSARY OF
SWAHILI WORDS

WHEN I WAS SEARCHING for the derivation of some Swahili words that did not appear in any of several dictionaries, or even online, but that I know just through using them, I received this helpful note and three definitions from Ian Parker. "There are three major versions and one minor version of Kiswahili. The classical Kiamu of Lamu in which most Swahili poetry and the Koran are written; Kimvitap—the Mazrui Swahili of Mombasa; Kiunguja—the language of Zanzibar, which is the most widespread version via the slave trade; and Kipemba of Pemba, which is the least comprehensible."

There is a fourth version, Kisettla, the grammar-butchering rendition of Kiunguja that has taken hold in Kenya's interior via the white settlers. As Edward Rodwell points out in *Coast Causerie 2*, the evolution of Kisettla is no different than the dialect developments of other languages, such as Creole from French and Afrikaans from Dutch. Most of my Swahili is of this variety, but it is definitely better than some of the amazing butchery done by some Kisettla users. A classic example of this from early settler days is told by Rodwell when he recounts how a "memsahib" told her gardener to go to the herb garden and bring some thyme. He translates her instructions as, *"To go bed* [as for sleep] *and bring time."*

The latest evolution in Swahili dialects is Sheng. Used mostly in Kenya by the university-educated young, it is virtually incomprehensible to me.

Following are words, meaning and some derivations of the Swahili used in this book.

SWAHILI	ENGLISH
askari	n. soldier, policeman
ayah	n. nanny or nurse, often for children, also spelt aya and (more recently) yaya; origin: Hindi
baraza	n. meeting
boma	n. corral, also castle or fort. In sensu stricto, a zariba is an enclosure of branches and scrub, usually of acacias. Once accepted throughout Kenya and Tanganyika as "a government station," use of this word can be traced to the early days when government officials conducted their business from within a zariba.
buibui	n. black garment worn by Muslim women (also spider)
chapli	n. sandal of particular form worn by Bengal Lancers and widely popular among Kenya settlers; origin: Hindi
ku-chinja (nitachinja)	v. to slaughter, cut the throat
chuma	n. metal, steel, also strong or dependable person
choo	n. lavatory
daktari	n. doctor
mwenyewe	pron. self (root is enyewe), as in mimi mwenywe, meaning "me myself"
faru (kifaru)	n. rhinoceros
habari	n. news, information
Habari yako?	What is your news?
Jambo/Hujambo	How do you do? Hello! Good morning! Hi!; the shortened version of Huna jambo? (Have you anything?)
kidonda	n. small wound, sore, ulcer; ki- is the diminutive; donda means "large wound" or "sore"
kima	n. monkey of Cercopithecus mitis group only; price or value
kupe	n. tick
lakini	but
lete	v. imperative form of verb kulete, to bring; most dictionaries state that lete should be leta, but lete is widely understood

SWAHILI	ENGLISH
luggah	n. seasonal watercourse; not found in any Swahili dictionaries, but widely understood. This word has the same etymological origin as *lak* in the Oromo tongue spoken by the Galla from Lake Tana in Ethiopia to the Tana Delta in Kenya. The Somali language shares many Oromo roots. In their guttural rendering, *lak* becomes *laggah*, which then becomes luggah. The spelling is not constant. These languages have similar roots to Hindi and the word literally means "flow" in Hindi, in which language it is also used to denote a seasonal watercourse. *Wadi* is now used for seasonal watercourse in modern Swahili dictionaries; origin: Arabic
makuti	n. thatch (coconut leaf for thatching); singular is *kuti*, which denotes one piece of coconut frond; a Kisettla term that is widely used and derived from Kiswahili
mambo	n. matters, things, affairs (but not material things); plural of *jambo*
mbwa	n. dog
mkono	n. hand
mkora	adj. rascal, bandit
munanda	n. crush and associated pens for livestock; not found in Swahili dictionaries. *Munanda* is of Bantu derivation and used widely in Kenya for what the North Americans and Australians would term "yards." It has entered the local language through Kisettla.
mzee	n. old man, elder; a term of respect.
ndiyo	adv. or pron. yes; literally "it is"; the most widely used term for "yes"
ng'ombe	n. cow, cattle
nyama	n. meat, animal; plural has prefix *wa-*
panga	n. machete
ku-piga sindano	v. to inject with a needle and syringe; literally "to hit with a needle"; definitely a coarse kisettlarism, but widely understood
piki piki	n. motorbike
plotti	n. *slang.* a plot of land
pori	n. bush (as in jungle, but not tree); wilderness
punju	n. snakebite
punyu	n. form of poison
safi	adj. clean, pure, bright, lucid; used *in sensu lato* for "classy" and anything of high quality and integrity
sana	adj. very
shuka	n. cloth; any piece of calico worn as a loin cloth or toga

SWAHILI	ENGLISH
siafu	n. safari ant of genus *Dorylus*
sindano	n. needle; in veterinary parlance usually implies needle and syringe
sumu	n. poison
vipi	*interrog. adv.* How? What? Which?
walipigwa	v. They were hit; from verb *ku-piga* (to hit) and in context refers to injection
wanyama	*n.pl.* plural form of *nyama*, meaning animals
Wapi?	*interrog. adv.* Where?
yote	*adj., n., adv.* All

SOURCES
AND
SUGGESTED
READING

INTRODUCTION

Adamson, Joy. *The Peoples of Kenya*. London: Collins and Harvill Press, 1967.

Bright, Michael. *Man Eaters*. London: Robson Books, 2000.

Dyer, Tony. *The Big Five*. Nidrum, Belgium: Hatari Times, 2003.

Kingdon, Jonathan. *East African Mammals: An Atlas of Evolution in Africa*. London: Academic Press, 1971.

"Lion killer is killed by hyenas." BBC website. http://news.bbc.co.uk/2/hi/africa/7105191.stm

Quammen, David. *Monster of God: The Man-eating Predator in the Jungles of History and the Mind*. New York: W.W. Norton and Company, 2003.

"The Rightly Guided Calpihs." http://www.usc.edu/dept/MSA/politics/firstfourcaliphs.html

1

Haigh, J.C. 1977. The capture of wild Black rhinoceros using fentanyl and azaperone. *South African Journal of Wildlife Research*. 7(1)11–14.

Haigh, J.C. 1975. Immobilization of bongo and other African antelopes. *Veterinary Record*. 98:237–39.

McWhirter, Norris and Ross McWhirter, eds. *The Guinness Book of World Records*. Enfield, UK: Guinness Superlatives Ltd., 1973.

2

Hofmeyr, Markus. *The African Wild Dogs of Madikwe: A Success Story!* Rustenburg, South Africa: North West Parks Board, 1997.

Legge, A.J. and P.A. Rowley-Conwy. 1987. Gazelle killing in stone age Syria. *Scientific American*. 257: 88–96.

Parkinson, Tony. "The Roan Story." *Africana*. 4:9 (1972): 15–16, 33–34.

Player, Ian. *The White Rhino Saga*. New York: Stein and Day, 1973.

3

Hedges, K. 1974. Acute pulmonary oedema at high altitude. *J. roy. Army med. Cps*. 120:102–108.

Jubb, K.V.F. and P.C. Kennedy. *Pathology of Domestic Animals*. 1st ed. Academic Press, New York: 1963.

4

De Laroque, Lucinda. *Paradise Found: The Story of The Mount Kenya Safari Club*. Nairobi: Camerapix, 1992.

Haigh, Jerry. *Wrestling With Rhinos: The Adventures of a Glasgow Vet in Kenya*. Toronto: ECW Press, 2002.

5

De Laroque, Lucinda. *Paradise Found: The Story of The Mount Kenya Safari Club*. Nairobi: Camerapix, 1992.

Hunter, J. A. *Hunter*. Long Beach: California Safari Press Inc., 1999.

Pavitt, Nigel. *Kenya: The First Explorers*. London: Aurum Press, 1989.

Thomas, Lowell. *India: Land of the Black Pagoda*. London: Hutchinson & Co., 1931.

6

Dyer, Tony. *The Big Five*. Nidrum, Belgium: Hatari Times, 2003.

7

House, Adrian. *The Great Safari: The Lives of George and Joy Adamson*.
New York: William Morrow and Company, 1993.

Noad, Tim and Ann Birnie. *Trees of Kenya*. Nairobi: T. Noad and A. Birnie, 1989.

Ricciardi, Mirella. *African Visions: The Diary of an African Photographer*.
London: Cassell & Co., n.d.

8

Lewa Wildlife Conservancy. http://www.lewa.org/

Mertz, Anna. *Rhino at the Brink of Extinction*. London: Harper Collins, 1991.

Paice, Edward. *Where Warriors Meet: The Story of Lewa Downs, Kenya*.
Illustrated by Sarah Elder. London: Tasker Publications, 1995.

9

Adamson, Joy. *The Spotted Sphinx*. San Diego: Harcourt Brace & World, 1969.

Haigh, Jerry. *Wrestling With Rhinos: The Adventures of a Glasgow Vet in Kenya*.
Toronto: ECW Press, 2002.

Kay, John. "Shootings threaten black rhino project." BBC website. http://
news.bbc.co.uk/2/hi/science/nature/7109429.stm

10 AND 11

Karesh, William B. *Appointments at the Ends of the World: Memoirs of a
Wildlife Veterinarian*. New York: Warner Books, 1999.

Kingdon, Jonathan. *East African Mammals: An Atlas of Evolution in Africa*.
London: Academic Press, 1971.

Makuchi. "The Forest Will Claim You Too." In *Your Madness, Not
Mine: Stories of Cameroon*. Athens, Ohio: Ohio University Center for
International Studies, 1999.

Roca, Alfred L., Nicholas Georgiadis, et al. 2001. Genetic evidence for two
species of elephant in Africa. *Science*. 293:1473–77.

12, 13 AND 14

Adow, Osei Kwadwo. "Wildlife: a source of medicine." *Green Dove*. Accra: Green Earth Organization, 2002. http://www.premioreportagem.org. br/index.php?pageId=sub&lang=pt_BR&currentItem=article&docId=506 &c=Ghana&cRef=Ghana&year=2002&date=outubro%202002

Anadu, P.A. 1987. Wildlife conservation in Nigeria: problems and strategies. *The Environmentalist*. 7(3):211–20.

Angelici, Francesco M. et al. 1999. Bushmen and mammal-fauna: a survey of the mammals traded in bush-meat markets of local people in the rainforests of south-eastern Nigeria. *Anthropozoologica*. 30:51–58

Auerbach, Paul. S., Howard J. Donner, and Eric A. Weiss. *Field Guide to Wilderness Medicine*. St. Louis: Mosby, 1999.

Avasthi, Amitabh. 2004. Bush-meat trade breeds new HIV. *New Scientist*. 183(2459): 8.

Baah, Vivian. "Confessions of a bush meat journalist." *The Evening News*. Accra. March 2001. http://www.premioreportagem.org.br/index. php?pageId=sub&lang=pt_BR&currentItem=article&docId=315&c=Ghan a&cRef=Ghana&year=2001&date=março%202001

Bakarr, M.I. et al. "Bushmeat utilization, human livelihoods and conservation of large mammals in West Africa." In *Links Between Biodiversity Conservation, Livelihoods and Food Security: the sustainable use of wild species for meat*, edited by Sue Mainka and Mandar Trivedi, 45–53. Occasional Paper Number 24. Gland, Switzerland: IUCN Species Survival Commission, 2002.

Barnett, Rob. *Food for Thought: The Utilization of Wild Meat in Eastern and Southern Africa*. TRAFFIC International, 2000.

Bonner, Raymond. *At the Hand of Man: Peril and Hope for Africa's Wildlife*. New York: Alfred A. Knopf, 1993.

Bowen-Jones, Evan, David Brown, and Elizabeth Robinson. *Assessment of the solution-oriented research needed to promote a more sustainable bushmeat trade in Central and West Africa*. Department for Environment Food and Rural Affairs. Wildlife & Countryside Directorate London. January 2002.

Brashares, J.S. et al. 2004. Bushmeat hunting, wildlife declines, and fish supply in West Africa. *Science*. 306(5699):1180–83.

Chardonnet, Phillipe et al. 2002. The value of wildlife. *Rev. sci. tech. Off. Int. Epiz.* 21(1):15–51.

"Conservation International Launches Second 'Biodiversity Reporting Award' for Ghanaian Journalists." Press release. February 22, 2002. http://www.conservation.org/xp/news/press_releases/2002/022202.xml

Cowlishaw, Guy, Samantha Mendelson, and J. Marcus Rowcliffe. 2005. Evidence for post-depletion sustainability in a mature bushmeat market. *Journal of Applied Ecology.* 42(3):460–68.

Denis, Armand. *On Safari: The Story of My Life.* London: Collins, 1963.

Driciru, M. "Predicting Population Viability Study of Lions in MFNP, Uganda." Master of Wildlife Health and Management thesis. Kampala: Makerere University, 2006.

European Parliament. Texts Adopted by Parliament. Provisional Edition. 14/01/2004. Illegal trade in bushmeat. P5-TA-PROV(2004)0019. A5-0355/2003. European Parliament resolution on Petition 461/2000 concerning the protection and conservation of Great Apes and other species endangered by the illegal trade in bushmeat (2003/2078(INI)). http://www.europarl.europa.eu/omk/omnsapir.so/pv2?PRG=CALDOC&FILE=20040114&LANGUE=EN&TPV=PROV&LASTCHAP=8&SDOCTA=4&TXTLST=1&Type_Doc=FIRST&POS=1

Fa, John E., Carlos A. Peres, and Jessica Meeuwig. 2002. Bushmeat exploitation in tropical forests: an intercontinental comparison. *Conservation Biology.* 16(1): 232.

Fa, John E. and Carlos A. Peres. "Game vertebrate extraction in African and neotropical forests." In *Conservation of Exploited Species,* edited by J. D. Reynolds et al., 203–241. Cambridge: Cambridge University Press, 2001.

Gao, F. et al. 1999. Origin of HIV-1 in the chimpanzee *Pan troglodytes troglodytes. Nature.* 397:385–86.

Hahn, Beatrice H., George M. Shaw, Kevin M. De Cock, et al. January 28, 2000. AIDS as a zoonosis: scientific and public health implications. *Science.* 287(5453):607–614.

Haigh, Jerry. *Wrestling With Rhinos: The Adventures of a Glasgow Vet in Kenya.* Toronto: ECW Press, 2002.

Hamburg, Margaret A., Joshua Lederberg, and Mark S. Smolinski. *Microbial Threats to Health: Emergence, Detection, and Response.* Washington: Institute of Medicine, National Academy Press, 2003.

Karesh, William B. and Robert A. Cook. "The Human-Animal Link." *Foreign Affairs*. July–August 2005. http://www.foreignaffairs.org/20050701faessay84403/william-b-karesh-robert-a-cook/the-human-animal-link.html

Karesh, William B., Robert A. Cook, et al. 2005. Wildlife trade and global disease emergence. *Emerging Infectious Diseases*. 11(7):1000–1002.

Kingdon, Jonathan. *East African Mammals: An Atlas of Evolution in Africa*. London: Academic Press, 1971.

Motkin, Miranda H., Elizabeth L. Bennett, and Danielle T. LaBruna. November 2005. "Wildlife farming: A viable alternative to hunting in tropical forests?" *Wildlife Conservation Society* working paper, 23:32 pages.

Parker, Ian. "Daunting Mission: Kenya's Taita-Taveta Wildlife Forum." *Swara*. 28:1 (January–March 2005): 48–50.

Parker, Ian. *What I Tell You Three Times Is True: Conservation, Ivory, History & Politics*. Kinloss, Scotland: Librario Publishing, 2004.

Parker, I.S.C. and A.D. Graham. 1989. Elephant decline: downward trends in African elephant distribution and numbers (part II). *Intern. J. Environmental Studies*. 35.

Peterson, Dale. *Eating Apes*. Afterword and photographs by Karl Ammann. Foreword by Janet K. Museveni. Berkley: University of California Press, 2003.

Pomerantz, David. "Dispute Over Monkey Meat Hits on Religious Freedom." *Special to the New York Sun*. August 20, 2007.

Rose, Anthony L. et al. *Consuming Nature. A Photo Essay on African Rain Forest Exploitation*. Photography by Karl Ammann. Los Angeles: Altisima Press, 2004.

Ryan, Oria. "Bushmeat boom benefits Ghana's farmers." April 3, 2006. file:///Users/admin/Desktop/06%20Book/Bushmeat%20pages/BBC%20NEWS%20Bushmeat%20boom%20.webarchive

Taylor, Louise H., Sophia M. Latham, and Mark E.J. Woolhouse. July 29, 2001. Risk factors for human disease emergence. *Philosophical Transactions: Biological Sciences*. 356(1411):983–89.

Western, David. *In the Dust of Kilimanjaro*. Washington, DC: Island Press/Shearwater Books, 1997.

Williamson, Douglas. "Wild meat, food security and forest conservation." In *Links between Biodiversity Conservation, Livelihoods and Food Security: The sustainable use of wild species for meat*, 19-22. Occasional Paper of the IUCN Species Survival Commission, No. 24. Sue Mainka and Mandar Trivedi. IUCN. 2002

Wolfe, Nathan D., Ananias A. Escalante, William B. Karesh, et al. April-June 1998. Wild primate populations in emerging infectious disease research: the missing link? *Emerging Infectious Diseases*. 4(2):149-158.

Woolhouse, Mark. 2002. Population biology of emerging and re-emerging pathogens. *Trends in Microbiology*. 10(10):3-7.

Woolhouse, Mark E.J., Louise H. Taylor, and Daniel T. Haydon. 2001. Population biology of multihost pathogens. *Science*. 292(5519):1109-12.

15

Aristotle. *Historia Animalium*. VI.XXXI-XXXII. Translated by A. L. Peck. Cambridge, MA: Harvard University Press, 1970.

Begg, Angus. "South Africa: Kruger National." *Travel Africa Magazine* (online). Edition 3. Spring 1998. http://www.travelafricamag.com

Frank, Laurence G. and Stephen E. Glickman. "The Mothers of Aggression." In *Encyclopedia Britannica Yearbook of Science and the Future*. 220-239. Chicago: Encyclopedia Britannica, 1996.

Glickman, Stephen E. 1995. The spotted hyena from Aristotle to *The Lion King*: reputation is everything. *Social Research*. 62(3):501-537.

Poole, Joyce. *Coming of Age with Elephants: A Memoir*. New York: Hyperion, 1996.

Poole, Joyce H. and Cynthia J. Moss. August 1981. Musth in the African elephant (*Loxodonta africana*). *Nature*. 292:830-31.

16

Adams, Douglas and Mark Cawardine. *Last Chance to See*. New York: Harmony Books, 1990.

Bradley-Martin, Esmond and Chrysee. *Run Rhino Run*. London: Chatto & Windus, 1982.

Martin, Esmond and Lucy Vine. January-June 2003. Trade in rhino horn from eastern Africa to Yemen. *Pachyderm*. 34:87.

P.P-H. But, Y-K Tam, and L-C Lung. 1991. Ethnopharmacology of rhinoceros horn. II: antipyretic effects of prescriptions containing rhinoceros horn or water buffalo horn. *J. Ethnopharmacology*. 33:45-50.

Milledge, Simon. *Rhino related crimes in Africa: an overview of poaching, seizure and stockpile data for the period 2000-2005*. TRAFFIC International, 2007.

Mills, Judy A. *Market Under Cover: The Rhinoceros Trade In South Korea*. A Traffic Network Report. TRAFFIC International, 1993.

Nowell, Kristin, Chyi Wei-Lien, and Pei Chia-Jai. *The Horns of A Dilemma: The Market for Rhino Horn In Taiwan*. TRAFFIC International, 1992.

Player, Ian. *The White Rhino Saga*. New York: Stein and Day, 1973.

17

Davies, Harriet T. and Johan T. du Toit. 2004. Anthropogenic factors affecting wild dog (*Lycaon pictus*) reintroductions: a case study in Zimbabwe. *Oryx*. 38:32-39.

Davies, Richard. *A Description and History of Madikwe Game Reserve*. Rustenberg, South Africa: North West Parks Board, 1997.

Hofmeyr, Markus. *The African Wild Dogs of Madikwe: A Success Story!* Rustenburg, South Africa: North West Parks Board, 1997.

Hofmeyr, Markus. *Operation Phoenix: The Restocking of Madikwe Game Reserve*. Rustenburg, South Africa: North West Parks Board, 1997.

Mertz, Anna. *Rhino at the Brink of Extinction*. London: Harper Collins, 1991.

Maugham, R.C.F. *Wild Game in Zambesia*. London: John Murray, 1914.

Woodroffe, R., J. Ginsberg, and D.W. Macdonald. *The African Wild Dog: Status Survey and Conservation Action Plan*. IUCN Canid Specialist Group. Gland, Switzerland: IUCN, 1997.

Woodroffe, Rosie and Joshua R. Ginsberg. 1999. Conserving the African wild dog (*Lycaon pictus*). I. diagnosing and treating causes of decline. *Oryx*. 33(2):132-42.

Woodroffe, Rosie, Peter Lindsey, Stephanie Romañach, et al. 2005. Livestock predation by endangered African wild dogs (*Lycaon pictus*) in northern Kenya. *Biological Conservation*. 124:225-34.

18

Welwitschia mirabilis
http://en.wikipedia.org/wiki/Welwitschia

19

Gale, F. Holderness, ed. *The Foreign and Colonial Compiling and Publishing Co.* Woking and London: Unwin Brothers/The Gresham Press, 1908, 1909.

Hill, M.F. *Permanent Way: The Story of the Kenya and Uganda Railway Being the Official History of the Development of the Transport System in Kenya and Uganda.* Nairobi, Kenya: East Africa Railways and Harbours, 1949.

Kingdon, Jonathan. *The Kingdon Field Guide to African Mammals.* London: Academic Press, 1997.

Patience, Kevin. *Zanzibar and the Shortest War in History.* Bahrain, Arabian Gulf: published by the author, 1994.

Rodwell, Edward. *The Sultan Said No!* In *Coast Causerie 2.* Nairobi: Heinemann, 1973.

Stevenson, Terry and John Fanshawe. *Field Guide to the Birds of East Africa.* London: Christopher Helm, 2002.

20

Driciru, M., L. Siefert, K.C. Prager, E. Dubovi, R. Sande, F. Princee, T. Friday, L. Munson. 2006. A serosurvey of viral infections in lions (*Panthera leo*) from Queen Elizabeth National Park, Uganda. *Journal of Wildlife Diseases.* 42:667–71.

Driciru, M. "Predicting Population Viability Study of Lions in MFNP, Uganda." Master of Wildlife Health and Management Thesis. Kampala: Makerere University, 2006.

Hugh-Jones, M.E. and V. de Vos. 2002. Anthrax and wildlife. *Rev. sci. tech. Off. Int. Epis.* 21(2):359–83.

Kock, Richard et al. 1998. Canine distemper antibodies in lions of the Masai Mara. *The Veterinary Record.* 142(24):662–65.

Roelke-Parker, Melody E., Linda Munson, Craig Packer, et al. 1996. A canine distemper virus epidemic in Serengeti lions (*Panthera leo*). *Nature.* 379:441–45.

de Vos, Valerius et al. 2001. The epidemiology of tuberculosis in free-ranging African buffalo (*Syncerus caffer*) in the Kruger National Park, South Africa. *Onderstepoort J. Vet. Res.* 68:119–30.

21

Hunter, J.A. *Hunter*. Long Beach, California: Safari Press Inc., 1999.

Lloyd, Albert B. *In Dwarf Land and Cannibal Country: A Record of Travel and Discovery in Central Africa*. London: T. Fisher Unwin, 1907.

Western, David. *In the Dust of Kilimanjaro*. Washington, DC: Island Press/Shearwater Books, 1997.

22

Adamson, Joy. *The Peoples of Kenya*. London: Collins and Harvill Press, 1967.

Corbett, Jim. *Maneaters of Kumaon*. Oxford: Oxford University Press, 1946.

Dyer, Tony. *The Big Five*. Nidrum, Belgium: Hatari Times, 2003.

Frank, Laurence, Seamus MacLennan, et al. "Lion killing in the Amboseli-Tsavo ecosystem, 2001–2006, and its implications for Kenya's lion population." May 18, 2006. http://www.lionconservation.org/LionKillinginAmboseliregion2000-May2006.pdf

Frank, Laurence. *Lions and Warriors: Conservation among Traditional Masai Pastoralists*. 6 pages. Berkley: Wildlife Conservation Society and University of California, Berkley, March 22, 2007.

Frank, Laurence. "Once there were lions." *Swara*. 26:3 and 26:4 (July–December 2003): 33–37.

Haigh, Jerry. *Wrestling With Rhinos: The Adventures of a Glasgow Vet in Kenya*. Toronto: ECW Press, 2002.

Hazzah, Leelah N. "Living Among Lions (*PANTHERA LEO*): Coexistence Or Killing? Community Attitudes towards Conservation Initiatives and the Motivations Behind Lion Killing in Kenyan Maasailand." M.Sc. thesis. University of Wisconsin-Madison, 2006.

Hill, Thomas and Richard Bonham. "Living on Borrowed Time." *Swara*. 28:4 (October–November 2005): 34–39.

Hunter, Luke. November–December 2006. The vanishing lion. *Wildlife Conservation*. 14(21)34–37.

Hunter, Luke and Gerald Hinde (photographer). *Cats of Africa: Behavior, Ecology, and Conservation*. Baltimore: The Johns Hopkins University Press, 2006.

Kraus, D. and L. Marker-Kraus. "The Status of the Cheetah (*Acinonyx jubatus*)." Report to the IUCN/SSC Cat Specialist Group. Postscript. 1991.

Loveridge, A.J., A.W. Searle, F. Murindagomob, and D.W. Macdonald. February 2007. The impact of sport-hunting on the population dynamics of an African lion population in a protected area. *Biological Conservation*. 134(4):548–58.

Paynter, David with Wilf Nussey. *Kruger: Portrait of a National Park*. Johannesburg: Southern Book Publishers, 1989.

Playne, Somerset, compiler. *East Africa (British): Its History, People, Commerce, Industries and Resources*. London: Foreign and Colonial Compiling and Publishing Co., 1908–1909.

Roosevelt, Theodore. *African Game Trails*. New York: Scribner's Sons, 1910.

Trench, Charles Chevenix. *The Desert's Dusty Face*. Edinburgh and London: William Blackwood & Sons Lts., 1964.

Turner, Myles. *My Serengeti Years: The Memoirs of an African Game Warden*. New York and London: W.W. Norton & Company, 1987.

Shelford, Frederic. "Notes on the Masai." *Journal of the Royal African Society*. 9:35 (April 1910): 267–69.

23

Churchill, Winston. *My African Journey*. London: Hodder & Stoughton, 1908.

24

Kahumbu, Paula and Peter Greste. "Chimps R Us—or are they?" *Swara*. 27:1 (March 2004): 19–20.

de Waal, Frans. *Chimpanzee Politics: Power and Sex among Apes*. New York: Harper & Row, 1982.

25 AND 26

Beuchner, H.K. 1961. Territorial behaviour in Uganda kob. *Science*. 133:698–99.

Haigh, J.C. 1975. Immobilization of bongo and other African antelopes. *Veterinary Record*. 98:237–39.

Kalema-Zikusoka, G., R.G. Bengis, A.L. Michel, and M.H. Woodford. 2005. A preliminary investigation of tuberculosis and other diseases in African Buffalo (*Syncerus caffer*) in Queen Elizabeth National Park, Uganda. *Onderstepoort J. Vet. Res.* 72:145–51.

Kingdon, Jonathan. *East African Mammals: An Atlas of Evolution in Africa*. London: Academic Press, 1971.

Kingdon, Jonathan. *The Kingdon Field Guide to African Mammals*. London: Academic Press, 1997.

27

Parker, Ian. *Jua Kali's Journey on the Jade Sea*. Kinloss, Scotland: Librario Publishing, 2004.

28

Kanuishiga, J.R. and M. Stahl, eds. *Park and People: Pastoralists and Wildlife. Proceedings from a seminar on environmental degradation in and around Lake Mburo National Park, Uganda*. Regional Soil Conservation Unit/ USDA. SIDA's Regional Soil Conservation Unit (RSCU), 1993.

Parker, Ian and Stan Bleazard. *An Impossible Dream*. Kinloss, Scotland: Librario Publishing, 2002.

EPILOGUE

Bonner, Raymond. *At the Hand of Man: Peril and Hope for Africa's Wildlife*. New York: Alfred A. Knopf, 1993.

"DR Congo rebel threat to gorillas." BBC News. Africa. http://news.bbc. co.uk/2/hi/africa/6677973.stm

"East African ban on plastic bags." BBC News. Africa. http://news.bbc. co.uk/2/hi/africa/6754127.stm

"Elite rangers take on rebels to end the slaughter of Congo's hippos." Special Report. Congo. http://www.guardian.co.uk/congo/story/0,,1977469,00. html

Frank, Laurence, Seamus MacLennan, et al. "Lion killing in the Amboseli-Tsavo ecosystem, 2001–2006, and its implications for Kenya's lion population." May 18, 2006. http://www.lionconservation.org/ LionKillinginAmboseliregion2000-May2006.pdf

Frank, Laurence. *Lions and Warriors: Conservation among Traditional Masai Pastoralists*. 6 pages. Berkley: Wildlife Conservation Society and University of California, Berkley, March 22, 2007.

Frank, Laurence. *Living with Lions: Laikipia Predator Project & Kilimanjaro Lion Conservation Project*. Annual Report. 2007

"Gospel According to Matthew." Chapter 7, verse 3.

Hunter, Luke. November–December 2006. The vanishing lion. *Wildlife Conservation*. 14(21):34–37.

Lawler, Andrew. "Raising Alexandria." *The Smithsonian Magazine.* April 2007. http://www.smithsonianmagazine.com/issues/2007/april/alexandria.php

"Massive Migration Revealed." http://www.wcs.org/353624/wcs_southernsudan

Osofsky, S.A., S. Cleaveland, William B. Karesh, et al. eds. *Conservation and Development Interventions at the Wildlife/Livestock Interface: Implications for Wildlife, Livestock and Human Health.* xxxiii, 220. IUCN. Gland, Switzerland and Cambridge, UK: IUCN, 2005.

Osofsky, S.A., R.A. Kock, M. Kock, et al. "Building Support for Protected Areas Using a 'One Health' Perspective." In *Friends for Life: New Partners in Support of Protected Areas*, edited by J.A. McNeely. 65-79. Gland, Switzerland and Cambridge, UK: IUCN, 2005.

Parker, Ian. *Around and About the Wildlife Fora.* A nine-part series of appraisals, wherein author and former game warden Ian Parker assesses progress made by the various Wildlife Fora that were established in 1990 amid efforts in Kenya to conserve wildlife living outside the country's protected areas. The entire series was published in *Swara*, the quarterly magazine of the East African Wild Life Society, between 2003 and 2005, in the following installments:

Parker, Ian. "The Shaping of a Game Plan." *Swara.* 26:1 (January-March 2003): 40-42.

Parker, Ian. "The Machakos Experience." *Swara.* 26:2 (April-June 2003): 48-50.

Parker, Ian. "A Formidable Institution." *Swara.* 26:3, 4(July-December 2003): 58-61.

Parker, Ian. "Nothing If Not Ambitious." *Swara.* 27:1 (January-March 2004): 56-58.

Parker, Ian. "Sleeping Giant?" *Swara.* 27:2 (April-June 2004): 48-50.

Parker, Ian. "A Radical Departure." *Swara.* 27:3 (July-September 2004): 78-82.

Parker, Ian. "In the Front Line." *Swara.* 27:4 (October-December 2004): 66-69.

Parker, Ian. "Daunting Mission." *Swara.* 28:1 (January-March 2005): 48-50.

Parker, Ian. "A 'tour de force.'" *Swara.* 28:2 (April-June 2005): 50-51.

Parker, Ian and Stan Bleazard. *An Impossible Dream*. Kinloss, Scotland: Librario Publishing, 2002.

Quammen, David. *Monster of God: The Man-eating Predator in the Jungles of History and the Mind*. New York: W.W. Norton and Company, 2003.

"Six wild elephants electrocuted in India after drinking beer, official says." Anon. Canadian Press: The Associated Press. October 23, 2007. http://www.msnbc.msn.com/id/21432722/

USEFUL WEBSITES

African Wild Dog Status Survey and Action Plan (1997)
http://www.canids.org/PUBLICAT/AWDACTPL/wldogtoc.htm

AHEAD (*A*nimal *H*ealth for the *E*nvironment *A*nd *D*evelopment Program)
http://www.wcs-ahead.org/

Karl Ammannn
http://www.karlAmmannn.com/about-site.php

Convention on International Trade in Endangered Species of Wild Fauna and Flora (CITES)
http://www.cites.org/

Committee on the Status of Endangered Wildlife in Canada (COSEWIC)
http://www.cosewic.gc.ca/

Fauna and Flora International (FFI)
http://www.fauna-flora.org/

Laurence Frank, *Living with Lions: Laikipia Predator Project & Kilimanjaro Lion Conservation Project* (Annual Report 2006)
http://www.lionconservation.org/

International Union for the Conservation of Nature (IUCN)
http://www.iucn.org/themes/ssc/

Jerry Haigh
http://www.jerryhaigh.com
http://www.jerryhaigh.blogspot.com

Kruger National Park
http://www.sanparks.org/parks/kruger/

Lewa Wildlife Conservancy
http://www.lewa.org/

Madikwe Game Reserve
http://www.madikwe.co.za/

Ol Pejeta Conservancy
http://www.olpejetaconservancy.org/

TRAFFIC: The Wildlife Trade Monitoring Network
http://www.traffic.org/Home.action

Uganda Wildlife Authority
http://www.uwa.or.ug/

Wildlife Conservation Society
http://www.wcs.org/

World Wildlife Fund
http://www.panda.org/

INDEX

Baah, Vivian, 155–56, 165
Babesiosis, 17–18
baboons, 195, 332, 337
Bagu, Edward, 314
Bailey, Jeremy, 318
Banyaruguru, 355, 357–59
Bao, 268–69
Barnett, Rob, 154–55
barracuda, 264
Barrie, J.M., 192
Basongora, 364, 365–66
Bastard, Seager, 167
Basuta, Gil, 335–37, **336**, 338, 339
bats, 179
Beard, Peter, 145
bears, 204, 289
Beatrice, Queen, 55
Beatrice (wife of Yonah Matojo),
    362–63
Begg, Angus, 238
Belgium, 175
Bernhard, Prince, 119
bin-Barghash, Seyyid Khalid-,
    257–58
birds, 36, 43–44, 333–35, **334**. See
    also specific names of birds
bittern, little, **242**
black rhinoceros, 111–12, 195–96,
    218, 220
Bleazard, Stan, 412
boma construction, 21–22
bongo, 12, 24
Bonham, Richard, 302–03
Bonner, Raymond, 149, 414
Borakalalo Game Reserve, 189–90,
    191, 192–93, 197–201, 206
Boran cattle, 39, 40
Born Free tv production, 76–78,
    80–88, 90

Botswana, 154, 240–44, 308
Botta, Andrew, 268, 269
Bowen-Jones, Evan, 177
Bowman, Kerry, 184–85
Bradley-Martin, Esmond, 202, 203
Brahim (guide), 73
Brashares, Justin, 157–58
Briggs, Mike
    camp style, 232–33
    field work, 225, 226, 227–28,
        235, 239
    friendship with, 228–29
    in Namibia, 192, 220
Brigid (student), 322
Britain, 175–76, 177, 178, 181,
    182–83
Brouwer, Koen, 180
brucellosis
    in cattle, 361–62, 364–65, 367
    as danger to vets, 362
    in kob, 361, 367, 369–73
    in Queen Elizabeth National
        Park, 342, 361–73
    students' study program for,
        362, **363**, 364, 367, 369–73
Buechner, Hans, 368
buffalo
    attacks by, 71–75
    as bushmeat, 156
    contact with, 273, 374, 404
    control, 68–71, 72
    cultural use of parts, 163, 205
    disease, 68, 109, 280, 354, 361,
        367, 401
    in Kasinga Channel, 376, 378, **381**
    as pest, 68, **69**, 295
    poaching, 354
    poisoning, 300

chimpanzees
attacks by, 337–38, 407
as bushmeat, 137, 161, 176
captive, **159**–60, 414
contact with, 137, 333, **340**
cultural use of parts, 129, 163
culture of, 335–37
disease, 55–59, 178
euthanizing, 62–63
Ngamba sanctuary, 406–07
at Sweetwaters Chimpanzee
Sanctuary, 168–73
treatment, 54, 55–59, **406**
China, 203, 204–05
cichlids, **402**, 404
CITES (The Convention on
International Trade in
Endangered Species), 169,
177
Claus (husband of Queen Beatrice),
55
Cleaveland, Sarah, 281–82
Cole, David, 40
Collins, Gary, 82
colobus monkeys, **81**, 82, 88–89,
179, 266–68, **267**, 333,
336–37
coltan mining, 184–85
Community Areas Management
Program for Indigenous
Resources (CAMPFIRE), 416
Congo, Democratic Republic of, 154,
161, 181–82, 184–85, 197,
203, 413
conservation
of lions, 301–07, 411–12
programs, 366–67, 412–13,
415–18

Conservation Through Public
Health, 366–67
Contagious Bovine
Pleuropneumonia, 366
The Convention on International
Trade in Endangered Species
(CITES), 169, 177
Cook, Bob, 121
Cook, Buster, 65, 71, 72, 94–95, 97
coral ear, 52–53
Corbett, Jim, 289
cormorants, 378–79
corridor disease, 68
Coverdale, Miles, 20
Cox, Debbie, 406
Craig, Batian, 112
Craig, David, 112
Craig, Delia, 112
Craig, Ian, 112, 113
Craig, Will, 113
cranes, 42–43, 44, 45–46, **47**, 53,
82, 89
crocodiles, 149, 151, **153**, 381
crows, **253**
cultural use of animal parts
by Banyaruguru, 355–59
big cats, 300–01
elephant, 163, 412
hippo, 355, 357
kob, 162, 352
and religious beliefs, 176–77
rhino horn, 202–05
widespread belief in, 162–64
wild dog, 216–17
Currah, Jen, **321**

Dahl, Merv, 319
Daiber, Bets, 247
Daiber, Michael, 247–48, 250, 251

Danhauser, Boet, 74
darting
  from airplanes, 106
  antelopes, 24, 369-72
  cheetahs, 66-67
  chimps, 56-57
  elephants, 125-26, 130-32,
    142-43
  for film, 12-13
  lions, 31, 225-26, 235, 350
  rhinos, 3, 6, 8-9, 106, 196-97,
    200-01
  wild dogs, 217-18
Davies, Harriet, 216-17
Denis, Armand, 160-61, 186
Denis, Michaela, 160-61
de Waal, Frans, 337
Dewar, David, 294-95
De Wildt Cheetah and Wildlife
    Trust, 221
De Wildt Endangered Species
    Breeding Centre, 212
dik-dik, **99**, 382
disease
  in antelope, 25, 27, 179
  in birds, 334
  in buffalo, 68, 109, 280, 354,
    361, 367, 401
  in camels, 17
  in cattle, 27, 35, 59, 68, 101, 330,
    366, 397, 401
  in chimps, 55-59, 178
  in dogs, 48, 95, 280-82
  in humans, 135, 319, 397
  in lions, 32, 228, 270, 278-83
  in rhinos, 15, 17-18, 92-93
  in roan, 24-25
  in rodents, 335

and settlement pressures,
    280-81, 283
transferred from animals to
    humans, 177-80, 182, 339
and translocation, 26-27
and vaccination programs,
    281-82
in wild dogs, 217, 218, 220, 221,
    222, 281
in zebras, 114. *See also*
    brucellosis; medicinal
    plants; medicinal use of
    animal parts
distemper, 217, 228, 270, 280-82,
    283
dogs, 48, 64-65, 74, 95, 280-82,
    299. *See also* wild dogs
Donna (student), 346
Dorper sheep, 254
Douglas, Frank, 68-71, 287, 288
doves, 19-20
Dranzoa, Christine, 314, 315-18,
    316, 325, 333, **334**, 335, 369,
    404, 416
Driciru, Margaret, 163, 282-83,
    300-01
Drongo, 266
duiker antelope, 24, 151, 152, 155,
    156, 179
Duncanson, Graham, 76,
    77-78
du Toit, Johan, 216-17
Dyer, Tony, xvi, 68, 292, 293-94,
    309-10

eagles, 243, 373, 378, **380**
East African Wild Life Society, 20
East Coast fever, 401

EAZA (European Association of
Zoos and Aquariums),
180–81, 183, 184
Ebola, 178–79
eco-tourism, 307
egrets, white, 242
Eileen of Drotsky's Cabins, 241
eland, 20, 398, 404
elephants
accidental deaths, 300
attacks by, 145–46, 345
in Cameroon, 124–25
collecting samples from, 132–33,
143
cultural use of parts, 163, 412
darting, 125–26, 130–32, 142–43
at Etosha, **244**, 246–47
in Kasinga Channel, 376, 378,
379–80
at Lewa Wildlife Conservancy, 113
in musth, **231**–32
numbers, 101, 398, 415
poaching, 135–36, 144
radio collaring, 132–33, 134, 136
snares, 158
in South Africa, 208
translocation, 102
in Uganda, 333, 345, 346–47
Elias (Cameroon crew member),
136, 144
Elkan, Paul
and antelope, 417
in Cameroon forest, 122, 123,
125, 127, 128, **129**, 133–34,
135, 142
darting elephants, 130–31
escape story, 144–45
out of forest, 137, 138

Elliott, Rodney, 23–24, 25, 30, 36,
37–39
Elsworth, David, 267
Etosha, 239, 244–47
Europe, 202–03
European Association of Zoos and
Aquariums (EAZA), 180–81,
183, 184
European Parliament, 181, 183–84
European Union, 158, 182
Evans, Jasper, 294
Exxon, 127

Fa, John, 155
Fauna and Flora International, 168
Fay, Michael, 418
Feline Respiratory Disease Complex,
283
Felix (elephant tracker), 127, 128,
131, 134, 136, 142, 143
Fernandes, Eddie, 68–71
Fischer's turaco, 266
fish eagles, African, 243, **380**
fishing
auction, 261, **262**
illegal, 185
and Kenyan fish plant, 393
in Lake Mburo National Park,
402, 403–04
study on, 157–58
in Uganda, 356–57, 381
in Zanzibar, 263–64
FIV immunodeficiency virus, 280
folk tales
and cultural properties of
animal parts, 162–64
and dik-dik, 382
and elephants, 126

disease, 179

treatment, 106. *See also* colobus monkeys

Moses (guide), 275, 276-77

Motkin, Miranda, 165

mountain lions, 289

Mount Kenya, **5**, 33-34, 35, 291-92

Mozambique, 287, 417

Mudumu North Complex (MNC), 416-17

Mugambi, Johnson, 269

Mugambi, Mutua

and birds, 43, 45

cattle pregnancy checks, 292, 293

and chimps, 58, 59

and dogs, 64

and horses, 61

and lions, 31, 32

and rhino capture, 107, 108

and rhinos, 4, 11, 15, 17

and roan, 24

Muhangi, Denis, **334**, 362, 363, 382-83

Muldaur, Diana, 82, 86

Muna, Joseph, 106

Munson, Linda, 281

Murchison Falls National Park, 282-83, 300

Murera River, 80

Murray, George, 48, 61-62, 287, 288

Murray, Irralie, 48, 59, 60, 61, 287, 288

Museveni, Yoweri, 414-15

Mushiga, Lawrence, **406**, 407

Mutuoto, James, 56, 57

Mwebi, Ogeto, 306-07

Mweya Lodge, 375-76

Mzee, Moses, 352-54

Nagana, 366

Namibia

camping in, 229-32, 234, 251-52

at Etosha, 244-47

history, 229

and hyaenas, 235-36, 239

and lions of Caprivi Strip, 224-28, 233, 239

M. Briggs in, 192, 220

and Mudumu North Complex, 416-17

Namib Desert, 253-54

ostrich farming, 250-51

and San, 247-51

searching for lions, 234-35, 238-39

Sussusvlei, 253-54

at Swakopmund, 252

Nathan (breeding station manager), 401

Neal, Andy, 8, 9

Neal, Christine, 97

Neal, Dick, 97

Neal, Jenny, 97

Neal, Mark, 97

Ngamba chimp sanctuary, 406-07

Ngarengare, Muthee, 74

Ngare Sergoi sanctuary, 112-13

Ngorongoro Crater, 270, 272-74

Nicholas, Chris, 48, 49, 51-52, 264

Nicholas, J.J., 51

Nicholas, Mary, 48, 49, 51, 52, 53

Nick (student), 345

Nigeria, 162, 175

Niven, David, 55

Nizeyi, JB (John-Bosco)

background, 317-18

and Basongora, 365, 366

on cattle, 360-61